THE DOCTOR WHO FOOLED THE WORLD

Brian Deer is a veteran British investigative journalist, best known for his inquiries into the drug industry, medicine, and social issues for *The Sunday Times* of London. Among his awards, Deer was twice named the UK's specialist reporter of the year, and in 2016 he was made Doctor of Letters (*honoris causa*) by York St John University.

THE DOCTOR WHO FOOLED THE WORLD

Andrew Wakefield's war on vaccines

BRIAN DEER

SCRIBE

Melbourne • London

Scribe Publications
2 John Street, Clerkenwell, London, WC1N 2ES, United Kingdom
18–20 Edward St, Brunswick, Victoria 3056, Australia

This edition published by arrangement with Johns Hopkins University Press
Published by Scribe in ANZ and the United Kingdom in 2020

For additional information about sources for quotations and facts cited in
the book, please see the Note to Readers on page 379.

Printed and bound in the UK by CPI Group (UK) Ltd, Croydon CR0 4YY

Scribe Publications is committed to the sustainable use of natural resources
and the use of paper products made responsibly from those resources.

9781911617808 (UK edition)
9781925713688 (Australian edition)
9781925938142 (ebook)

Catalogue records for this book are available from the National Library of
Australia and the British Library.

scribepublications.co.uk
scribepublications.com.au

O what a tangled web we weave,
When first we practise to deceive!

WALTER SCOTT, *MARMION*

CONTENTS

- - - - - - - - - - - - - - - - - - -

Prologue: Resurrection   1

BIG IDEAS

1. The Guinness Moment   13

2. It Must Be Measles   22

3. Quests Collide   32

4. The Pilot Study   42

5. Child Four   51

6. A Moral Issue   61

SECRET SCHEMES

7. Everybody Knows   75

8. First Contact   86

9. The Deal   94

10. Trouble in the Labs   104

11. Spartanburg Science   113

12. Asked and Answered   123

13. Turn of the Century   134

14. On Capitol Hill   146

15. Letting Go   156

16. The Bridge   167

17. Unblinded   177

EXPOSED

18. Assignment   191

19. Cracking the Coombe   201

20. The Spoiler 211

21. Texas 223

22. Nothing As It Seems 233

23. Sesame Street 245

24. Enterocolitis 255

25. We Can Reveal 268

26. Cry Smear 283

27. An Elaborate Fraud 293

AVENGED

28. Rock Bottom 305

29. Payback Time 315

30. Vaxxed 327

31. Wakefield's World 339

32. Cause and Affect 349

Epilogue: A Wonderful Doctor 361

Timeline 373

Note to Readers 379

Acknowledgments 381

Index 387

Resurrection

On the first night of the Donald Trump presidency, a video went up on the World Wide Web that sent a shudder through medicine and science. It featured a sixty-year-old man in a black tie and tuxedo, grinning into his phone under blue and white lights from a ballroom in Washington, DC.

"Sorry about that, guys," he says, in a mellow British accent that would suit James Bond or a Harry Potter wizard. "I don't know whether people are back on. Yeah?"

Then he repeats himself. "Sorry about that."

Below medium-brown hair, his face glistens with sweat. White light flashes on gray eyes. As he talks, he walks: first in brightness, then shadow, pursing full lips as if searching for a thought. Then raising a fist to cough. "Just looking round to see if there's anyone important here," he says, unzipping a smirk at his proximity to power. "If I can prevail upon them."

The picture is shaky and doesn't last long: two-and-a-half minutes of sideways-turned images, streamed live on Periscope, a self-broadcasting app, from that night's most exclusive event. A muffled beat thumps. Spotlights blaze. Secret Service agents take up positions.

To some of us watching—as I was, from London—he looked like the perfect party guest. People once said he was "handsome," even "hot," with a sportsman's physique, a charismatic charm, and a confidence that led others to trust him. That night, in a winged collar and pretied bow, he might have passed for a diplomat, a knighted stage actor, or a retired major league baseball star.

But to others around the world, his appearance provoked gasps. You'd think the Prince of Darkness had stepped onto the dance floor. For this was Andrew Wakefield, a disgraced former doctor who'd been booted from his profession on charges of fraud, dishonesty, and a "callous disregard" for children's suffering.

"Too much to comprehend," sneered a Texas gastroenterologist, in a flurry of Twitter posts fired that night. "I need anti-nausea meds," moaned a chemist in Los Angeles. A Dutch autism researcher: "Scary times indeed." A Brazilian biologist: "An administration for charlatans." And from a PhD student on the North Island of New Zealand: "I hoped he'd just crawled under a rock."

No chance of that. This man reveled in infamy. His nature and predicament required it. Not since the 1990s and the arrest of one Harold Shipman—who serially murdered two hundred of his patients—had a British medical practitioner been so scorned. The *New York Times* described Wakefield as "one of the most reviled doctors of his generation." *Time* magazine listed him among history's "great science frauds." And the *Daily News* spat that he'd been "shamed before the world," under the headline:

Hippocrates would puke

His fall wasn't recent, or easily missed by Trump's team tasked to check the night's guest list. By now, his disrepute was both acute and chronic, absorbed into popular culture. He'd been drawn as the villain in a cartoon strip ("The Facts in the Case of Dr. Andrew Wakefield"), sweated over by students in high school exams ("Was Dr. Wakefield's report based on reliable scientific evidence?"), and his name embraced in public conversation as shorthand for one not to be believed.

The Andrew Wakefield of biology

The Andrew Wakefield of politics

The Andrew Wakefield of transportation and planning

Yet here he was at the Liberty Ball, on Friday, January 20, 2017, at a little after seven in the evening. Behind him, on Level 2 of the Walter E. Washington Convention Center, the first of the night's revelers to pass through security rustled in their finery toward fluorescent-fronted bars. And Trump would later shuffle here with the first lady, Melania, to Frank Sinatra's 1960s classic "My Way."

"So, uh, yeah, very, very exciting times," Wakefield gushed. "I wish you could all be here with us."

Me too.

Four days later, I got the call. Could I file eight hundred words on this development? For thirteen years, on and off, I'd tracked him for the *Sunday Times* newspaper in London. With national press awards, and even an honorary doctorate, I'd become the Abraham Van Helsing to our subject's Count Dracula, who now appeared to be climbing from his grave.

He'd originally acquired profile on my side of the Atlantic, in the United Kingdom of Great Britain and Northern Ireland. Back in the day, he'd been nobody: a doctor without patients at a third-rate London hospital and medical school. He'd been a laboratory gastroenterologist, a former trainee gut surgeon, most relevantly defined by what he *wasn't*. He wasn't a virologist, immunologist, or epidemiologist. He wasn't a neurologist, psychologist, or psychiatrist. He wasn't a pediatrician or clinician.

As time passed, however, he became a global player—a man with his fingerprints on nations. But he didn't offer healing, or scientific insight. He brought epidemics of fear, guilt, and disease.

These he exported to the United States, and from there to everywhere that humans are born. As a stinging editorial from the *New Indian Express* put it:

> Can one person change the world? Ask Andrew Wakefield.

I'd first heard his name in February 1998, on the occasion of a report, or "paper," he published in a top medical journal, *The Lancet*. In a five-page, four-thousand-word, double-columned text, he claimed to have discovered a terrifying new "syndrome" of brain and bowel damage in children. The "apparent precipitating event," as he called it on page 2, was a vaccine given routinely to hundreds of millions. He later talked of an "epidemic" of injuries.

In time, he'd take aim at pretty much any vaccine, from hepatitis B to human papillomavirus. But, in the beginning, there was one in his crosshairs. This was a three-in-one shot against measles, mumps, and rubella (MMR), which he argued was the cause of a rising tide of "regressive" autism, in which infants lost language and skills. "Sufferers have to live in a silent world of their own unable to communicate," he warned.

Across Britain, no surprise, young families were petrified. From the hospital where he worked—and more particularly, from its medical school—he launched a crusade, triggering a public health crisis unrivaled since the early years of AIDS. Immunization rates plummeted. Killer diseases returned. And countless parents of children with developmental issues, who'd followed doctors' orders and vaccinated their kids, endured the horror of blaming themselves.

> It has made me so bitter and twisted. I feel so guilty.

> Eight years ago I made a tragic mistake as a parent.

> We'd convinced ourselves it was nothing we had done. Now we knew it was our fault.

At the time, I ignored him. I'd looked into vaccines, and I thought that his paper stank. His findings were too cute, too eerily familiar. But I assumed they were impossible to check. Among my bigger stories had been medical investigations (especially chasing fraud and drug industry scams), and I reckoned that the proofs of what Wakefield had done would take more than a lifetime to unearth. They'd be buried in the vaults of patient confidentiality, as accessible as Trump's tax returns.

But then, five years later, all that changed with a topical feature assignment. By then, the "MMR doctor" was so celebrated in Britain that anything new would get a "good show," as journalists used to say in the golden age of ink on paper. So I interviewed the mother of a developmentally challenged boy whose details were anonymized in that *Lancet* report. And there began Wakefield's end.

Nothing came easy. He refused to be interviewed, and ran away when I approached him with questions. *The Lancet* defended him. The medical establishment protected him. Other journalists waged war on me. But, as I pressed on, asking questions, gathering documents, and resisting lawsuits that he brought to try to gag me, his report was retracted as "utterly false," and his doctoring days were done.

"Many people have had papers in *The Lancet*," I'd quip (with shameless immodesty, yet impeccable timing). "But *I* have had one *out*."

It was what reporters like me would call a "result." So I planned to move on to other projects. What I'd long looked forward to was to take a pop at statins—the uberblockbuster, anticholesterol class of drugs—including what was in those days the top prescribed medicine. Not because I knew anything that nobody had spotted, but because with Big Pharma there's always *something* going on, and like with Mount Everest, it *was there*.

But unlike the killer Shipman, who died in his cell, Wakefield wouldn't leave the stage. He'd labored since the beginning to make it in America: appearing on *60 Minutes*, addressing congressional committees, and schlepping round a network of anti-vaccine-tinged conferences.

And now he'd been noticed by "the Donald."

"When I was growing up, autism wasn't really a factor, and now all of a sudden, it's an epidemic," the future forty-fifth president of the United States had declared, while still a mere billionaire property developer with a slot on reality TV. "Everybody has a theory," he told a local newspaper, before unleashing a one-man Twitter storm on the subject. "My theory—and I study it because I have young children—my theory is the shots."

It wasn't *his* theory. He'd gotten it from Wakefield, whether or not he knew of its provenance. And just three months before the election that stunned the world, a Republican chiropractor and high-dollar donor who ran a combined medical and legal service for people in car crashes brought them fender-to-fender. They huddled for nearly an hour in Kissimmee, central Florida, then posed for photographs beside a furled state flag: Trump mouth open, as if unable not to talk; Wakefield grinning, hands clasped near his groin, in a black suit jacket, blue denim jeans, and tan boots, scuffed at the toes.

They had so much in common. And I'm sure Wakefield sensed this. In many ways, they were two of a kind. At the time, both were frantically crisscrossing the country (one in a bespoke Boeing 757, the other with a black recreational vehicle) pursuing uncannily similar objectives. The candidate's priority was the white working class. Hurt. Angry. Neglected. The ex-doctor, meanwhile, sought a subset of parents—parents of children with autism and similar issues—who were hurt, angry, and neglected.

People sometimes spoke as if being on "the spectrum" was fashionable: a quirk of hard wiring. And it can be. But for mothers and fathers of kids with no-quibble autism, its first symptoms often heralded a desperate quest through a labyrinth of hope and fear.

If you haven't this experience, just pause to imagine it. The most precious thing in life, born so perfect, now with first words and steps. And then, sometimes subtly or sometimes so suddenly, there's a *difference*. There's *something wrong*. A son or daughter won't speak, doesn't want to be held, or obsessively watches their fingers. Maybe they have seizures, which seem to come out of nowhere. Possibly, they have a profound disability.

Then along comes a hero, with what sounds like solutions to riddles that others can't solve. As one Wakefield associate told the *New York Times*, "To our community, Andrew Wakefield is Nelson Mandela and Jesus Christ rolled up into one."

Others compared him to the Italian astronomer Galileo, who battled the Roman Catholic Church. "One of the last honest doctors in the western world . . . a genius . . . a beacon of scientific integrity . . . a brilliant clinical scientist of high moral character . . . incredible courage, integrity and humility."

On such versions of the affair, this man was a visionary, crushed in a cynical conspiracy. The way he told it, *he'd done nothing wrong.* Every complaint leveled against him was a lie. Rather, he'd fallen foul of a hideous plot—by governments, drug companies, and especially by *me*—covering up horrific injuries to kids.

"It was a strategy," he declared of the revelations that ruined him. "A deliberate strategy. A public relations strategy to say, 'we discredit this man, we isolate him from his colleagues, we destroy his career, and we say to other physicians who might dare to get involved in this: *this is what will happen to you.*'"

But while Trump spoke of hope—with a campaign slogan to "make America great again"—as Wakefield had trekked around the United States that year, he'd only brought shades of suffering. Just weeks before the ball, a YouGov opinion poll found that nearly one third of Americans now feared that vaccines "definitely" or "probably" caused autism. Immunization rates were falling as parents hurried to pediatricians to seek exemptions from the shots for their children. And not three months after that inauguration night, a resurgence of measles would explode around the planet, as what I thought I'd snuffed out reignited.

Reports began in Minnesota, where Wakefield had campaigned. Then more poured in from Europe, South America, Asia, and Australasia, as a disease once slated for universal eradication returned to sicken and kill. And by the time the new president would seek reelection, the United States had experienced its worst outbreaks in three decades, while international agencies described "vaccine hesitancy" as one of the top ten threats to human health.

It wasn't just one man. Other gurus were available—most notably an actor, Jenny McCarthy, and a lawyer, Robert Kennedy—with their own critiques of vaccines. Controversy stretched back at least a thousand years to when the Chinese learned to protect against smallpox. But it was Wakefield who stepped up to seize the modern crown as the "father of the anti-vaccine movement." And, like with L. Ron Hubbard who invented Scientology, or Joseph Smith who received the Mormon golden plates, to evaluate the merits of the creed he preached, you didn't need sermons on -isms and -ologies. You needed to know the man.

To me, his story is like *The Wizard of Oz*: a story in more ways than one. Here's the protagonist on a twisting road, with real people and specific facts that should amaze, or anger, any right-thinking reader. And here, too, is another story, a *"We can reveal,"* laying bare how the tricks were done. The curtain is lifted, and the machinery displayed. The wizard himself is exposed.

He knew what he was doing. He felt it was his right. Rules were for suckers. He was *special*. But his road to Trump's ball had been his own desperate quest: through a sinister side of science that threatens us all. If he could do what he did—and I'll show you what he did—who else is doing what in the hospitals and laboratories that we may one day look to for our lives? And who else is out there, fooling the world, behind charisma and talk of conspiracy?

Laughing into his phone at the Liberty Ball, Wakefield signed off with glee. "I'm just going to bring some pictures of Donald," he promised.

The ex-doctor without patients was back.

BIG IDEAS

- - - - - - - - - - - - - - - - - - - -

ONE

The Guinness Moment

In some imaginary universe, he might be revered as Professor Sir Andrew Wakefield. Two decades before his invitation to Trump's ball, the destination that he felt beckoned, like a big bony finger, wasn't Washington, DC, or anywhere in America, but a concert hall in downtown Stockholm. Dressed like Fred Astaire, in white tie and tails, his dream, people said, was to collect a gold medal from the hands of the King of the Swedes.

"You'd hear them in the canteen," a former colleague of his tells me. "They'd be talking about the Nobel Prize."

But to that, or any, universe, the gateway was the same: the portal to all his possibilities. It stood then—and stands now—on Beacon Hill: high above the city of Bath, in the county of Somerset, ninety minutes by train west of London. Here you'll find the entrance to his childhood home, and the exit to all roads he will travel.

It's no picket gate. This isn't *Tom Sawyer*. I'd guess the frame weighs more than a ton. Embracing two ten-foot Doric columns and matching pilasters, with an ornately carved frieze across a multilayered architrave, it resembles the entrance to a Victorian mausoleum, or a side door to the Colosseum of Rome. It speaks of wealth, class, authority, and entitlement. In uppercase, the lintel is lettered:

HEATHFIELD

The "Heath" in question was James Heath, an entrepreneur, who patented his own "Bath chair." This was a delicate hand-pushed, or horse-drawn, minicarriage, with a folding hood or sedan-like enclosure. Profits paid for a house (although it's said he never lived here) on a rugged escarpment of fossil-rich moraine, with slopes to match the best of San Francisco's. It looked out, and looks out, across the Avon River valley to a pale yellow city, built in oolitic limestone, that's today a United Nations site of world heritage.

The six-bedroom stone residence—an "Italianate villa"—was completed in 1848. Beneath its blue slate roof and tall, tall chimney stacks were two floors of high-ceilinged, big-windowed, family rooms, and below them, a half floor, dug into the moraine, once quartered by parlor maids and cooks. These two societies were linked by hidden networks of wires, connected at one end to metal levers on fireplaces, and at the other to jangling bells. By the mid-twentieth century, these contraptions had rusted. But you could never forget they were there.

During the 1960s and 1970s, the Wakefield family—two adults and five children—lived here, by all accounts happily. As a home it was mayhem, with a swing hanging from a doorframe and the tap-tap of dog paws on parquet. But amid the rough and tumble, the mother, Bridget Matthews, later remembers her second son—the future crusader—as an island of calm and compliance.

"He was the least troublesome of my children; he's a conformist really," she tells me, in tones that betray a struggle to explain this. "When he was a child, if you shouted at him, and said, 'Your room's untidy,' he'd look at you and say, 'I'm sorry, Mum.' But he would never, like the others, say, 'Oh, I haven't got time to clean it up,' or this, that, and the other. And it took the wind out of your sails."

Both parents were doctors—as were Bridget's father and grand-father—which made Andrew a fourth-generation medic. And if such a fine pedigree didn't *guarantee* greatness, it at least vali-dated the ambition. In England's stubborn class culture, he would reside above stairs: granted permissions to pull life's levers, and exemptions from answering its bells.

Role model number one was his father, Graham Wakefield, a patrician and physically imposing neurologist who rose to the National Health Service's top rank—consultant—at the Royal United Hospitals across the valley. He'd trained in brain doctor-ing before the advent of scanning, and some thought this lent his character an inclination to certainty before all of the facts were in. Without computerized tomography or magnetic resonance im-aging, his formative diagnoses were rooted less in medical sci-ence than observation, interrogation, and guesswork.

Consultant neurologists were gods among gods. Ward rounds were stately processions. "He would quiz you very precisely," a former junior doctor recalls. "But it was never to humiliate, or em-barrass. He took time to explain. Every patient would be another chance to teach. 'What does this mean?' 'At what level is the lesion?' 'What do you think is the cause?'"

Graham was a busy clinician but briefly dabbled in research, including a study published in *The Lancet*. In October 1969, he was the second of three authors of a three-pager on vitamin B_{12} and the neurological complications of diabetes. It included tables reporting on eight Royal United patients, plus a stop-press "addendum" of four late cases. Home-delivered, it would have dropped onto the Heathfield doormat when young Andy was aged thirteen.

Bridget d'Estouteville Matthews (also styled "Mrs. Wakefield") was yin to her husband's yang. She was a firm family physician, or "general practitioner," with a no-nonsense manner and a strong sense of mischief, who met Graham when they were students at St. Mary's Medical School in the Paddington district of west London. She had nerves of titanium and knew a thing about grit, having been evacuated to New Mexico during World War II, sailing with her three sisters, at the age of ten, to return four years later on a troop ship.

"She has no fear of anything, a determined chin, a strong will and piratical temperament," her father, Edward Matthews, warned her wartime hosts, in advance of his children crossing the ocean. "She has a streak of cruelty in her which she uses to cover her sensitivities and can devise the most malignant remarks with which to crush opponents."

But it wasn't only his parents in whose image Wakefield grew. A yet taller tree towered over Heathfield. His grandfather Edward ("call me Ted") became a psychiatrist at the Royal United and retained a room at the house for consultations. He also trained at St. Mary's (like his father before him), and as his son-in-law matured as a doctor of the brain, Edward flourished as a man of the mind.

His big project was a two hundred–page book for boys titled *Sex, Love and Society.* Published in 1959, when he'd just turned sixty, it professed to be "an attempt to discover the basic patterns of the mind." But that mind, for the most part, was his own. As the Swinging Sixties loomed, he used his pages to campaign: against copulation before marriage, prostitution, homosexuality, and the "increasing aggressiveness" of women.

"It was Helen of Troy's face which launched a thousand ships," he explained in a topical passage, trawling Greek myth, "not the violence of her tongue, or the strength of her biceps." And his book, dedicated to grandsons Andrew, Charles, and Richard, was an antidote to idle pleasures. "The boy who masturbates is always fed up and tired," he warned. "If you feel that you must masturbate in spite of your good intentions, get on with it and get it over with as quickly as possible."

Young Andy was nearly three when such nuggets were handed down. What heed he later paid isn't clear. Andrew Jeremy Wakefield was born on Monday, September 3, 1956, at the Canadian Red Cross Memorial Hospital, near Taplow, Berkshire—forty miles west of London. Built on land donated by the Astor family of New York, and paid for by the Ottawa government, it was a North American contribution to Britain's titanic struggles during the First and Second World Wars.

At the time of his birth, his parents were junior doctors and had already started a family with a son. They shared a Gloucestershire cottage, before relocating to Bath: to eventually pass through Heathfield's mighty gateway, when a period of serenity began.

Education was local: King Edward's School, Bath, an exclusive independent, founded in 1552, where Andy showed no special smartness. Indeed, his mother confides that to follow her family into medicine at St. Mary's, he sat his final school tests twice. "I won't say he excelled in his exams," she tells me. "He actually had to re-do."

But one signature quality that surfaced at King Edward's was a natural "charisma" that people would speak of, and which equipped him for what was to come. With a remarkable ability to win the hearts of others, it first manifested most dramatically in sport. "When he got to secondary school, he was captain of rugby really," Bridget remembers. "And then," she appends, "head boy."

The story was the same on his admission to St. Mary's: academically unmemorable but socially brilliant, again showcased as captain of rugby football. He led the team and took a featured position, in the coveted number "8" shirt. Other players had titles—say, "prop" or "fly-half"—but "Wakers," as he was dubbed, occupied the only role designated simply by a number. This was a marauding forward, in the heart of hostilities, needing huge raw strength, fitness, agility, and the fearlessness to smack into an enemy.

"He's a typical Mary's man," snarls the crusty old author of the rugby club's history, when I phone for the lowdown on the player. "Read Lord Moran's book."

"Oh, right. What's it called?"

"*The Anatomy of Courage.*"

"I see."

Courage Wakefield had. And courage he would need: to survive two weekends in the "8 man" position, let alone two decades trashing vaccines. But courage that's powered with the fuel of ambition can hurl a character into the path of worldly winds. Success or failure. Praise or blame. Fame or disrepute. Pleasure or pain. A life may blow this way, or that.

His career Plan A was professor of surgery. "If in doubt, cut it out" and all that. Here was medicine's most self-regarding branch, still clinging in England to a quaint medieval custom of distinguishing surgeons from mere "Dr." physicians with the prenominal "Mr." or "Miss." They'd nurtured this snobbery since their days of blood and gore when, should you need any part of your body removed, your loved ones took you to the barber.

"Andrew always wanted to be a surgeon," his mother tells me. "Even as a little boy he used to sew patches on his trousers, and they were always beautifully sewn on. And he *always* wanted to be a surgeon. He never said he wanted to do anything else."

He would crave that professorship. And had he stuck with surgery, I can't conceive he wouldn't have gotten one. But when he watched the craft closely, as first a student, and then a junior doctor, even the most heroic of slashing and stitching lacked something he knew his life needed. Resecting intestine would make a difference to patients. But his dreams were bigger than that.

The fracture with a timeline featuring scalpels and clamps didn't come until he was thirty years old. After graduating St. Mary's in 1981, he finished a string of training jobs, mostly around London, and then turned up in Canada on a two-year fellowship at the Toronto General Hospital.

At the time, "the General's" top surgeons were buzzing. Its big beasts were racing for a first. They aimed to beat rivals to a whole-bowel transplant, the most heroic item left on their bucket list. Wakefield, however, sloped off into lab work—a switch that his mother calls "just the way things went"—which offered prospects of achievement beyond swapping organs: not merely for the patient, but the world.

He was the seventh of eight authors on his first journal article, about poisoning from mercury batteries. And the next saw him fourth of seven sharing credit for a study of immunity issues in rats. "He did a lot of very good research," Zane Cohen, professor of surgery, told the *Toronto Star*, years later. "He is definitely not a corrupt individual."

But then—and this was back in 1987—the legacy of Heathfield kicked in. For reference, I'll call this his "Guinness Moment," when the worldly winds first howled at his door. He only talked of it once publicly, as far as I'm aware: in an interview with a London journalist named Jeremy Laurance, with whom I once briefly shared an office.

The location of the moment was a bar in downtown Toronto, on a freezing winter night. Wakefield was sitting, it was said, with a pint of Ireland's favorite black beverage, when—alone, and missing his young wife, Carmel—he had the first in a string of life-defining ideas, from which the rest of this story unfolds.

At the time, the Holy Grail of gastroenterology lay in the field of inflammatory bowel disease. Classically, there were two—ulcerative colitis and Crohn's disease—of which the latter would become his main target. Named after the sharp elbows of one

Burrill B. Crohn, and first systematically described in the 1930s, it could sometimes get so bad that it ate through the GI tract. And yet scientists couldn't agree on the cause. Most thought it started as an autoimmune reaction, perhaps triggered by bacteria or food.

But an ocean away from home, and facing a creamy Guinness froth, Wakefield experienced an epiphany. "What if inflammatory bowel disease was not a bowel disease at all," Laurance captured the thought-line from this vital moment, "but a vascular disease, caused by damage to the blood supply?"

That's bigger than you think. In fact, it's *epic*. And in Canada, Wakefield went further. He hypothesized that the ultimate culprit was a *virus*, causing inflammation and cell death in blood vessels. It was a brave speculation that would shape his life. But, if right— and especially if he could *name that bug*—then the white tie and tails might be his.

A virus? Why not? This was the 1980s. This was the age of AIDS. Although trying to link mystery illnesses with proposed infectious agents had stymied visionary doctors and scientists for centuries, whoever stepped to the plate and proved the cause of Crohn's disease would deserve some of life's gold medals.

It wasn't even that Crohn's affected huge numbers of people; estimates said less than six per one hundred thousand in any one year. Rather, its fascination lay in the riddles of a foe that had defeated some of the bravest and brightest. It was geographically more prevalent in the north than the south; commoner in cities than in rural areas; more frequent among cigarette smokers; often ran in families; and, most enticingly, likelier to be found in those whose first home was plumbed with a hot water tap.

Now came courage. At the end of his fellowship, he forsook the scalpel forever. And in its place he was issued a lab researcher's coat at one of the least regarded medical schools in London. Embedded within the fabric of a hospital—the Royal Free—it would be there that, for the next thirteen troubled years, he would seek to fulfill a promise to himself on that icy Toronto night.

Looking back, on the face of it, he had much on his side. There was the double helping of confidence, and the personal charisma to build teams and run with the ball. Medical science is a mix of inspiration and collaboration, most productive when its leaders show courage. He had all of that behind him—plus a calm determination to prove that his ideas were right.

But courage in science isn't proving yourself right. It's in your efforts to prove yourself wrong. And there Bridget's son had an issue with himself that would scar more lives than his own.

- -

TWO

It Must Be Measles

The Royal Free hospital and medical school, Hampstead, squatted on the slopes of one of London's biggest hills, four miles north of Trafalgar Square. Squeezed between eighteenth-century townhouse terraces, nineteenth-century brick-and-mortar churches, and with views across the meadows and woodlands of Hampstead Heath, it brooded over the neighborhood like a concrete castle, in fourteen stories of modernist brutalism, seen from the air as an irregular cross.

Like *USS Enterprise*, "Royal Free" was a nameplate that had moved from ship to ship. Unveiled at a different location in the 1830s, "Royal" was the gift of a young Queen Victoria, and "Free" a recognition of its no-cost treatments, one hundred years before the National Health Service. For much of its early life, it was the capital's only institution that trained female doctors, with what was the London School of Medicine for Women.

But in the late 1980s—when Wakefield joined the staff—this wasn't any center of excellence. The medical school was nearly bankrupt, according to its dean, and the hospital (which leased it one quarter of the building) was admired for its liver unit, and little else.

Wakefield arrived here in November 1988. He was then thirty-two years old. In that year, the world saw George H. W. Bush elected to succeed Ronald Reagan in the White House. Hollywood brought forward its first portrait of autism in an Oscar-winning movie, *Rain Man*. Just months into the future, a Brit—Tim Berners-Lee—would invent the World Wide Web.

Two years before his arrival, Wakefield married Carmel. That's Carmel Philomena O'Donovan: a diet-conscious, blonde-haired Zelda to his Scott, whom he met when they were students at St. Mary's. Like him, she wasn't wedded to caring for patients, and quickly switched to a desk job with the Medical Defence Union, which shielded doctors against their mistakes. "She seems like the kind of person you want to take into a knife fight," one admirer assessed her charms.

At the time, the couple lived with their first baby, James Wyatt Wakefield, in a flat-fronted, two-story, mid-terrace house, near a tidal stretch of London's River Thames in the west side district of Barnes Bridge. This was eight miles by train from the new father's place of work, and the journey gave him hours to ponder his mission: to find the undiscovered culprit for Crohn's.

These were exciting times in his chosen field. Although the inflammatory bowel diseases weren't yielding many secrets, further up the GI tract, in the stomach and duodenum (the uppermost part of the small intestine), two Australians were rocking the specialty. At the Royal Perth Hospital, Robin Warren, a pathologist, and Barry Marshall, a clinician, were publishing claims about a spiral-shaped bacterium (eventually named *Helicobacter pylori*), which they argued wasn't merely the main cause of peptic ulcers but could be cured with cheap antibiotics.

They were right and would later share the Nobel Prize. But at the time, they were as popular with the medical establishment as a hair in an after-dinner brandy. Any general practitioner would have told you that ulcers were caused by excess stomach acid, stress, bad diet, smoking, drinking, or the legacy of awkward genes. They would then prescribe you a fistful of antacid tablets that, if you took indefinitely, might relieve your symptoms and bring a smile to the manufacturers' share price.

The Perth pair, however, were fêted by *The Lancet*: the world's number two general medical journal. Founded in London in 1823, by a rabble-rousing surgeon-politician named Thomas Wakley, it was proud of a legacy of contentious propositions and wasn't shy of Warren and Marshall's. It had delivered their big break in June 1984: a four-page paper in its most prestigious research slot, underneath the main dateline near the front.

Unidentified Curved Bacilli in the Stomach of Patients with Gastritis and Peptic Ulceration

Wakefield had watched Warren and Marshall for years. Like him, they asked big questions. And only weeks after settling into a small second-floor office, next to the Royal Free's gruesome pathology museum, he thumbed through *The Lancet*'s Christmas double-issue and feasted on more from the Aussies. They now had a five-pager, with seven coauthors, again in the journal's top slot.

Heathfield . . . the Guinness Moment . . . Warren and Marshall . . . thus, the beginnings of the Wakefield story. Years later, all manner of armchair commentators would look for overarching explanations in media, sociology, or a mystical zeitgeist for why millions became exercised over vaccines. But there were only real people, and specific facts, in a cascade of cause and effect.

Next came reaction—only eleven months later—when, inspired by the Australians, a Wakefield-led team seized *six* pages in the journal's top position. Using electron microscopes to photograph resin casts of archived samples cut from Crohn's patients' intestines, they reported inflammation, blockages, and tissue death in blood vessels supplying the gut wall.

Six pages in the number two general medical journal. Wakefield walked on water. Publishing was the first of two metrics of his performance, and *The Lancet* could transform a career. More important to the Royal Free's dean and managers (and shaping their behavior in what was to come) was its potential for their profile and accounts. At the time, the medical school competed in a national "Research Assessment Exercise." Using a scale, mainly based on success in high-impact journals, activities at institutions of higher education were ranked in steps, from 5 down to 1, to decide the share-out of hundreds of millions in government grants. University College London, three miles south, was assessed with straight 5s in two vital areas. The Hampstead school: 2 and 3.

Those pages on Crohn's were therefore money in the bank. But Wakefield needed to name that virus. Then the dean, a virologist by the name of Arie Zuckerman (whose role in the scandal would have to be seen to be believed), might join him for drinks at Buckingham Palace, after one or both of them knelt before Her Majesty the Queen.

Some researchers stumble upon their signature achievement. Others test everything that moves. But Mr. Wakefield—still styled and self-described as a surgeon—employed a technique so simple for the next step on his path that his lack of science training proved a boon. As he later explained to the journalist Jeremy Laurance, who quoted this line in a nine-hundred-word feature:

> I sat down with two volumes of a virology textbook, and worked through it.

Simple as that.

When I took up the story, I mimicked Wakefield's approach. The book was *Fields Virology*. Two red-and-silver tomes, each weighing half a brick. An encyclopedia of viruses. Second edition. It grouped these microbes into eighteen families, with members profiled alphabetically, across double-columned pages: histories, clinical features, epidemiology, and genetics. A *who's who* and *what's what* of what he sought.

But Laurance had the quotes. And we should be grateful for his diligence in capturing them for posterity. "I got to measles virus," Wakefield told him, "and it described how it gets into the gut, causing ulcers and inflammation. You could have been reading an account of Crohn's disease."

Measles virus. In the *Morbillivirus* genus of the paramyxovirus family of single-stranded RNA bugs. The thirty-two-page chapter pointed to origins, possibly, in ancient Rome or China, evolving from the cattle plague rinderpest. History's pioneering Greek doctors Hippocrates and Galen never noted it, and the symptoms—fever, cough, rash, and telltale white "Koplik spots" in the mouth—seemed to take hold with the evolution of cities, as a roughly ten-day illness of childhood.

"In the mucus membranes of the mouth, the necrotic epithelial cells of the Koplik spot slough, leaving a tiny shallow ulcer," noted the passage that quickened Wakefield's pulse.

> Lesions equivalent to Koplik spots have been found during the prodrome and first day of the rash on mucosal surfaces throughout the body, including the conjunctivae; the oropharynx; the nasopharynx; the lining of the larynx, trachea, bronchi and bronchioles; the entire length of the gastrointestinal tract; and the vagina.

The entire length of the GI tract. That's just how Crohn's could be. Although most typically found in the ileum (the part of the small intestine that's furthest from the stomach), the condition may manifest from mouth to anus. And *lesions equivalent to Koplik spots.* So . . . the nasty ulceration of the inflammatory bowel disease was like measles of the gut.

Eureka.

So here was the first great Wakefield hypothesis: measles virus caused Crohn's disease. And now, announcing formation of what he called the "Inflammatory Bowel Disease Study Group" at Hampstead, he began drawing in others with technical skills, whom he led onto the field of battle, like in rugby.

"I thought he was a man who had a good idea, or what seemed like a good idea at the time," says Philip Minor, then chief of virology at the British government's National Institute of Biological Standards and Control, on the northern fringe of London. "And he was looking round for scientists to help him."

Wakefield knew that his path wouldn't be easy. Naysayers preened like parakeets. Some pointed out that his photographs were mere snapshots and didn't prove inflammation began *outside* the gut, rather than *inside*, as they assumed.

Whispers went round that maybe the ex–bowel surgeon *just didn't get* the science. "He gave a seminar in my department," recalls one senior academic over lunch. "And there were a lot of people in my department, basic scientists, very, very smart, whose whole life was working on blood vessels. And he came and gave this talk—and this was the first time I heard him talk real science. And I sat there, and it was a sort of hour-long seminar, and after about three sentences, I had no idea what this guy was talking about."

You just heard a voice from the medical establishment: an establishment that had been wrong before. "Everybody knows the stomach is sterile," was how the Australian Robin Warren would recall of the naysayers later, when in Stockholm collecting his medal. Such was gastric acidity, experts assured him, that the bugs couldn't survive the environment. And even if they could, *somebody else* would have noticed. "Why has not anyone described them before?"

Repelled by such complacency, Wakefield was encouraged. Like the Aussies, he'd keep his nerve. Still barely recognized among the school's staff of seven hundred, he coauthored papers in the journals *Gastroenterology* and *Gut* in which his team continued probing blood vessels. Then, in April 1993, he broke big again in the *Journal of Medical Virology*. Known to its readers as *J Med Virol*, it was edited by Zuckerman, the medical school's dean.

"These studies suggest that persistence of measles virus in intestinal tissues is a common event," Wakefield summarized, amid nine dense pages of text and images, "and a consistent feature of tissues affected by Crohn's disease."

In his career résumé, that would be paper twenty-seven (with the one that would make and break his career numbered eighty), adding a feather to his professional cap. *J Med Virol* wasn't great for impact. But with a team of six associates, whose names followed his, he reported impressive results. Probing for evidence of the virus in surgically removed Crohn's tissues, they used three methods (all laboratory standards), each of which came up trumps. One scored positive in thirteen of fifteen patients, another likewise in nine of nine, and the third in ten out of ten.

One technique—known as "immunohistochemistry"—looked for signs of proteins from which the virus is built: coded, as measles is, in RNA. Another—called "in situ hybridization"—hunted for a segment of the RNA itself, deep within the bug's genetic core. Neither was foolproof. But his third was box office: using an electron microscope, magnifying specimens up to eighty-five thousand times, his team appeared to *photograph* his quarry.

There was measles—or there it was reported—smudgy shadows in a moonscape of craters, blobs, swirls, and spots, which he described in a 260-word caption. He noted objects "consistent with densely packed viral nucleocapsids," with "virus particles" and "infected" cells. He gazed on the face of his destiny.

The second metric of his performance was the money he raised: whether in grants from the government's Medical Research Council, from charities in the field of inflammatory bowel diseases, or, more often, from the pharmaceutical industry. In Toronto he was funded by the Wellcome Trust: at the time the grant-giving arm of a British-American drugs empire, founded by a Wisconsin-born salesman, Henry Wellcome. But after an extension of that award through 1993, his begging bowl was out for more.

Economics were also under review at home. He and Carmel had moved to a bigger west London house: in a short terraced street of bay windows and brick, beside a rail line from Waterloo station. They now paid out as parents of two young boys, with the second, Samuel Ryder Wakefield, named after his great grandfather (Edward Matthews's father), a St. Mary's graduate of 1896.

Much of Wakefield's work was routine, even boring, compared with the excitement to come. But the clock was ticking. He needed results. And the naysayers pecked at his heels. Not only was he listed on the medical school's budgets, but critics pointed out that while his hypothesis proposed that Crohn's was caused by measles and, in developed countries at least, Crohn's diagnoses were rising, cases of measles had fallen through the floor with the advent of immunization.

A lesser-driven man might have slapped his forehead and spent three weeks in a bar. But the way Wakefield told it (although I'd later bring a different light) was that this apparent contradiction inspired him. Measles vaccines contained weakened, but functional, measles virus. Therefore, he reasoned, these might also cause Crohn's and so explain its rising prevalence.

Proving that hypothesis would definitely need money. And he knew he'd the skill to get it. Time and again, I heard of this quality: a remarkable attribute that, to be frank, nearly everyone lacks. "Charisma . . . charisma . . ." Like a drumbeat through his life: an astounding psychological power.

Now he applied it to pharmaceutical executives, along with charities and not-for-profits. He lured Upjohn of Michigan, Searle of Illinois, the Swiss giant Hoffmann-La Roche, and the London-based Glaxo (later GlaxoSmithKline, or GSK) to lob more than coins into his hat.

Such support would sit uneasily with his claims, years later, that he was a victim of Big Pharma scheming. And, yet more irony, the next link in the chain of specific facts that led him toward what became his war on vaccines was in part funded by Merck of Rahway, New Jersey, the world's number one vaccine manufacturer. "It was kind of basic work," a retired executive shares the joke with me. "But he did take money from Merck."

Now switching from virology to epidemiology, his team followed up two unrelated British studies executed in the 1950s and 1960s. One was a child health survey before measles vaccines were introduced, and the other an early trial of the shots. By writing to participants (at least those who could be traced), Wakefield concluded that Crohn's was *three times more common* in those who'd been immunized compared with those who weren't.

His target for publication was, again, *The Lancet*, with its cherished crowd-pleasing inclinations. As a general medical journal, it sought to appeal to readers from disparate specialties with big-brush, sometimes frankly tabloid, topics that everyone would remember from medical school. So, in April 1995, it printed his study in a three-page paper, with four authors listed, including the Royal Free's professor of gastroenterology, Roy Pounder, and a Wakefield sidekick named Scott Montgomery, who were both to feature in supporting roles as hagiography would give way to disgrace.

The Lancet took chances. But it guarded its name with specially commissioned winks to the wise. For specialist readers, who might otherwise complain, it often printed extra articles—effectively editorials—to pull the sting of extravagant claims. And, in this case, two scientists at the US Food and Drug Administration were invited to file a "commentary."

Wakefield, they pointed out, had compared incomparables: like trying to match plums against mangoes. "There were fundamental differences in the ways in which the study cohorts were recruited and interviewed," they wrote of the 1950s and 1960s sources, "and in how their constituents were ultimately classified according to exposure and disease."

To be fair, the team's paper owned up to shortcomings. It was speculative. Nothing was *proved*. Measles "may" persist in gut tissue, they said. Early exposure "may" be a risk. People with Crohn's "may" have an altered immunity. And so weak was any link with immunizations that their report's title was flagged with a question mark.

Is measles vaccination a risk factor for inflammatory bowel disease?

The caveats were glaring. They leapt from the page and provoked a few titters of amusement. Some branded the title as a case of "Hinchliffe's rule" (known in journalism as "Betteridge's law of headlines"): that when a title is a question that can be answered yes or no, the correct answer is invariably no.

Nevertheless, Wakefield's sights were now set on *vaccines*—not merely on measles found wild in nature—as the cause of Crohn's disease.

But *where*—he wondered—could he find the evidence to *prove* such a big idea?

THREE

Quests Collide

The way Wakefield would tell it, his adventures in autism began with a phone call from a mother.

Narrowly framed, it's true. This was May 1995. Friday, May 19, to be specific. In his second-floor office, a telephone rang. A lady recounted the story of her six-year-old son. And nothing would ever be the same.

She was also the mother who triggered my investigation. So, you might say, she brought us together. I'll call her "Ms. Two," and her son "Child Two": anonymized with the number he'd be given in the research project for which Wakefield would never be forgotten. But nothing about this mother and boy was secondary. They were emphatically, irrevocably, first. The then doctor would describe them as the "biggest influence" on his life. Child Two was his "sentinel case."

The boy was born in late July 1988—full-term, the due date—weighing 8 lb. 10 oz. (3.9 kg)—with not a hint of anything wrong. His mother's pregnancy was uneventful. She needed no drugs in labor. And four or five minutes after a snag-free delivery, her new baby scored a perfect 10 on the APGAR scale (Appearance, Pulse,

Grimace, Activity, and Respiration), against which the condition of newborns was logged.

Carried home from the hospital in the county of Cambridgeshire, northeast of London, Child Two was all set for the best life could bring to a middle-class twentieth-century English family. His father was a computer specialist, employed in engineering, and Ms. Two an information manager and business analyst for a top travel agency in the capital.

Thus began infancy as good as it gets. The boy's gaze sharpened. He rolled, babbled, and laughed. He began to crawl, then cruise, gripping furniture. He pointed, shaped sounds—"*mama . . . dada*"—and, one amazing day, rose to his feet unsupported and took his first steps, before tumbling. In this child was a reason, an ultimate fulfillment, a crowning existential achievement.

Second year: looking good. Blond hair. Blue eyes. He splashed toys in the bath, pulled a toy dog with a waggy tail, and built towers of bricks to match the best.

But, sadly, horribly, it wasn't to last. His parents' desperate quest would begin.

Medical records pinned the change after the middle of that year—a few months before his second birthday. He became "withdrawn and inaccessible," with "nightly screaming bouts" and, at some point, episodes of "head banging." You'd be surprised how many infants go through such phases, and snap out of them, no worse for wear. But Child Two didn't. He began ignoring his parents. And such speech as he'd gained slipped away.

There'd been a time when Ms. Two could hold up a ball, and the little boy—her second son—would name it: "ball." She could point to a book, and he'd say "book." But then "ball" became "all," and "book" became "ook," until his vocabulary dissolved into nothing. "The very last word that he lost was 'juice,'" she tells me when we meet at her home, eight years after the phone call to Wakefield. "It went from 'juice' to 'uice' to 'ooo.' And then it went."

No cause or explanation was ever agreed on. Over a period of years, he experienced several regressions, losing speech, play skills, and regard for others, leaving specialists using labels such as "autistic" and "retarded." But, while regression is sometimes a feature of autism, doctors balked at a precise diagnosis.

Few parents dawdle in the face of such nightmares. And, marshaling professionals like a Japanese tour guide, this mother wasn't shy to seek help. Before she called Wakefield, there was a Professor Dryburgh, Dr. Hunter, Professor Neville, and Dr. Tuck. There was a Professor Warner, Dr. Rolles, Dr. Cass, and Ms. Moore. There was a Dr. Richer, Dr. Silveira, Professor Davies, Mr. Martin, Professor Goodyer, Dr. Bhatt, Dr. Cavanagh, and Dr. Wozencroft.

And now there was the doctor without patients.

The inciting event that led to the phone call was publication of Wakefield's question-marked *Lancet* paper that tried to link vaccines with Crohn's. Notwithstanding the holes in this comparison of incomparables, the dismissive commentary from FDA scientists, and that telltale "?" at the end of its title, two institutions, as trusted as the journal, also forgave its obvious deficiencies to bring it to the public's attention.

One was the Royal Free medical school. As part of a shake-up in the capital's health system, it was scheduled to merge with its more successful near-neighbor: University College London. With hopes for the top job in the resulting combined faculty, Hampstead's dean, Arie Zuckerman, seized on Wakefield's appearance in the journal to showcase the talent he led. So, despite thirty-five years of research experience, the dean agreed to chair a press conference.

Years later, he would call this decision "a disaster." Seated amid ranks of lawyers and doctors at Britain's longest hearing into medical misconduct, he voiced his "regret" for what he described as an "almost dramatic" fall in the uptake of MMR. And though the twelve-month decline was only point three of one percent (from 91.8 to 91.5 of children getting the shot by the age of two), this small drop would be the start of a slide that wouldn't fully recover to pre-Wakefield levels for nearly twenty years.

In medicine, press conferences were traditionally reserved for breakthrough treatments, or infectious disease outbreaks, not a mid-rank lab researcher's speculations. But, in a prelude to something similar, far bigger, yet to come, on the morning of Friday, April 28, the hospital's wood-paneled Marsden Room was laid out with rows of soft-backed chairs, facing a narrow trestle table for speakers.

Wakefield took his place in a light jacket, patterned tie, button-down shirt, and dark pants. His hair looked oddly thick, as if gelled into a helmet. And, clipped to a pocket on the left side of his chest was a photo ID bearing a Maltese cross logo with, at its center, a lion looking backward.

His right hand grasped controls for a mechanical projector, which clanked slides to a fabric screen. "Hypothesis," said one, in white on blue.

Crohn's disease is caused by a cell-mediated immune response to persistent virus infection of the mesenteric microvascular endothelium

This virus may be measles

That wouldn't be listed as the day's top news. *The Guardian* ran three hundred words, on page 8; the *Times*, ninety-six, on page 4. But that evening, a second institution—the British Broadcasting Corporation—also had talent to showcase. A new science correspondent, schooled in physics and computers, was granted thirteen minutes on medicine by *Newsnight* on BBC2.

"A report in the medical journal *The Lancet* today suggests that people who get vaccinated run a higher risk of developing debilitating bowel diseases," declared the show's anchor—an acerbic, dark-haired interviewer named Jeremy Paxman, whose script exaggerated almost everything. "The implication that vaccination may not be good for everyone in all circumstances flies in the face of a policy which—as our science correspondent, Susan Watts, reports—has become an article of faith."

An "article of *faith*"? Not science, or public health? And Watts's package tiptoed further down that path. Instead of looking into the mouth of the *Lancet* report, she stretched her story by adding *brain damage* to *bowel disease*. And she fingered MMR (which Wakefield's paper never mentioned) as a possible cause of both.

Ms. Two tells me later that she never saw the broadcast. But along with footage from the Hampstead event and a few talking heads, Watts, thirty-two, conflated a group "against vaccinations" (in a meeting that I think was staged for the camera), government warnings over the risks of measles, a segment about an eight-year-old (without saying what was wrong with him), and a studio interview with a woman named Jackie Fletcher, wearing a lens-popping scarlet dress.

"Now Mrs. Fletcher," Paxman addressed her. "Your son, Robert, was vaccinated when very small. What were the side effects?"

"Well, exactly ten days after his MMR," she replied, "he became extremely ill, and his whole life changed."

Apart from the dress, most striking was her hair—dark, shoulder-length, combed sharply from the center—and a piercing, brown-eyed gaze. She explained how her three-year-old, at the age of thirteen months, suffered a seizure and later developed severe epilepsy and learning issues (but not bowel disease, or autism).

She argued that parents needed more information about such matters and obliquely referred to a group she'd launched sixteen months before, with an ambiguous acronym: "JABS." This was slang in much of Britain for an injected vaccine, and would cleverly spell out, should anyone ask, as "Justice, Awareness, and Basic Support."

But Fletcher, thirty-eight, a former bank clerk, wasn't 100 percent free of mixed motives. Upon launching JABS, her personal ambition was to sue the vaccine's makers. But she'd no chance of going it alone. Such a colossal shitfight could only be paid for in Britain by a free legal aid scheme, run by the government. And the rules for this meant that she would need to find hundreds of families with complaints like her own to justify the cost.

At the time, the triple vaccine wasn't controversial. Fletcher hoped to disturb that calm. So, after appearing in the same *Newsnight* package as Wakefield, she got in touch with him at Hampstead and advised others to do the same.

Ms. Two was the first to get through.

Ms. Two was then aged forty—two years older than Wakefield—and had grown up in Preston, a once-noted mill town two hundred miles up-country from London. When he answered his phone, she talked quickly in the voicetones of the English Northwest (*was* sounded "wooz"; *some* sounded "soohm"), with a confident, insistent style.

"Please listen to me," she ordered.

And listen he did. The call lasted about two hours.

"She was an extremely articulate woman," he'd recall years later. "She told a story which made a great deal of sense."

At the outset, however, her approach confused him. Had she even got through to the right number? Child Two had been diagnosed on the autistic spectrum—then a fast-evolving cluster of developmental definitions involving peculiarities, deficits, or sometimes frank handicaps in thinking, communication, and behavior.

But why was she calling a gastroenterologist—and a laboratory researcher to boot? The way he'd tell it, he reacted with surprise. Although schooled in general medicine before specializing in surgery, when he studied at St. Mary's in the early 1980s, "autism" wasn't even taught.

"I'm sorry, I have no idea how to help you," he later said he responded. "I know nothing about autism."

So, then she said (or, at least, *he* said *she* said), "My child also has terrible bowel problems. And I believe that the bowel problems and the behavioral problems are related. When one is bad, the other is bad; when one is good, the other is not so bad."

And so they continued (reconstructed in hindsight) with a conversation that united their quests. Both remembered that, at some point early in the call, she insisted that her son was vaccine damaged.

"She said to me, in very clear terms," Wakefield explained later, in one of countless retellings, "that her normally developing child had received his MMR, and within several weeks he'd started to develop regression."

Regression. A word no parent would want to hear in connection with a son or daughter. At the time, it was reckoned that between about a quarter and a third of children with autism were affected by this distressing variant. An infant (usually a boy) appeared to develop typically for around twelve to twenty-four months, but then lost language and skills. Experts linked it to rapid brain expansion and the expression of genes playing out.

Ms. Two was gobsmacked by the doctor's attention. She'd never gotten such a hearing before. But Wakefield's employment contract excluded patient care, so that Friday, he'd plenty of what clinicians lacked: *time.* He'd no waiting room, ward, or list to attend to. His days were planned much as he pleased. He did next to no teaching and had but one preoccupation: to prove that measles virus, now especially in vaccines, was the undiscovered cause of Crohn's.

Ms. Two didn't know he was a doctor without patients, but Fletcher had briefed her on his interests. The JABS campaigner talked not only of the question-marked *Lancet* paper but also about his earlier work, in *J Med Virol*, which claimed the discovery of measles in bowel disease.

"*That* was the moment of epiphany," Ms. Two tells me, when we meet. "I *knew* when Jackie said that, that I had the mechanism, potentially. *That* was the turning point."

Wakefield listened, ever more eagerly. What she told him dovetailed with his goal. Her son, *he* said *she* said on the phone, suffered from abdominal pain and diarrhea—both possible symptoms of inflammatory bowel disease. And these, she deduced, were caused by vaccination, which she also felt was at the root of the boy's behavior.

"It happens that I believe he was affected by the MMR," she tells me she told him. "It happens that he's now autistic. And it happens that I believe the brain comes secondary to the gut problem."

Now *that* was some conjecture. Wakefield loved it. But then, like him, she was a doctor's child. Her late father had been a Preston general practitioner, bequeathing her a mind for big ideas, which, that Friday, she rehearsed on the phone.

Confronted by riddles she was anxious to solve, her quest had led her to ply her son with every kind of remedy. She tried alternative supplements. A hospital staff member suggested the Feingold diet, which sought to eliminate food colorings and additives. She persuaded doctors to give her son massive shots of vitamin B_{12} ("I tried it out, and it worked," she tells me). And she joined a parents' group called Allergy-Induced Autism, where she was introduced to a notion called "opioid excess": that certain substances in foodstuffs, especially bread and milk, could cause autistic behaviors.

"It was presented in a cool, lucid way," Wakefield remembered. "She had clearly thought through the problem very carefully."

He listened to her voice. And then he listened more. She talked about "metabolic disease," "sulfation," and "pathways." And the parents' group, she explained, had many families like her own.

She sounded too good to be true.

This mother, it appeared, had everything he sought. So much of it chimed with his thinking. Even the vitamin B_{12} (mostly absorbed from food in the small bowel's ileum) chimed intriguingly with his hypothesis. Forget electron microscopes, musty tissue samples, or question-marked epidemiology from ancient research projects, Child Two, and the other kids that this mother's group knew of, might be *living proof* that vaccines caused Crohn's.

There and then he responded by proposing that she ask for a specialist medical opinion. "My only concern at that stage was for the clinical well-being of this child," Wakefield argued later, at the same disciplinary proceedings where the dean was questioned. "It is my duty as a physician, and as a human being, to respond to the plight of this mother."

So he recommended an Australian named John Walker-Smith—then at another London hospital, four miles south, called St. Bartholomew's or, more commonly, "Barts." He was fifty-eight years old, a professor of pediatric gastroenterology, and (after more than two years of being lobbied by Wakefield), was set to move, with his team, to Hampstead. He would bring two consultants skilled in colonoscopy, transforming opportunities for research.

Energized by the mother's call, Wakefield phoned Walker-Smith. And on a bright August Tuesday in 1995—ten weeks after the two-hour conversation I've described—Ms. Two traveled with her son, then aged seven, eighty-five miles south to London.

At Barts, the Australian gathered a history from the mother.

Normal pregnancy, normal delivery . . . Breast fed until 20 months . . . Begun to have diarrhea at 18 months . . . MMR injection at 15 months . . . went downhill ever since

His account of what she told him was longer and more detailed. But, after examining the boy, Walker-Smith added to his notes a repeated string of three letters.

Abdomen NAD . . . Anus NAD . . . Mouth NAD

This meant "nothing abnormal detected." His final verdict:

No evidence of Crohn's disease.

"The child was referred to me via Andy Wakefield of the Royal Free because of mum's perception of the child's illness really began with MMR, and in view of the possible link of measles with Crohn's disease," Walker-Smith dictated into a letter to another doctor. The patient's story, he added, sounded like multiple food allergy, or irritable bowel syndrome. "On examination there is absolutely nothing to suggest the diagnosis of Crohn's disease."

Good news for Child Two. Bad news for the hypothesis. But Wakefield was only getting started. Most doctors are delighted if they don't find disease. Not this one. He couldn't let go.

"She was clear, she was intelligent, the story made so much sense," he'd say of her phone call, many years later. "She wasn't anti-vaccine. She'd taken her child to be vaccinated. But he was clearly vaccine damaged, profoundly injured. And that was the sentinel case."

FOUR

The Pilot Study

John Walker-Smith didn't want to move to the Royal Free. But he felt that he'd run out of options. As part of the same London shake-up that would see medical schools merge, his department at Barts was threatened with closure. So, at Wakefield's suggestion, and after years of being schmoozed, the Australian cut a deal, gathered his team, and hit the road north to Hampstead.

The way he saw it, there was only one hospital: only one in the world at which to practice. Barts. *Barts*. It had to be Barts. Founded by monks in 1123 and the place that, as the child of a surgeon in Sydney, he heard called "the mother hospital of the Empire." If he hadn't found a job there—in 1972—he would have stayed in Westmead, New South Wales, at the Royal Alexandra Hospital for Children.

"There is," he'd explain, "a kind of 'apostolic succession' from the ancient origins of western medicine on Cos" (a Greek island) "to the Isola Tiberina in Rome" (another island) "and then to Barts in London."

Some thought he was a snob. More English than the English. *"Plus Anglais que les Anglais,"* as they say. Others reckoned he had a touch of the cultural cringe that masked a more intimate insecurity. He maintained, for instance, that it was "improper" and "unacceptable" for Britain to have "abandoned" its colony, Australia, by cutting it adrift with independence.

He didn't come cheap. To woo him to Hampstead, they really rolled out the rug. In a six-story zone at the back of the hospital, new offices and a laboratory were built to receive him. A personal ward—Malcolm Ward—was refurbished for his patients. And to lead a new, and magnificently titled, University Department of Paediatric Gastroenterology, his status was dialed up to eleven.

In conservative dark suits and with scrupulous courtesy, into this domain he strolled, in September 1995, struggling to restrain a vulnerability of character. His appointment was "an event of international significance," he trilled in the privacy of his autobiography, *Enduring Memories.* "I was to be a full professorial head, taking my place at university committees with the professors of medicine and surgery."

From a second-floor office near the pathology museum, the welcome was no less generous. Ms. Two's phone call had heralded, in Wakefield's later words, "the opening of the floodgates" as families with links to Jackie Fletcher's JABS group, and Ms. Two's affiliation with Allergy-Induced Autism, spread news about the doctor who *listened.*

What he wanted from Walker-Smith and his squad of pediatricians was to do research on these families' children. Here was an unprecedented opportunity to learn of any impact from persistent measles virus in the gut. Conventional wisdom said the bug came and went within weeks, but could it chronically linger to cause Crohn's disease? And, even bolder, was there a link between the bowel and autism? Ms. Two's ideas *were* intriguing.

Walker-Smith leapt at the chance to find out. Research had long been a passion. At Barts, his department boasted the only lab in Britain dedicated to the subspecialty of pediatric gastroenterology, and he was anxious to keep his hand in. His new collaborator, moreover, was a favorite of *The Lancet*, which had just appointed a new editor-in-chief—Richard Horton—who'd worked at Hampstead in the 1980s, with a room on the same corridor as Wakefield.

The professor's step had a spring for another reason too: the extent to which he looked up to Wakefield. This was a literal fact, since Walker-Smith was short and barely two-thirds of the other man's bulk. But colleagues also recalled him hailing a "true prince." And when the Australian came to publish his autobiography (a few weeks before I arrive in his life), he was so under the influence of the doctor without patients that he spoke of "shades" of England's Princess Diana.

> He is tall, handsome, fluent, charismatic and above all a man of conviction. He is a man of utter sincerity and honesty. In reality the out of fashion term "crusader after truth" would best describe him.

Meetings were convened, more clinicians enlisted, and a battery of investigations agreed. "Andy Wakefield was keen to organise a research study of this group of children," Walker-Smith wrote afterward. "My own role in all this was permissive as Andy Wakefield was the research leader, the conductor of the orchestra, a classical role in research for a gastroenterologist. A team was assembled, an ethical committee application was obtained and a pilot study went ahead."

The initial plan was to investigate ten such children, either with Crohn's or a related inflammation. If Wakefield's hypothesis about the virus was correct, he expected to find it in the *terminal ileum*—the last few centimeters of the small intestine—the most common seat of the disease.

Under a template doctors dubbed the "Wakefield protocol," each child would be admitted on a Sunday afternoon and discharged the following Friday. In the meantime, they'd undergo a daunting regime, including sedation or general anesthesia; magnetic resonance imaging brain scans; wires-to-the-head electro-encephalograms; blood and urine tests; lumber punctures to draw cerebrospinal fluid; barium drinks and abdominal x-rays; a radio-active Schilling test for vitamin B_{12} absorption; plus, most crucially, a colonoscopy with ileoscopy (often compressed into the term "ileocolonoscopy"), intubation to the small intestine.

No hospital had ever embarked on such a project. The management described it as "unique." With a speculative premise concerning measles in vaccines, even to perform a colonoscopy for developmental issues was an exceedingly unconventional approach. Senior doctors questioned how any ethical review could have approved such a problematic venture.

"In our research planning meetings, we had all these referrals," explains Simon Murch, a consultant pediatrician who transferred from Barts with Walker-Smith's team, discussing it with me later in the school. "And so that was prospectively planned research to a defined number of children, just in terms of assessing the limits of what we're having."

To begin, the kids' parents needed referral letters from local doctors: the only route to non-emergency admission. The first was solicited, in February 1996, from a general practitioner on the outskirts of Liverpool, two hundred miles northwest of London. "Thank you for asking to see this young boy," she wrote to Walker-Smith of a six-year-old patient, "who developed behavioural problems of an autistic nature, severe constipation and learning difficulties after MMR vaccination."

That start was promising, and before long the Royal Free would become the Mecca, or Lourdes, for desperately questing families of developmentally challenged children. As one mother wrote of Wakefield, before any were admitted:

He said that there is a test which [my son] could have which will either connect or eliminate his condition to the measles vaccination.

What parent in her shoes wouldn't say yes if the ordeal might glean that information? So they traveled to Hampstead by road, rail, and air, including from the United States. Nor did Wakefield forget his sentinel case. Notwithstanding Walker-Smith's belief that the boy didn't have Crohn's, this child would be "pivotal" (to use the professor's term) and among the first to undergo the procedures.

In fact, he was second (hence "Child Two"), after his mother phoned Walker-Smith in May of that year and entered her son for the protocol. Wakefield backed her, putting an argument to the professor that, whether or not the boy had Crohn's, his bowel might still have some "subtle" inflammation, and so benefit from colonoscopy, or "scoping."

Walker-Smith agreed and saw the mother and child again at a Friday food allergy clinic. He ordered blood tests for inflammation (which came back normal), and two months later—on the afternoon of Sunday, September 1—admitted Child Two to Malcolm Ward.

This was five weeks after Child One had been and gone: a three-year-old boy ferried one hundred miles from an air force base, but who proved a disappointment to doctors. Even after a strong laxative "bowel prep" drink, he was so rock solid with constipation that the endoscopist couldn't reach his small intestine—even failing again, three days later.

Next, Ms. Two's son was processed in accordance with the protocol. Upon arriving at the ward on the hospital's sixth floor, a junior doctor, David Casson, took the child's history from the mother, and a link with vaccination was noted.

Mum does recount that at 13 months of age he had had his
MMR immunisation, and 2 weeks following this had started
with head banging behaviour and screaming throughout the night.

She said the same to a child psychiatrist, Mark Berelowitz, who supported young patients on the wards.

[Ms. Two] reiterated that [Child Two] started head-banging about 2 weeks after the MMR and hasn't looked right since.

The morning after the boy's arrival, he was trolleyed to the endoscopy suite, four floors above Malcolm Ward. And, as midazolam and pethidine sedation kicked in, he was rolled onto his left side to be scoped.

According to ethical codes, the procedure was "high risk," but much of Walker-Smith's career had mirrored the evolution of flexible fiber-optic endoscopes sufficiently delicate to use on children. This didn't always pan out, though, and after the initial admissions to the Wakefield protocol, a five-year-old's bowel would be perforated in twelve places, prompting a half million pound settlement by the hospital.

To reach the lattermost portion of the small intestine (where only a few centimeters are accessible to scoping), the instrument has distance to travel. It must first pass the rectum and the slightly S-shaped sigmoid colon, then journey up the descending colon, on the left side of the body, to a bend: the splenic flexure. There it turns across the transverse colon, which sags horizontally behind the rib cage, to another bend: the hepatic flexure. Now on the right side of the body, it turns again, into the ascending colon, then down to the cecum (about three fingers from the hip bone) where the dead-end appendix branches off.

Now came an even trickier maneuver: at the ileocecal valve. This is where the large bowel (a.k.a. the colon, or large intestine; the job of which is mainly removing water from feces) transitions to the ileum—the first stretch of the small bowel—where nutrients from food are absorbed. Here is the stretch that takes up vitamin B_{12}, and where Crohn's most typically does its worst.

Generally, Walker-Smith ordered the procedure. But he didn't scope children himself. For Child Two it was Murch who navigated the route, observing progress via a video monitor mounted on a rack at face height in the endoscopy suite. Murch had recently turned forty and, like his colleagues, was a gentleman possessed of the grand manner. His hobby was rowing, and he was proud to explain that he could successfully intubate a child's small intestine on nine attempts in ten.

Murch assumed the position, with his shirt and tie safe behind a green disposable plastic apron, and was ready to scope Child Two. With hands snugly gloved in skintight cream latex, his left clutched the controls, and his right the body of a Fujinon pediatric colonoscope. This was about one and a half meters long, and ten to twelve millimeters in diameter, built of steel mesh wrapped in smooth polymer.

Embedded throughout the instrument were "angulation wires" to steer its head like a snake. Under the doctor's gentle pressure, it traveled glistening pink corridors, scored with arteries and veins, inside the unconscious boy (now aged eight). At the front peered a lens, with a light source, air blower, and water supply, as well as channels for suction and tools.

To Murch's right stood two nurses. Watching the monitor from behind the participants was Ms. Two and Wakefield, and also nearby, a fair-haired young scientist named Nick Chadwick. He was the "coordinating investigator—molecular studies," waiting for tissue to take away and test for measles.

Upon reaching the valve, Murch felt relief. This was where he'd been blocked with Child One. And, with a final maneuver of twisting and pushing, the scope blazed into the ileum of the sentinel case, like a torch into Pharaoh's tomb. Here was the goal: the repository of treasure. At least, so Wakefield hoped.

I guess we'll never know his reaction to what they saw. But watching on the monitor, Ms. Two felt horror as the instrument reached its limit. In the light of the scope, patches of nodules glistened: pale and swollen, protruding through mucosa. They looked vile, malignant, *wrong.*

She'd never seen, nor heard of, anything like this. She felt shock, and more: *vindication.* "The doctors said these were evidence of inflammatory bowel disease," she told Lorraine Fraser, the *Mail on Sunday* newspaper's medical correspondent, who, two and a half years before, had also reported the launch of Jackie Fletcher's JABS group. "I felt such relief. At last we had found what we knew to be there."

Crocodile-jawed forceps stretched from the head of the snake and bit off a tiny chunk of flesh. Then the scope retreated, snatching five more—from the cecum, ascending colon, transverse colon, descending colon, and rectum—which would be cut into pairs for analysis. One set was dispatched, fixed in formalin preservative, to the histopathology department on the hospital's second floor, where it would be sliced, mounted on slides, and stained for study under a microscope. The other went with Chadwick to a tenth-floor lab to be frozen in liquid nitrogen at minus 70°C and probed for any fingerprint of the virus.

More tests followed over the rest of the week. Trolleyed back and forth from Malcolm Ward, Child Two would undergo the lumbar puncture, MRI brain scan, B_{12} investigation, electroencephalogram, blood and urine tests, and so forth.

All of these procedures yielded normal results. But the hospital's pathologists, studying Child Two's biopsies, reported subtle signs of inflammation. Their craft was "histology" (the microscopic study of tissues), which in this case would be reviewed, and reviewed, and reviewed, as Wakefield's career rose, and fell.

"The mild patchy generalised increase in inflammatory cells with lymphoid aggregates and follicles is not very specific," the pathologists reported, three days after the scoping, "but could be in keeping with low grade quiescent inflammatory bowel disease."

Another *eureka*? Wakefield's team thought so. Marrying that finding with the swollen glands, the provisional diagnosis from Walker-Smith was Crohn's. It would seem that they'd found what they were looking for.

Crohn's in an eight-year-old. A somber diagnosis. The outlook would likely be bleak. Not only would Child Two struggle with developmental issues, but his guts would likely burn and blister. Regarded as lifelong (characterized by spells of remission and relapse), Crohn's most often required long-term hardcore drug therapy and repeated rounds of surgery.

How would a profoundly autistic person cope with that? And the prognosis was sometimes worse. Crohn's also raised the risk of a host of other conditions, including depression, arthritis, eye diseases, and cancer. Some treatments caused bones to become brittle.

But Ms. Two later tells me—*her* impression, not mine—that the professor couldn't disguise his excitement. "He skipped into that room like a two-year-old," she says of Walker-Smith's visit to Malcom Ward to break news that her child might have Crohn's disease. She says he said, "Mrs. [Two], you were right."

FIVE

Child Four

Years later, an American group, Moms on a Mission for Autism, seized a chance to interrogate Wakefield. His favorite movie? *Doctor Zhivago*. His favorite actor? *Jack Nicholson*. His favorite song? *"Your Tiny Hand is Frozen."* And the "song that reminds you of the happiest time in your life?" *Andrea Bocelli sings "Con Te Partirò."*

The latter was an oily pop operatic: lush with strings and sweeping cadence. Four minutes. Romantic. With a tune you could whistle. Translated, "With You I'll Leave." Bocelli, a tenor, first sang it publicly in February 1995 at a festival in Sanremo, northern Italy. Then it took off majorly over the next two years, bastardized under the title "Time to Say Goodbye" (breaking German sales records in February 1997) as a duet with a midmarket soprano.

That dubs the soundtrack of as good as it gets to the time of Wakefield's pilot study. This was the project that was to make his name, and would later enter his profession's annals of shame as among the most unethical, dishonest, and damaging medical research to be unmasked in living memory.

A dozen children were scoped for it—numbered 1 to 12—with the results to be published in *The Lancet*. The first was admitted in July 1996, and the last the following February. They were aged between two and a half and nine and a half years. Eleven were boys. All were white. Nine came from England; one from Wales; one from the British island of Jersey, near France; and one from the Bay Area of California.

All were rendered unconscious, scoped, and tested for evidence of measles virus in their guts.

By this time, the Wakefields had moved house again: to 43 Taylor Avenue, Kew. This was a prosperous, leafy, west London neighborhood made famous by Kew Gardens, a renowned botanic park, under the flightpath into Heathrow Airport. With his wife, Carmel, he snagged a six-bedroom, three-bathroom interwar villa for themselves and now a brood of three young children: the latest, Imogen Marie.

Child Two would forever be the sentinel case. But the *best* at that time was another little boy, whose mother approached Wakefield in April 1996, three months before the first was scoped. He was nine years old, from a town in Tyneside—a region once famous for coalfields and shipyards—280 miles north of Hampstead. He was the next big catch: yielding what Wakefield would describe as the "most compelling case history" of vaccine damage.

I'll call him "Child Four," and his mother "Ms. Four," who, writing on three pages of flower-patterned notepaper, requested information about the research.

> Dear Dr Wakefield
> I was advised by Jackie Fletcher the JABS coordinator to contact you. I have a son [Child Four] aged 9 who is diagnosed Autistic. Recently I have been to see [a lawyer] in Newcastle as I believe the measles injection and the MMR injection may be responsible for my son's condition.

In a small, neat script, Ms. Four summarized the story before concluding with the purpose of her approach.

Could you tell me what you think of all this and whether there are any tests [my son] can have to help in confirming that the injections may have caused his problems?

Those problems were many, and of a similar severity to those of Child Two's. But, unlike the happily born Cambridgeshire boy, Child Four had struggled from the start. His mother's womb was unusual—so-called "bicornate"—where the uterus is heart- or Y-shaped. Following a pregnancy five weeks short of average, her son presented, not headfirst, but in the trickier breech position. And, although Ms. Four recalled that a C-section was proposed, no doctor was available to perform one. Concern was then raised about the baby's features, and it was later discovered that a gene commonly associated with learning challenges, Fragile X, had "a very small deletion" of unknown import.

"It was a terrible birth," she says when we meet years later, after she emails me offering help.

I should have done this years ago but at the time I was stressed with other things to do with my sons care and I was loyal to Dr Wakefield as I believed at the time he was right and telling the truth.

She was a lightly built woman, a residential home assistant, who, after a two-year course in preschool social care, had for sixteen years worked in mental health and disability. Straight off I liked her style. We meet in a bar at Newcastle train station, where she arrives in black leather, clutching a metal-studded handbag, like she'd skipped off the back of a motorbike.

But, as she talks of her first child—in the warm "Geordie" accent of the English northeast—I can't imagine the wind in her hair. "My son progressively regressed from being a happy, normal little boy, to slowing down, to losing every single skill," she says. "The only skill he had left in the end was—which he still has—is using a spoon."

Child Four, she recalls, had initially learned about a dozen words, before, at the age of approximately fifteen or sixteen months, his development slowed, then plateaued. Until he was four, however, he still played with toys and had yet to adopt the repetitive behaviors that often helped to define childhood autism.

Somewhere between four and four and a half years, she says, he disappeared into a world of his own. "He just started banging his head off the wall, running backwards and forwards," she tells me. "He didn't know who I was anymore. He started making little noises. Just everything went. He didn't have any skills, like. He couldn't do anything anymore. He couldn't play. He was playing with cars and garages and things when he was two years old. All that went. You couldn't hold him anymore. You couldn't do anything."

Her life was shattered. She'd no explanation. And that of the boy's father was devastating. "He blamed me," she volunteers of a partner in such pain that he upped and walked away from his family. "He actually blamed me. Thinking it was something to do with me."

Unlike Ms. Two, she didn't claim to have answers. Like most parents, I found, who fell into Wakefield's orbit, she relied on *him* to tell *her*. "I hadn't thought about the MMR," she says of the time when her son's issues had first arisen. But, five months after *Newsnight*, she did. The occasion was a visit to a community center, where she spotted a local newspaper clipping, pinned to a noticeboard, headlined:

Jabs safety fear folk flood hotline

It gave the phone number of a local mother from Fletcher's group, explained that this mother's son had regressed after a shot, and named a lawyer, one Richard Barr.

"There was a story on the board," Ms. Four remembers of the moment she first suspected the three-in-one, when her son was eight years old. "It was basically the same as [my boy's] story. They had been totally normal, had regressed, with loss of skills, and everything."

She phoned the number on the clipping and, months later, wrote the letter introducing herself to Wakefield. Ten days after she posted it—and to her surprise—he phoned her at home, and they talked. She minuted the conversation at the time, in blue ink, later giving me a copy of what she wrote.

> He told me to ring him or write in 3–4 months as he is now recruiting people to do research into bowel problems caused by measles & that it will show up if measles injection caused it so I can get legal aid.

Child Four, she told him, had no significant bowel issues, except (if she let her son have fruit juice or yogurt) an occasional bout of diarrhea.

But, what made Child Four's case so compelling to Wakefield was an oddity in his medical history. He was born in January 1987, more than twenty months before MMR was launched. Although the triple shot was first licensed in the United States in 1971, it didn't reach Britain until October 1988. So, at fifteen months, the boy received a *single* measles shot (which had been around in the UK since at least 1968) and then the three-in-one at four years and one month.

So here were *two* immunizations with measles-containing vaccines, which could be matched against the boy's development. Pediatricians generally said that any perception of a link between vaccines and autism was the result of a simple coincidence. The first dose of MMR was almost always given in the second year of life, and this was the same window in which the first symptoms of autism were most typically recognized by parents.

But, in this child, the history offered extra ammunition. Given two measles-containing shots (first a single, then the three-in-one), not only was his MMR *outside* the usual window (and hence not prey to the traditional wisdom), but Wakefield could posit a "double hit," or "rechallenge" effect, strengthening the impression of a *cause*. Although Child Four's story isn't one that Wakefield ever told, the mother's letter and their conversations set him thinking. And when two months later the mother wrote to him again—reporting that her son experienced diarrhea on cod liver oil—he suggested she ask her family doctor for a referral letter. Then he phoned that doctor to make sure.

Thus it was that on a Sunday in September 1996—three weeks after Child Two had been and gone—Ms. Four and her son set off from their home, an affordable little house in a brick-and-stucco terrace, to spend six days at Hampstead.

Four hours later, they stood at a pair of locked doors on the sixth floor of the Royal Free Hospital. Here was Malcolm Ward: an airy, friendly space, with around a dozen beds in two bright bays, plus en suite side rooms big enough for an extra bed, where a parent could sleep by their child. Toys for all ages lightened the mood, with a circular play table and blue springy mat, laid out for patients' recreation.

But despite the ward's comforting appearance and welcoming staff, Ms. Four remembers her son's stay as a nightmare. "You believe in doctors," she tells me, remembering the ordeal. "I just knew they'd do a test to try and find out if the MMR caused autism. That's why I went. If I'd known they were going to be so invasive with [my son], I wouldn't have went."

It made nothing easier that she arrived in distress. By the time she met Simon Murch, who was to perform the ileocolonoscopy the following morning, she was so drained by the journey, and so hopeful for his help, that he would remember she broke down sobbing.

The regime was the same as it was for Child Two. A history was taken from the mother, and the boy's bowel prepped. Then, at

8:30 a.m. Monday, he was trolleyed to the endoscopy suite, four floors up, and sedated for the vital procedure.

Rectum . . . colon . . . valve . . . ileum.

And there they were again: *those swellings*.

Protruding through mucosa, so visible on the monitor, glistened those nodules that had shocked Ms. Two. "Hyperplasia" was the word that doctors used. "Ileal lymphoid nodular hyperplasia."

Ms. Four noted in a diary that the scoping took an hour. Then she documented days of misery. As the battery of tests Wakefield wanted was attempted, staff documented Child Four's "inconsolable crying." He fought with nurses. Blood was found in his stools. He pulled the mattress from his bed, repeatedly vomited, and was "tearful throughout" a procedure.

> Wed morning. 9.15 to xray for barium meal, but [my son] wouldn't drink the chalky drink. Back to ward tried holding him down & using syringe—but [he] fought them. Tried tube in nose no good so gave up. Then they decided to sedate him for it then changed their mind. Called off.

Such was an example of the experience families went through in this phase of their desperate quests. They would have done anything for answers about their kids. And Child Four had it bad: two days after scoping, this profoundly autistic nine-year-old collapsed.

"He collapsed in the corridor," Ms. Four tells me. "There was nobody around, and I was trying to get back to the lifts. I'd gone down a couple of floors, I think, to get a paper, or something like that. He was walking along and, all of a sudden, just collapsed. There was nobody around, and I couldn't get any help. I was panicking a bit, and then, I can't remember how much further, he collapsed again."

In all, he collapsed three times that day, she remembers. Other children in the study also suffered. It took three people, for instance, to hold down Child Two, merely for a standard blood draw. A four-year-old experienced such headache after lumbar puncture that, following discharge, his mother called an emergency doctor. And Child Five, aged seven, fared so badly from the same test (which had taken cerebrospinal fluid under general anesthetic) that he was rushed by ambulance from his home to a local hospital and kept for two days' observation.

The mother of that last boy initially contested that a spinal tap was even needed. "We said, 'No,' you know, we thought that it was not relevant," she says. "It was only because they sort of *begged* that we decided to."

Child Four escaped the needle into his spine. After electroencephalogram and magnetic resonance imaging—both performed on the Thursday, under sedation—the attempt at lumbar puncture was abandoned. The boy was so ill, and repeatedly vomiting, that on Friday he was bundled with his mother into a taxi, and driven 280 miles home.

That Friday evening, Wakefield addressed a JABS meeting in London, with *Newsnight*'s woman in scarlet—Fletcher—and Barr, the lawyer in the newspaper clipping that alerted Ms. Four to MMR. "I found your short discourse both informative and interesting," the mother of a six-year-old wrote to Wakefield afterward, before bringing her son, Child Twelve, to be scoped.

Two weeks later, back in Tyneside, Ms. Four received good news. Notwithstanding the ileal lymphoid hyperplasia, blood tests for bowel disease came back normal. And the hospital's pathologists (strictly, "histopathologists," since the study of tissue under a microscope is histology), who'd examined her son's biopsies for evidence of disease, found "no histopathological abnormality."

So that was that for Ms. Four and her son, she thought. But then something peculiar occurred. Nearly six months later, John Walker-Smith, *changed* the boy's diagnosis.

Although Child Four hadn't returned for any further tests, and the findings of normality had been reviewed, and agreed upon, between pediatricians and pathologists, the Australian professor reclassified the results: from apparent bowel *health* to *disease*. Now, he said, the boy suffered from "indeterminate colitis," which to gastroenterologists meant a serious, potentially life-changing condition, but at the specific time-point couldn't be positively diagnosed as either ulcerative colitis or Crohn's.

The little boy, however, didn't have either. And neither, it was realized, did Child Two. Despite the excitement after the sentinel case's scoping, he'd been sent away for two months on a special liquid diet, scoped again by a doctor not involved in the research, who reported a "complete return to normal." Like Walker-Smith had concluded, while still at Barts Hospital, Child Two suffered from a food intolerance.

Nevertheless, on a Tuesday in March 1997, Walker-Smith wrote to Child Four's local doctor. In light of the "histological finding of a colitis," he explained, he recommended prescription of a powerful anti-inflammatory drug—mesalazine—often given to patients with Crohn's.

Facing charges of misconduct eleven years later, Walker-Smith would admit that he couldn't explain the provenance of his revised diagnosis. He'd made no entry in the boy's clinical records. And mesalazine was by no means a trivial pharmaceutical, carrying special "black box" warnings in drug reference manuals of potentially serious or life-threatening reactions. They were reactions, moreover, of which a nonspeaking, developmentally challenged child could hardly communicate concern.

The [Committee on Safety of Medicines] has recommended that patients receiving mesalazine, olsalazine or sulphasalazine should be advised to report any unexplained bleeding, bruising, purpura, sore throat, fever or malaise that occurs during treatment. A blood count should be performed and the drug stopped immediately if there is suspicion of a blood dyscrasia.

Ms. Four wasn't convinced that the drug treatment was even necessary. She says a good diet prevented diarrhea. But, as recorded in her documents contemporaneously, she checked her feelings with a doctor at the hospital: a man who at that time she trusted.

> Dr Wakefield told me the medicines would dampen inflammation [and] it also reduces behaviour & Autistic problems. I was not willing to give [my son] the medicines as I am so against them. He advised me strongly to try & get 2 other mothers to talk to me about results.

In the end, she gave in to what was evidently an experiment. But when given the drug, her son developed abdominal pain, and his behavior didn't improve. Mesalazine was a "total disaster," she tells me. "I was quite shocked," she says of her reaction when she saw the package information. She says, "It had 'colitis' on it . . . where has that come from?"

Back at Hampstead, however, Wakefield's team was euphoric. If not close to collective hysteria. He was now speculating that autism itself was an inflammatory bowel disease, while Walker-Smith was prescribing mesalazine, olsalazine, or sulphasalazine to almost every child enrolled in the project.

SIX

A Moral Issue

To unleash epidemics of fear, guilt, and disease should be expected to require preparation. From the concrete castle overlooking Hampstead Heath, the ground was laid for Wakefield's signature accomplishment—aided, incredibly, by a hospital and a medical school—many months before his study of eleven boys and one girl was formally presented to the world.

Since the *Newsnight* broadcast, his profile had soared. The *Sunday Times Magazine* led the national press with a five-page feature ("A Shot in the Dark"), showcasing him, Jackie Fletcher, and the lawyer, Richard Barr. The ITV network ran a thirty-minute prime-time *Big Story* report on his claims linking MMR with Crohn's. And at the *Mail on Sunday*, Lorraine Fraser, who'd covered JABS's launch and Child Two's scoping, began a determined campaign as Wakefield's champion.

But all this would melt away as historical small change. By the summer of 1997, he was riding high on the results of the pilot study scopings—especially the frequency of the swollen glands—and what parents had reported at the hospital. In case after case, they'd told John Walker-Smith's team that their children had developed behavioral problems and bowel complaints shortly after they received MMR.

By convention, research findings were meant to be kept confidential until peer reviewed and published in a journal. But after being seeded by leaks to a doctors' magazine, *Pulse*, a barrage of media coverage erupted from Hampstead in August, linking the three-in-one with both autism and Crohn's.

Kill or cure?

Both of my little boys are autistic and my wonderful marriage is in tatters

Crying shame of the vaccination victims

Wakefield was quoted, speaking of *five* "forthcoming" papers. He said they "clearly confirm our suspicions." And further boosting interest in the study's results was a more senior figure, from the purple of the medical establishment. This was the professor of gastroenterology Roy Pounder, fifty-three, who was a council member of the Royal College of Physicians and harbored medicopolitical ambitions. Ten years before, he'd hired the doctor without patients, and he'd mentor him through the rest of his career.

"I am very convinced," Pounder told BBC television that August. "Almost all" the data were "biologically plausible," he said, demonstrating that "the virus is there."

That was in public. Meanwhile, in private, not one, but *two* papers were submitted to *The Lancet*, reporting the pilot study's results. One was clinical, titled "A New Syndrome: Enterocolitis and Regressive Behavioural Disorder," with "neuropsychiatric diagnoses," "findings," and suchlike from Wakefield and eleven coauthors. The other was "scientific," mostly immunohistochemistry, with a splash of molecular data thrown in.

The performance was bravura. He'd done it again. Even the *H. pylori* pioneers, Robin Warren and Barry Marshall, never had a pair of papers in *The Lancet*. Now, as the father of four children (the latest, Corin John Ogilivie, aged four months), Wakefield waited on the journal's decision.

There wasn't much doubt about what was to follow. The worldly winds were all at his back. Should the *Lancet*'s traditions not prove sufficient, the summer's burst of publicity was sure to grab Richard Horton, its ex–Royal Free editor-in-chief. Vital calculations of his journal's impact—based on its performance in attracting citations by researchers—had shown it slipping against the market leader, the *New England Journal of Medicine*.

Then more luck, in the desk editor Horton assigned to wrangle the manuscripts into print. This was a waggish family doctor, John Bignall, fifty-four, who was then on a roll after fast-tracking a case series of a rare brain disease (new-variant Creutzfeldt-Jakob). He was the champion of a policy that colleagues called "Bignall's rule": that if a submission was discussed for more than ten minutes, then it had "interest" and ought to be run.

For every manuscript accepted, however, scores were spat back. Success couldn't be taken for granted. Much would depend on the peer review process. And, once again, Wakefield's winds blew warm. In mid-November 1997, Bignall posted both submissions to a professor of pediatric gastroenterology named David Candy, eighty miles southwest of London. He'd never reviewed papers for *The Lancet* before, and his career mentor was John Walker-Smith. "I knew," Candy tells me, "that anything by John would be well written and reliable."

Small world.

The hospital and medical school were already preparing. This would be their biggest moment in decades. Wakefield and Pounder met with managers from both and persuaded them to recommend another press conference, even bigger than for the question-marked paper. "Dr. Wakefield says that he was contacted by every major news organization," the hospital's press officer, Philippa Hutchinson, told Arie Zuckerman, the dean, in the wake of the summer storm of publicity.

A tall, broad man, with owl-sized glasses and the stiff demeanor of one striving for eminence, Zuckerman, sixty-five, wasn't only a professor of microbiology and editor of *J Med Virol*. He was also a director of the World Health Organization and a pioneer of hepatitis B vaccines. So to be, in his own mind, on the safe side, he ruled that the event shouldn't be described as a "press conference" but a "briefing," focusing the media on certain "gastrointestinal changes" reported in the clinical study.

He would regret that colossal misjudgment forever. He assumed that, as dean, he should command the media, placing Wakefield's contributions in context. And he assumed that a press release his school issued in advance, describing the findings as "controversial," would dampen the ardor of reporters. "Until and unless the appropriate national and international authorities and the World Health Organisation decide to review the policies relating to MMR immunisation," this said, "the Royal Free will continue to support the current programme."

Even as Zuckerman stressed caution, however, a PR company was hired and months of planning went forward. To hit the ground running (in an era when battery size still limited the convenience of mobile phones), extra landlines were installed for reporters to call their desks. Mechanical answering machines were ordered to field the public reaction. A rehearsal was scheduled to smooth the choreography. And an unprecedented twenty-one-minute package of video clips was ordered to maximize TV impact.

Nobody involved could seriously argue that they couldn't foresee what would happen. Public fear in the wake of the question-marked paper had now shaved one point from the uptake of MMR: a big figure when compounding year on year. Within days of the *Pulse* report, the hospital was "inundated" (Wakefield's word) with families asking about tests. And, in the video clip package, commissioned by the hospital, he claimed that what he'd found in the dozen scoped kids warranted the triple vaccine to be "suspended" by the government, in favor of single shots.

"There is sufficient anxiety in my own mind for the long-term safety of the polyvalent—that is the MMR vaccination in combination—that I think it should be suspended," he said in one of four variations of the same message in the video. "My own opinion, again, is that the monovalent—the single vaccines; measles, mumps, rubella—are likely, in this context, to be safer."

His mentor, Pounder (hoping for advancement at the college of physicians), warned the government of what was coming. Although the second, "scientific," study was rejected by *The Lancet* (in a later lawsuit Wakefield claimed that he never even kept a copy), the clinical paper was certain to provoke uproar. "We believe there is only a limited amount of monovalent measles vaccine available at the present time," Pounder wrote to England's chief medical officer, Kenneth Calman, "and your department may wish to investigate this potential problem."

But the professor of gastroenterology also had concerns closer to home: not least any advantage to be gained for his department as a result of his protégé's publication. Under the national Research Assessment Exercise, government money was meant to filter to the most successful units—with publishing, again, a key measure. In short, that paper might not only mean money for the medical school, but money for gastroenterology. Indeed, years later, when I ask a scientist who'd worked at the Royal Free, "what explains the phenomenon" I was by then investigating, she replies with two words: "Roy Pounder."

And so it was that all was ready—with an overflow pressroom, and coffee and biscuits for fifty—when on Thursday, February 26, 1998, at shortly after 10:00 a.m., the latest Wakefield paper was released.

The location for the event was what the hospital called the Atrium, on Level 1, near the building's main entrance. Fifty feet by one hundred, with no natural light, it rose a mere twenty feet to a white neon ridge that a moth wouldn't mistake for the sky. A blond oblong of hardwood, three-quarters of the floor, was edged with seven pillars and surrounded by carpet, like the ballroom of a midpriced hotel.

By ten o'clock, reporters, producers, and camerapeople were gathered on ranks of hard-backed chairs. They faced a blue-clothed table, where the platform party was to sit, and a wooden lectern, where Zuckerman would stand. The *Times*, *The Guardian*, the *Daily Telegraph* and *The Independent* were there. So were the *Mail on Sunday*, *The Express*, and *Practice Nurse*. There was Channel 4, Channel 5, the BBC, and Sky News. There was the Press Association and Reuters wire services. *Pulse* sent two people; *The Lancet* three. Team Wakefield totaled nearly a dozen.

During the months that had passed since its first submission to the journal, the paper had significantly changed. There was the addition of an author—a consultant pathologist named Susan Davies—taking the total now credited to thirteen. And, after discussions, a new title had been devised: placing in journalists' hands and scattering on chairs five double-columned pages under a two-line gothic heading:

Ileal-lymphoid-nodular hyperplasia, non-specific colitis, and pervasive developmental disorder in children

Hardly any non-doctor could unravel that mouthful, and even many who could wouldn't get it. But the paper's conclusions, in a section headed "Interpretation," were plain enough for all to grasp.

We identified associated gastrointestinal disease and developmental regression in a group of previously normal children, which was generally associated in time with possible environmental triggers.

The text made clear that nothing was *proved*. But those triggers—described as the "apparent precipitating events"—practically phoned themselves into the news.

As a facing pair, on the second and third pages, were two three-inch-deep tables, each across both columns, itemizing apparent facts about the children. The patients were anonymized, numbered 1 to 12: the eleven boys and one girl, described as aged three to nine. None were diagnosed with Crohn's.

Table 1 was complex. Even seasoned medical journalists would struggle to decode its terms. In three columns, set against the patients' numbers, were strings of "abnormal laboratory tests" plus "endoscopic" and "histological" findings. Nearly every line contained the same arcane phrases. Almost all included "chronic nonspecific colitis"—inflammatory disease of the large intestine—and "ileal lymphoid hyperplasia," the ugly swollen glands in the small intestine.

Table 2 was simple. It was as easy to read as a big fat sign screaming, "DANGER." This page-wide rectangle was labeled "Neuro-psychiatric diagnosis," with the first column headed "Behavioural diagnosis" and the second "Exposure identified by parents or doctor." Below these were listed the reported diagnosis for each of the children, and the apparent precipitating event:

Autism . . . Autism . . . Autism . . . Autism . . .
MMR . . . MMR . . . MMR . . . MMR . . .

People got what this paper was about.

Nine of the diagnoses were reported to be "Autism" (although one, Child Four's, was given as "Autism? Disintegrative disorder?").

In eight cases, the "exposure" was "MMR."

Turning back to page 1, an opening "Summary" gave the first of the paper's "Findings"—apparently based on what parents, such as Ms. Two and Ms. Four, told John Walker-Smith and his team.

Onset of behavioural symptoms was associated, by the parents, with measles, mumps and rubella vaccination in eight of the 12 children.

Eight of twelve? That's two out of three. So . . . two out of three families of children with autism blamed it on MMR.

More startling information lay at the foot of the next page: reporting a terrifying sudden onset of the problems. The "first behavioural symptoms" (also described as "behavioural features" and "behavioural changes") were said to follow the shot within *days*.

In these eight children the average interval from exposure to first behavioural symptoms was 6.3 days (range 1–14).

So, up to *fourteen days* to onset—two weeks, maximum—the very figure that was given by Ms. Two to the hospital's doctors for when her son's head-banging began. The shortest times, meanwhile, were a mere "24 h" and "immediately" after MMR.

Last came the wordiest section, headed "Discussion." Among other things, this hypothesized mechanisms of damage, including vitamin B_{12} issues and "opioid excess," both raised by Ms. Two in her phone call. And, at the end, unusually, was a stop-press "Addendum"—just like there had been in the 1969 paper by Wakefield's neurologist father, Graham. Forty more patients had been "assessed," it said, with *thirty-nine* having what it called "the syndrome."

At the blue-clothed table, four speakers took their seats: Wakefield (who, it transpired, had alone written the paper), Pounder (who wasn't listed among its authors), Simon Murch (listed as second author), and a smooth-domed child psychiatrist, Mark Berelowitz (credited as the seventh of thirteen).

Presiding from the lectern, to their left, facing the press, Zuckerman strove to reassure. "Hundreds of millions of doses of these vaccines have been given worldwide," he declared. "They've been shown to be absolutely safe."

But if Zuckerman presided, Wakefield commanded. He was the reason why everybody came. Wearing a soft-shouldered black suit, white shirt, and patterned tie, he spoke into the glare of television lighting, every inch the honest doctor and surefooted guide on a perilous frontier of science.

"The association—the temporal association—between MMR and autism was initially made in the United States," he said. "We have confirmed that temporal link in our small cohort."

As he spoke, dozens of hands around the Atrium twitched. Reporters scribbled quotes. Producers logged sound bites. The press officer, Hutchinson, took minutes.

> Selection criteria: 1, Normal development; 2, behavioral regression; 3, bowel symptoms.
> Average time 6.3 days, 1–14 days range.
> Lymphoid nodular hyperplasia and chronic colitis.

Four times the paper referred to a "syndrome," said to be a constellation of bowel and brain issues. "This particular syndrome that we are describing is very new," Wakefield explained from his chair at the front. "It appears that it may have come into being beyond 1988, when MMR first originated."

The dean fought back with measles statistics. During the previous year in Romania, he said, there were twenty thousand cases, and thirteen children died.

But Wakefield heaved such background aside and called for the triple shot to be suspended. "It's a moral issue for me," he announced. "And I can't support the continued use of these three vaccines, given in combination, until this issue has been resolved."

Those words alone would have been enough—even billed as the opinions of one doctor. But sitting to Wakefield's right, sometimes adjusting the microphone, Pounder endorsed the message.

The professor's visual tell was a curious kind of gaze, with the hoods of his eyes curved like crescent moons, which he projected on the assembly like a bird. "Now, my feeling about vaccination goes more along with Andrew Wakefield," he said. "It does seem that this unique combination of having three viruses in the same day may be an unnatural, unusual, event."

That should do it. And that day, it did. After months of planning, Wakefield, Pounder, and a minor medical school shouted "bomb" in a crowded place.

Independent Television News hit the note that night:

Questions were raised today about the safety of the combined mumps, measles, and rubella vaccine . . .

Channel 4:

New research showing a possible link with a bowel disease which could lead to autism . . .

Channel 5:

Claims there could be a link between a common childhood vaccine and autism . . .

Trucks and trains hauled the story through the night, pounded onto paper for news vendors and mailboxes. And, the next morning, the nation woke to coverage such as the *Guardian*'s. It ran three reports, kicking off on page 1.

A MEDICAL study suggests today that there could be a link between the measles, mumps and rubella vaccine (MMR) given to children in their second year of life and inflammatory bowel disease and autism.

Dr Andrew Wakefield and colleagues at the Royal Free Hospital in Hampstead, London, report in the Lancet that children referred to them with signs of autism and gut problems had a hitherto unknown bowel syndrome and that treating it alleviated some of the symptoms of autism.

They also found that the behavioural changes in the children which are typical of autism, such as forgetting the basic language they had just learned, began within days of their MMR vaccination.

Naysayers squawked like Hitchcock ravens. The study was too small. Twelve children meant nothing. There were no control subjects (without autism, or MMR) to check if the "syndrome" was unique. Parents were susceptible to "recall bias." The pathology wasn't evaluated blind.

The Lancet, too, would come under fire. Surely, it was irresponsible to raise doubts without proof. And to publish on just *twelve* children? But like three years before, with the question-marked paper, the journal had covered itself. Two scientists from the US Centers for Disease Control and Prevention—including an epidemiologist, Frank DeStefano—had been invited to contribute a twelve-hundred-word rebuttal, dumping on Wakefield's work.

"A first dose of MMR vaccine is given to about 600,000 children every year in the UK, most during the second year of life, the time when autism first becomes manifest," they noted. "Not surprisingly, therefore, some cases will follow MMR."

But these were public health doctors preaching to the choir. The national congregation wasn't listening. If it was true there was a hospital where, in the space of a few months, a string of parents surfaced in a bowel clinic's caseload saying their child got the MMR and showed behavioral symptoms within days, then surely that needed explaining? Maybe elsewhere, at hospitals throughout the world, less vigilant doctors had missed the first snapshot of a hidden epidemic of injury.

And *twelve not enough? No controls? What?* The naysayers should have known better. Crohn's disease was first systematically reported, in 1932, on gut specimens from just *fourteen* patients.

Autism was classically described, in 1943, in a mere *eleven* children. And what became known as AIDS was initially published, in 1981, on *five* gay men in Los Angeles. Should those observations have passed without comment, for fear of triggering alarm?

Nothing was written in the paper, or said in the Atrium, about the role of Jackie Fletcher and JABS. Or that the children had been brought to take part in research and weren't merely routine referrals. I'd discover all that, to trigger uproar, years later. But, if the study's subjects and findings were as they appeared to be, then surely they were worth a few pages of *The Lancet*.

If they were as they appeared.

SECRET SCHEMES

- - - - - - - - - - - - - - - - - - - -

SEVEN

Everybody Knows

I'm pretty sure I cried when I discovered vaccination. Well, whoever knew a baby that didn't? And the hypodermic syringe that punctured my skin, at a clinic on Raglan Street in Kentish Town, north London, was scary enough to hold up a bank. Here was a reusable glass barrel, practically as thick as an oboe, a nickel-plated brass plunger, with sufficient suction to clear drains, and a beveled steel needle (heat sterilized between stabbings) that my mother might have paired to knit sweaters.

Memory plays tricks. But that was then the standard kit: ten years after World War II. Thirteen years more, and my mother was dead of breast cancer, leaving me a portable typewriter, a judgmental disposition, and a folder of paperwork (birth certificate, school reports . . .), including records of my immunizations. The first was a shot against the diphtheria bacterium, which, according to a four-inch by three-inch green card, I was given on Wednesday, May 4, 1955. I was fifteen months and twelve days old.

From that you can age me. And I'm now much older: so old, I confess, that when I joined the *Sunday Times*, the paper was set in lead. As a smartass twenty-something in black suede winklepickers, I'd begun in the 1980s on the business section, as a rewrite man and "stone sub" editor, sweating over slugs of back-to-front type that were locked into a flat steel tombstone (called a "forme") to be pushed away on wheels by the printers.

What set me on collision with Andrew Wakefield, however, were just sixteen published words. At the time I wrote them, I was the paper's social affairs correspondent and had recently run a campaign to get an act of Parliament giving new rights to people with disabilities. On the day in question—Friday, April 1, 1988—I held forth in a thousand-word opinion column sideswiping a vaccine controversy. This was over a shot against *Bordetella pertussis*, the bug that caused whooping cough, that, for most of the 1970s and 1980s, was thought (by doctors, as well as many parents) to sometimes, if only rarely, cause brain damage.

A generation later, this saga was forgotten, superseded by anxiety over MMR. But only two days before I wrote the piece in question, a judge, sitting in the magnificent gothic palace of London's Royal Courts of Justice, near the River Thames embankment, had issued a landmark ruling. After a sixty-three-day hearing, with evidence and experts from all over the world, Lord Justice (Sir Murray) Stuart-Smith, a sixty-year-old father of three boys and three girls, had read aloud to a breathless, creaking courtroom, a fourteen-chapter 273-page opinion, largely bringing the controversy to an end.

His answer was no. On the balance of probabilities, the pertussis shot *didn't* do the harm that many people thought. "I was ready to believe that this belief was well founded," read the former cavalry officer, whose hobbies included shooting and playing the cello. "But over the weeks that I have listened to, and examined, the evidence and arguments, I have become more and more doubtful."

I didn't agree. And, two and a half miles east, near the Tower of London, I set aside his lordship's opinion. That Friday, I'd conducted my own inquiry, swiveling in my chair in the *Sunday Times* newsroom, snapping rubber bands, and riffling manila folders stuffed with yellowing newsprint clippings. The evidence was overwhelming—even a *Sunday Times* campaign later accorded its own logo: "The Vaccine Victims."

Vaccine victims win round 1 in fight for compensation

Whooping cough vaccine risks concealed, say victims' parents

Whooping cough: the facts parents have not been told

Bundles of the stuff. Beyond a doubt. A "special investigation" by our medical correspondent had even concluded that the risks from vaccination were greater than from pertussis itself. "The government is presenting its case with misleading figures," he found. Experts' opinions were "concealed."

The picture wasn't simple as I flicked through the clippings. As parents became alarmed, vaccination rates slumped. On one measure, notifications of whooping cough jumped from 8,500 to 25,000 a year. And, in just one of many outbreaks, near the end of the 1970s, three dozen kids coughed themselves to death, with another seventeen left brain damaged.

Vaccinations decline "may lead to epidemic"

32,463 hit by whooping cough after vaccine scare

Four children die of whooping cough

Great stuff for newspapers: two scares for the price of one. And the concern that lurked behind my sixteen words was merely to point out that the struggling families of brain-impaired children needed help, whatever the cause of their issues. "When need outweighs blame" was the headline I was given, with a twenty-two-word "standfirst," as we called them:

After a "vaccine-damage" ruling last week, children will not get help. BRIAN DEER says all disabled people should have equal rights.

I still think that, but the piece was hardly memorable—apart from the sixteen words. From the court of Her Majesty's Press I decreed for printing, 1.2 million times:

Everybody knows there is a rare association between the whooping cough vaccine and severe brain damage.

In those happy days before universal email, nobody wrote in to complain. But I think my statement put down a marker among some to certify a particular interest. And, a few years later, I got a call from a woman in Ireland, who was then the queen of vaccine campaigners.

Her name was Margaret Best. She lived near the city of Cork, in Ireland's ceaselessly rainswept south. She'd famously won a huge financial settlement—£2.75 million, plus her lawyer's bills—from the Wellcome Foundation drug company (which coincidentally funded Wakefield's early career) over her neurologically challenged son, Kenneth. In September 1969—when Margaret was twenty-two, and her son four months—she'd taken him for immunization against the whooping cough bug, combined, as it was, with those against tetanus and diphtheria, in a three-in-one DTP, or DPT.

Within hours, she said later, she phoned the local doctor after Kenneth suffered a terrifying seizure. "His face got very red and his eyes turned in to the right," she said. "Both his arms came up to his chest, and it was as if his whole body was stiff."

In November 1996, she invited me to go see her. She was forty-seven years old: short, energetic, with tight black curls, and a rolled-up-sleeves kind of manner. Separated from her husband, Ken, she lived with a boyfriend, Christy, in a freshly built house with electric gates, gravel drive, barking dogs, and furniture that looked like it was bought at one department store in a matter of an hour or two.

Kenneth, twenty-seven, occupied an annex. He didn't speak, but sometimes screamed. His greatest pleasure was to blend balls of knitting wool into big soft bundles of color.

Margaret and I talked at her kitchen table, where I tried to visualize events. Between us lay a transcript of her evidence to a Dublin court, and a little blue magnetic-tape microcassette voice recorder that spared me the distraction of making notes.

"So, where did you phone the doctor from?" I asked after maybe thirty minutes, in the hope of reconstructing the awful night of which she spoke.

Margaret got up, and fumbled at the stove. Tape *off*. Then *on* when she returned. "Well," she said. "There was a neighbor whose phone I sometimes used."

That made sense. Phones were scarce. The incident occurred in the year of the first moon landing, in a poor fishing village called Kinsale.

"So, is that what you did?" I pressed, keen for color.

Margaret got up again, moved back to the stove, and paused before responding. "No."

Again, I waited. Tape *off*. Tape *on*. "So, what, you used a phone box?"

"Yes."

It was no big deal. Or so it felt at the time. But when I got back to London, and replayed the tape, my chin sank and my eyebrows rose. Why mention the neighbor if she used a pay phone? Why the walkabout, delay, and terse responses? Surely the night when her child's life was wrecked was indelibly etched on her mind?

And that's what would set me on my path to Wakefield. A week after my trip to Ireland, I ordered the transcript of *Best v. Wellcome*—and a big box of spiral-bound binders arrived, reporting every day of a thirty-five-day trial that, I thought, was riddled with anomalies. There were medical records contradicting Margaret's account, for instance, and she'd even taken her son for a second DTP, despite the apparent reaction.

"I am not suggesting for a moment that Mrs. Best is telling lies," Wellcome's leading counsel, Henry Hickey, had told the presiding judge in June 1989. "What I am saying is her recall is wrong, and that the events of which she talks occurred six weeks to two months *after* the time she thinks they did."

Who could say, so many years later? But the judge wasn't easily persuaded. "I think it goes further," replied Justice Liam Hamilton, president of Ireland's High Court, sitting among benches nearly as creaky as Stuart-Smith's. "I am satisfied, if her account isn't accurate, she is *lying*."

The drug company, however, maintained its stance—and this was where the case got interesting. Although the boy's doctor had made all kinds of notes ("snuffles," "eczema," "chesty," and so forth), he wrote nothing about seizures, which, on Margaret's evidence, were occurring up to twenty times a day.

Hickey insisted that the mother was "confused," and he persevered with his argument. "People can convince themselves of the truth of events in retrospect," he said. "We see it every day of the week in road traffic accidents."

But that submission only helped to seal Wellcome's fate, allowing the Supreme Court of Ireland to have a say. Margaret's story was so intricate—recounting daily seizures and visits to the doctor—it deduced that, if her account *wasn't true,* she *must be* lying. Therefore, given the company's position that she *wasn't* lying, then logically, she was telling the truth.

"They could have kept their mouths shut," Margaret tells me later, of a victory celebrated in a minor media festival. "If they'd said nothing and just conducted their defense, and didn't open their mouths about whether they thought I was lying, or whether I was telling the truth, or whether I was confused—it didn't matter a damn—if they had said nothing they might have been better off."

There, I confess, was *my* Guinness Moment. I thought: *Could* she? *Would* she? *Why not?* Here was an icon of much that I valued. She was a working-class mother. She left school at twelve. And she'd defeated a drug company. *Fantastic.*

But when I gave it more thought, the clichés dissolved. She hadn't earned her triumph in a bubble. It mattered to other families, facing choices over shots, trying to balance the benefits and risks. Besides, I was journalist. I wasn't a campaigner. I believed that in truth lay freedom.

So, I dug a little further. Well, a year's work further. And I discovered the story—real people, specific facts—behind that difference of opinion between a High Court judge and a Sunday newspaper reporter.

Incredibly, that story began with a doctor: a doctor at a London hospital. He published a research paper in a medical journal that was pounced on by TV and newspapers. It was a case series of children who, within fourteen days of a three-in-one-shot, were said to have suffered a neurological injury. An epidemic of fear circled the globe.

But this doctor wasn't Wakefield. His name was John Wilson, a consultant pediatric neurologist. The hospital was the Hospital for Sick Children, at Great Ormond Street, London: one of the world's top pediatric centers. It was three and a half miles south of the Royal Free, Hampstead. The journal was the midrank *Archives of Disease in Childhood*. And the media alarm was launched on a show called *This Week*—when Britain had only three TV channels.

I ordered the video and watched it many times.

"Are you satisfied that there is a link between the whooping cough vaccine and brain damage?" Wilson was asked, in April

1974, by *This Week*'s reporter, who wore a big-collared pink shirt, chunky spectacles, and sideburns trimmed to his jawbone.

"I personally am," the neurologist replied. "Because now I've seen too many children in whom there has been a very close association between a severe illness—with fits, unconsciousness, often focal neurological signs—and inoculation."

"What do you mean? You've seen a lot?"

"Well, in my time here, the last eight and a half years," he recalled of his tenure at Great Ormond Street, "I personally have seen somewhere in the region of *eighty patients*."

Wilson was a contemporary of Wakefield's father, Graham, and like him, was a god among gods. He wore his black hair oiled, flashed cuff links from dark suits, and spoke in the meticulous, languid tones of a less-than-passionate Christian bishop.

He'd gotten interested in immunization early in his career, before the then dreaded smallpox was vanquished. England blazed the trail in beating that disease, dating back to the late eighteenth century, when a physician, Edward Jenner, invented "variolation": credited as the first true vaccine. And catching the tail end, in the 1960s, Wilson had a sideline with personal injury lawyers, assisting claims of damage from the shots.

He published his DTP paper in January 1974, three months before starring on *This Week*. That was twenty-four years before Wakefield's twelve-child study, when, with two trainees—a German, Marcia Kulenkampff, and a Brazilian, José Salomão Schwartzman—Wilson authored four pages in the *Archives*.

"Between January 1961 and December 1972 approximately 50 children have been seen at the Hospital for Sick Children, London, because of neurological illness thought to be due to DPT inoculation," Wilson explained in the text. "There were 36 children in whom there was adequate data on the timing, and only those neurological illnesses occurring up to 14 days after DPT inoculation were included."

Wilson had gotten his two juniors to trawl the hospital's vaults for children's records implicating the vaccine. Then he used the two-week timeframe, which he picked himself, to segregate vaccine victims. "It was a very naive study," says Schwartzman, more than forty years later, when I visit with him in São Paulo, Brazil.

Before the TV broadcast, 79 percent of England's kids got DTP. But by 1978, after newspapers joined the furor, the figure had slumped to 31 percent.

Litigation followed. As I probed the history, I found reports of massive lawsuits, in Canada, the United States, and two test cases in London—both presided over by the cello-playing Stuart-Smith. And it was from *those* that I learned a few lessons in life that later would help in peeling the rancid onion from which the Wakefield story tumbled out.

The first English DTP case concerned a developmentally challenged boy by the name of Johnnie Kinnear. According to the evidence of his mother, Susan, he suffered "five or six" seizures on the night of his shot. Then more, every day, after that. But, despite doctor appointments for a string of minor ailments, the boy's medical records revealed nothing serious being raised for the next five months.

She lied.

The scene was tragic. Susan snarled at the court, like a lioness defending her cub. "You see, you are trying to confuse me now. You are trying to confuse me."

But they weren't.

Stuart-Smith ruled that she "was not telling the truth," and it was Johnnie's own lawyers who pulled the plug. "Anybody who was in court and heard the relevant witnesses," his counsel addressed the judge, in May 1986, "and saw the discrepancies between their accounts and the medical records, can be left in no doubt that his prospects are effectively nil."

Then came the second test, involving Susan Loveday, a developmentally challenged girl. This time, however, the parents weren't allowed to give evidence (for fear of a second collapse, with huge costs and delay), unless the science alone favored their claim. Most notably, the trial analyzed a landmark British study, which reported the "attributable risk" of permanent brain damage from DTP as *1 in 310,000 shots*.

That research (named the National Childhood Encephalopathy Study) ran for three years, included two million doses of DTP, and was the most definitive such inquiry anywhere. Its top line would be quoted in product data sheets and by doctors all over the world.

But when the judge went to work, he found the calculation ultimately rested on just *seven* key patients. So, overruling objections from the researchers responsible, he ordered the records of the seven to be produced and went through them, child by child. One had Reye's syndrome, which isn't caused by vaccines. Three were afflicted by viral conditions. And the files on the remainder showed their outcomes were "normal": cutting the attributable risk to *nil*.

Stuart-Smith galloped on, looking at more kids' cases, and concluded that even the saddest accounts weren't necessarily dependable.

> Case 1473: The parents' account is inconsistent with a previous account given by them.

> Case 1509: Onset of symptoms was in the previous October; it was changed to an onset of less than 24 hours on the basis of the parents' account given many months later.

> Case 1215: The parents' claim, as recorded in the documents, that the child was normal before vaccination, is plainly incorrect.

He also found what looked like fraud. It's hard to think what else could explain it. Two different printouts were discovered of tests of children's skills, showing that scores inexplicably *changed*.

Although they referred to the same patients, and the same examinations, the more recent results were erratically lower, dumbing down certain borderline patients.

"Bizarre," said the judge, "because it is difficult to see how the same data can give rise to different scores."

It was Wilson, however, who came off worst, along with his study claiming three dozen victims. Stuart-Smith reviewed them all. The neurologist admitted that in *eight* there was *no link* between the vaccine and illness. In *fifteen*, he accepted there was a reasonable alternative cause. He only stood his ground on twelve. And of this remaining third, a mere *three* were instances in which enough information was available to understand the circumstances, and even a role in those couldn't be proved.

Surprisingly, some kids on whom Wilson reported suffered their first symptoms *before* vaccination. But the most striking in his series was a pair of identical twin girls who weren't only diagnosed with a genetic condition, but—despite their function in triggering a twentieth-century health panic—never received DTP.

Unforgettable. My investigation bore fruit in almost seven thousand words, across six elegant pages of the *Sunday Times Magazine*. It taught me that, when it comes to vaccine victims, you can't *simply believe* either parents or doctors. And, after mastering arcane topics that I'd never need again (from the "mouse weight gain test" to the "tenets of Arlwyn Griffith"), it also taught me that vaccines as a field of inquiry was too difficult to be tackled on a whim.

So that was on my mind—literally, *right then*—when on Friday, February 27, 1998, I picked up *The Guardian* in a doctor's living room and read its page 1 from Hampstead. I was still on the road over DTP when Wakefield hit the news with MMR.

"You should investigate *that*," the doctor suggested as I left.

"No way." I laughed. "*Not a chance.*"

EIGHT

First Contact

So where did it begin? *Really* begin. Was it the phone call from Ms. Two, as Wakefield would say, introducing him to the story of his sentinel case? Was it the formation of JABS by *Newsnight*'s woman in scarlet, as she sought allies to help her sue for compensation? Or had it started decades before, at Great Ormond Street, with a different doctor and a different three-in-one?

I'll peel the rancid onion, so you don't have to, for what headlines would later shout:

THE TRUTH

At the start there *was* a phone call. But it wasn't *to* Wakefield. It was from him to a British civil servant. This was a man by the name of David Salisbury, forty-six, the government's top official on vaccines. He was a beige kind of character, never prone to indiscretion, and a pediatrician who once worked under the neurologist John Wilson: an experience that shaped his life.

He'd been there, on the wards, during the whooping cough crisis, greeting blue-light transfers to Great Ormond Street and its specialist kid-size ventilators. He saw babies cough for their lives as they were carried from ambulances, parents crying, nurses scurrying, and patient histories that didn't end well. He saw congenital rubella syndrome, which can lead to brain damage, deafness, blindness, and heart disease in babies. He saw the horrors of SSPE.

Subacute sclerosing panencephalitis: caused by measles virus attacking the brain long after initial infection. It usually began with mild memory loss, then falls, fits, coma, and a vegetative state, with death after one to three years. He even traveled with Wilson to break the news to parents of a young boy given the diagnosis.

"I'll always remember John explaining to them, very gently and sensitively," Salisbury tells me on the phone one evening, "how their child was going to die."

At the time of Wakefield's call, Salisbury worked at Friar's House: an anodyne oblong office building at the Elephant and Castle, a run-down neighborhood surrounding a complex traffic system a little more than a mile south of the River Thames. Here was a cluster of government outposts—pensions, welfare, social services—and few staff got better than Salisbury's office, room 388, overlooking a parking lot.

This was two and a half years before Ms. Two phoned Wakefield, and two months, to the day, before Jackie Fletcher's son, Robert, was vaccinated, as she said on *Newsnight*. It was Wednesday, September 23, 1992, when, from outside Salisbury's office, his secretary buzzed with a call that would herald the beginning.

At the time, Salisbury's big project was rolling out a new vaccine: against *Haemophilus influenzae* type b. He was chasing supplies with pharmaceutical companies, catching snags in transportation by Department of Health contractors, and fielding endless inquiries from physicians.

"*I've got a Dr. Andrew Wakefield. Royal Free medical school. Something about MMR.*"

More MMR. Salisbury was getting a lot on that, due to news of a safety issue. Only a week last Monday, Kenneth Calman, the chief medical officer, had written to every doctor in England and Wales, announcing that two brands of the vaccine were being dropped. One was called Plusarix, from the British company SmithKline Beecham. The other was Immravax from France's Pasteur-Merieux. This would leave only one—Merck's M-M-R II—if supplies from the United States were sustained.

The reason was simple, Calman explained in his letter. Crudely, the mumps component was running too hot, sporadically breaking through to cause illness. Like measles and rubella, mumps was included in the triple shot as a modified "live" virus. And the strain in the two products, called Urabe AM9, was sometimes causing symptoms of the disease it should prevent, presenting usually as a mild meningitis—inflammation of the lining of the brain.

Canada and Japan had already acted. But British government laboratories had now calibrated the risk: at 1 in 11,000 injections. "This rate," however, Calman's letter stressed, was "appreciably lower" than from natural infection.

For nine days, Salisbury had monitored press coverage, delivered each morning to his desk. The *Times* was first, with 140 words on Tuesday, September 15. Coverage was low-key, and since the brands were withdrawn, public concern over the issue was minimal.

Salisbury had never heard of the doctor without patients. And when his secretary flipped a button to connect him with the caller, and a broad-chested voice introduced itself, the civil servant was initially perplexed. As Wakefield would experience two and a half years later when Ms. Two got through to his place of work, Salisbury wondered over the reason for the contact.

In the light of what followed, it would be unwise for a journalist to rely on one party's recollection. So I'm indebted to Wakefield, who summarized the conversation in a two-page follow-up letter. At the time, he was waiting for publication of his *J Med Virol* paper on the virology of Crohn's disease. This was where he'd reported finding measles virus and his team photographed what he'd seen.

"So I'm thinking," Salisbury tells me, "why do we need to take this seriously? We have a very good vaccine program. We have no measles."

But in the phone call that day, Wakefield was blunt, citing *J Med Virol* as his credential. While acknowledging that the paper was nothing to do with vaccines (or, for that matter, mumps, or the brain), he explained his purpose: he wanted a meeting. And, more, he wanted *money*.

If I could split screens, like an early Quentin Tarantino movie, now would be the moment to do it. Because Wakefield wasn't the only player to spot an opportunity in the government's repudiation of the brands.

Another was a lawyer. This was Richard Barr, who would later be featured in the *Sunday Times Magazine*, and whose name would appear in the clipping on the notice board that led to Ms. Four's suspicions.

Dark-haired with wide-set eyes and flattened rural vowels, Barr might have passed for a piano tuner, a carpet salesman, or the landlord of a real-ale pub. Then aged forty-two, his main claim to fame was coauthorship of a book: *Which? Way to Buy, Sell and Move House*. And before that November, when the Urabe brands were discontinued, his career was less than downtown.

"A jobbing solicitor," he describes his work at that time, when we meet, nearly twelve years later. "Magistrates court in the morning, conveyancing at lunchtime, probate in the afternoon."

He practiced in King's Lynn, near the Norfolk coast, almost halfway up the east side of England. But, like "royal" in Royal Free, "king" in King's Lynn wasn't a pledge of anything classy. The town (population forty thousand) had largely turned its back on a medieval heritage, and since the 1960s had been blighted by lax planning, the lack of a university to brighten its evenings, and a doggedly white monoculture.

Nevertheless, Barr longed for what most lawyers long for. And, apart from that, he'd an abiding ambition. He wanted to bring a trial to the Royal Courts of Justice, the nation's cathedral of disputes. His father was a lawyer, his mother a doctor, so all came together in him wanting more than most things to get a pharmaceutical class action going.

After the first *Times* report, he moved like a greyhound. He was talking to journalists within hours. Eight years before, by the kind of luck you make yourself, he'd carried out the conveyancing for a commercial caterer named Angela Lancaster, who bought a four-bedroom bungalow near the Sandringham Estate, one of the Queen's many properties, ten miles northeast of King's Lynn.

The purchase was one-off, of no great value. But then, one day, his client reappeared. In May 1990—two and a half years before the brand withdrawals—Lancaster's son, Richard, aged thirteen, came down with mumps meningitis. At an exclusive private school, he'd been lined up with his friends, and vaccinated with MMR.

"It was horrendous," Angela remembers of the acute phase in the hospital, where her son was stretchered with headaches, light sensitivity, fever, vomiting, a stiff neck, and lethargy. "They were taking his temperature every ten minutes."

She asked Barr about the prospects of suing the doctor. She'd heard from another mother that general practitioners earned bonus payments for meeting immunization targets. So, the way she saw it, the one who came to the school had profited from a risky procedure.

For Barr, step one was to claim legal aid: taxpayer cash to fund representation for people who can't afford to pay. In the British system, minors were always eligible, so Barr completed a green form for step two: an expert's report and a statement from the mother on what happened to her son and when. The case looked promising, and the government's Legal Aid Board would pay the lawyer's bill, win or lose.

But, after five weeks in a darkened room, the boy completely recovered. He'd not lost income. He'd no dependents. And, if anything, his mother had gained the impression that Urabe might have done him some good.

"It probably transformed my son," she tells me, laughing at the idea that maybe a touch of inflammation may have sharpened his mental focus. "He just read computer magazines. And, at the age of thirteen, he basically said he wanted to work for NASA, and at the age of twenty-three, he turned them down."

Fast forward to the brand withdrawals of November 1992—Barr remembered the Lancaster's case. When Angela got home at around four o'clock on the Tuesday afternoon of the *Times* report, she found messages from the lawyer asking for permission to give out her phone number to reporters. Her son's story was now news: a perfect anecdote to make the most of the government's action.

The mother tells me she spoke with the midmarket *Daily Mail*, but the journalist missed a deadline to file. Faring better was the upmarket broadsheet *Independent*, whose medical editor, Celia Hall, was a veteran of the DTP scare. She hammered out not one but *two* reports that evening. Barr had connections with both.

One tie was oblique, possibly a coincidence in a country with a population then of 58 million. Hall interviewed a family doctor in a village near Wisbech, thirteen miles from King's Lynn. Wisbech was a town where Barr's firm had a branch, and where his father had long practiced as a solicitor.

Hall's first story was headlined across three columns of page 2, "Children received vaccine despite meningitis link," and rested on criticism from the family doctor of a lack of speed by the Department of Health.

One GP accused the department of choosing administrative neatness over maximum safety. "They wanted the MMR II supplies to be in place before they told us," Dr David Bevan, of Outwell, near Wisbech, Cambridgeshire, said.

Not exactly the most trenchant objection, or source, to warrant a national news story. Especially when the doctor also acknowledged, as he did, that the Urabe brands were better than nothing. But, having scored a half page of controversy over vaccines, Hall did the business for Barr.

"'Horrific' experience leads some to take legal action," ran the headline of the *Independent*'s second story, underneath. The only case identified was the long-abandoned Lancasters', with four paragraphs on how Angela had planned to sue. Then came a sentence with the rasp of scratched backs:

> But their solicitor, Richard Barr, of King's Lynn, a specialist in
> compensation cases, is representing another family, from the
> North of England whose five-year-old son was left profoundly deaf
> after meningitis following MMR vaccination.

Barr . . . a *specialist in compensation cases*? Hall, it appeared, was a prophet. For then, as it was, in the early 1990s (before every Indian restaurant had its menu on the web), getting named in a newspaper was the bait of choice for lawyers fishing for clients.

And so it would be that the otherwise unmemorable solicitor emerged from the undergrowth of his chosen profession to win a contract from the legal board to represent families hoping to sue over MMR. It was a contract that would blossom over the next twelve years, as he and Wakefield nurtured a crisis over the vaccine that one day would be felt everywhere.

The lawyer and the doctor had yet to meet. But by the time of the phone call to the civil servant, Salisbury, it seemed that Wakefield's big idea had evolved. Now it wasn't *measles virus*. It was measles *vaccine virus*. And while this had "not been addressed" in *J Med Virol*, he warned "this will be the first question that is raised."

In his third-floor office, Salisbury sensed a dog whistle. He'd seen the downside of such speculations before. He remembered the wards during Wilson's DTP scare, the retching babies, the SSPE, the telling parents how their child would die.

"My concern," Wakefield told him, "is that although measles, and in particular the vaccine, may ultimately have no association with Crohn's disease whatsoever, what will be picked up by the press is the apparent association between the increasing incidence of disease and the vaccine."

Picked up by the press? Why should that be? The caller's insinuation hit the spot.

Wakefield's career had taken a different path to Salisbury's. Patients were never high on the agenda. "Therefore I think it would be imperative for us to meet in the near future and discuss the way forward," the voice insisted, as minuted by letter. "However, adequate funding is crucial to this research programme and this is an issue which must be discussed when we meet."

More than a decade passes before I speak with Salisbury. But he remembers that conversation like yesterday. "Even his very first phone call rang alarm bells," he tells me, admitting that he's paraphrasing what he took to be a shakedown. "The tone, the sort of blackmailing, bullying, 'You will want to take notice of this. You will want this. *There might be consequences.*'"

NINE

The Deal

Richard Barr was born where medicine met the law and the United States met the United Kingdom. His mother, Marjorie, was a pathologist from Scottsbluff, Nebraska, who met his father, David, a British solicitor, amid the wreckage of Nazi Germany. It should thus come as no surprise that long before their son's coup over the MMR brand withdrawals, he yearned for one of those epic, crusading, may-we-approach-the-bench class actions in which, at last, big business comes unstuck.

According to another lawyer—who tells me she checked records—Barr first contacted Wakefield in about October 1995. That was three years after the brand withdrawals, six months after *Newsnight*'s bowel-brain conflation, nine months *before* the first of the twelve children was scoped at the Royal Free, and more than two years before the *Lancet* paper was unveiled. It would begin a collaboration that was to echo down the years to haunt parents not even born. Two months later, the two men shared their "shot in the dark" triumph in the *Sunday Times Magazine*, where they appeared alongside Jackie Fletcher. And, by January 1996, Barr was claiming seventy cases of alleged injuries from vaccines containing measles virus, and hundreds more "in the pipeline," he said.

Although never revealed until I expose it years later, in the first of the revelations to tumble from my inquiries, they were already hand-in-glove. "As you may have read in the *Sunday Times*," Barr wrote that January, in the fourth of a string of campaigning "newsletters" mailed out by post to clients and contacts, "Dr Andrew Wakefield has published some very disturbing material which indicates a clear link between the measles element of the vaccine and Crohn's disease."

Well, no it didn't. There was never a "clear link." But the newsletter (rescued for me by Angela Lancaster, the mother who helped Barr get his name in the press) listed what he said were "signs to look for." These included weight loss, diarrhea, "unexplained low level fever," mouth ulcers, and aching joints. "If your child has suffered some or all of these symptoms," he requested, "could you please contact us and it may be appropriate to put you in touch with Dr Wakefield."

Here were activities that would remain unknown to almost everyone who would gather in the Atrium. Not only Fletcher, but also Barr, sent Wakefield clients and contacts: talking up symptoms so vague, or common, that practically any parent might wonder if their child was suffering from an appalling inflammatory bowel disease and so benefit from referral to the hospital.

Two weeks after the mailshot, Barr took a train and sped south through the winter green of England. No more would he rely on representing shoplifters, scratching out house deeds over a ploughman's sandwich, or reading wills to the happily bereaved. After two hours to London, and a ten-minute taxi ride, he'd be ensconced in a magnificent Georgian brownstone to confer with Queen's Counsel (a senior trial attorney), and the charismatic Royal Free doctor.

At Barr's side that day was his assistant, Kirsten Limb. Five years later, they would marry. With straight brown hair, sometimes worn waist-length, she was ten years younger than the man she accompanied, to whom she'd originally come as a client. Her daughter, Bryony, had suffered severe brain damage in a medical accident, over which Limb had hoped to sue.

To his MMR clients, Barr advertised Limb as his "Scientific and Medical Investigator," "scientific expert," or more often simply "Scientist." As the *Independent* reported, with no mention of Wakefield:

> Mr Barr, who refused to let his children be vaccinated, said their research was being helped by having an in-house scientist working on the cases.

But Limb wasn't quite the scientist that some parents might have expected. According to her first husband, Robin Limb, they met at university, each graduating with a bachelor of science degree in *agriculture*. And I obtain their curriculum: it wasn't quite farming. Then they worked at an experimental sugar beet farm, on flat landscapes, east of Cambridge.

The main man that Barr and Limb traveled to meet that day was Augustus Ullstein, forty-nine. He was a jovial, blue-eyed, relatively new Queen's Counsel, specializing in personal injury, clinical negligence, and product liability disputes. "A genuine gentleman who is prepared to go the extra mile," he would be praised in a consumer guide.

He didn't come cheap. But, then, did they ever? By the time he finished over vaccines, years later, Ullstein would be reported in a document I obtain to have cost the taxpayer £360,000 (about £595,000 or US $744,000 at the time I write this).

Wakefield would be there: Barr's then only expert, so thin was any evidence against the shots. There wasn't even agreement on the scope of the injuries that MMR was supposed to inflict. Although Limb would claw together a mountain of paper, there were no convincing data (except concerning the withdrawn brands

issue), and the overwhelming consensus in medicine, if not agriculture, was that the product's safety profile was good.

The doctor's assignment from Barr was to disrupt that consensus: in a deal so secret, especially its timing, that even many
years after I reveal it, to public anger, Wakefield would deny when
it really began. The way he told it was that the children came to
Hampstead as purely in need of the bowel unit's care, and only
after was he asked to help lawyers.

"Now let's be very clear," he'd say, for instance, to the NBC network's correspondent Matt Lauer, in a *Dateline* show focused on
my reports. "They were admitted to the Royal Free for investigation of their symptoms. Nothing to do with research. Nothing to
do with class action. Nothing to do with vaccines."

And with regard to his relationship with the Norfolk solicitor,
he'd tell a conference in Brussels, Belgium, "When the children
were approached by a lawyer, I was asked—and this is after they
had been seen at the Royal Free Hospital—I was asked if I would
help as a medical expert in determining whether there was a legal
case against the manufacturers of the vaccine."

In fact, he agreed to work for Barr *before*, *at*, or *within days*
of meeting Ullstein—when *not one child* had crossed the Royal
Free's threshold for the project that would make it into *The
Lancet*.

"Thank you for your kind comments following our meeting
with Counsel last week," Wakefield wrote to the solicitor, confirming their relationship, on Monday, February 19, 1996: six weeks
before the first of the twelve kids attended an outpatient clinic in
a first floor suite at the hospital. "I would be happy to act as an expert witness on behalf of your clients for £150 per hour plus expenses" (about £248 or US $310 at the time I write this).

That would be another thing that he would say over the years:
that he'd *just been an expert*, and how "many, many, many doctors,
during the course of their work, act as medical experts."

But he wasn't just an expert. Experts gave opinions, helped courts with science, and represented fields of medicine for litigants. His role was unprecedented: commissioned, as he would be, to *create the evidence* against the shot.

Hundreds of phone calls would pass between the solicitor and the doctor. Crates of records would be trucked back and forth. And an assistant from Barr's firm, named Adele Coates, would be seconded to work from a cramped garage office, beside Wakefield's Taylor Avenue home.

Together they fashioned what Wakefield predicted would be "the biggest medical litigation case in history."

It started small: first with what Barr called a "detailed scheme" from Ullstein—which they borrowed from the DTP lawsuits. At the end of the second trial, in the name of Susan Loveday (before I volunteered my "everybody knows" opinion), Lord Justice Stuart-Smith had set out a checklist of the kinds of evidence that would be needed to convince a court that a vaccine caused an injury.

The judge's first heading was, "A distinct and specific clinical syndrome."

Next, "A specific pathology."

Third, what he called a "temporal association" between the time of vaccination and symptoms.

Fourth, "Plausible mechanisms" (or "Biological mechanisms").

Fifth, of least significance, "Animal experimentation."

And finally, "Epidemiological evidence."

Wakefield would attempt to create all of these (bar the animals) while employed in his deal with Barr. The Royal Free was to become a litigation factory, processing at least one hundred children that I can prove (whose parents were listed in a court register I obtain), and numbered by other sources at more than twice that. With pediatric gastroenterology allocated four slots a week in the endoscopy suite, that was the equivalent of full capacity—receiving no other patients from John Walker-Smith's unit—for possibly much longer than a year.

But first, Barr asked Wakefield to design a study, covering both clinical evidence (symptoms, signs, histories, and suchlike) and scientific, or laboratory-type, tests. Then, five months after the meeting with Ullstein—but still before *any* of the kids were seen for scoping—they asked the Legal Aid Board to pay for it.

If I didn't have the documents, I wouldn't believe the manifesto they submitted that summer. But in a three-page "Proposed Protocol and Costing Proposals," plus a seventeen-page "Proposed Clinical and Scientific Study," they set out plans for the grueling regime the children would undergo, giving the names of eight staff who would later appear on the *Lancet* paper, an itemized estimate of how much would be charged to the board, and the purported upshot (you might think surprisingly): *a test for vaccine damage.*

"The children will come into the Paediatric Gastroenterology Ward under the care of Professor John Walker-Smith," Wakefield specified in the submissions. "Costs for four nights stay for the child and their parent plus colonoscopy will be £1,750."

Naming as his "coordinating investigator–molecular studies" the young scientist Nick Chadwick, who would be waiting at the endoscopy suite to freeze tissues in nitrogen, the documents offered (at £500 a pop) "strain-specific" sequencing of measles virus: meaning reading its genetic code to discover where it came from—a vaccine, nature, or a lab.

Two groups of five kids were proposed at this time. The first had Crohn's disease, Wakefield said. That was still his primary focus. The rest would take him into a new field of inquiry, central to Barr's ambitions. As in the DTP trials, the lawyer's target was the brain, and particularly involving children with autistic spectrum

disorders: an increasingly common group of developmental diagnoses, inevitably appearing in Fletcher's client lists.

These patients, said the protocol, formed part of a "new
syndrome"—Stuart-Smith's checklist item 1. This married bowel
inflammation and "symptoms akin to autism." And (addressing
the checklist item 2) the evidence, the document said, was "un-
deniably in favour of a specific vaccine-induced pathology."

> It is of course not possible to anticipate the conclusions that will be
> reached, but the indicators are that it should be possible to establish
> a clear causative link between the vaccines and the two sets of
> conditions.

In other words, they decided what the research ought to find, before they set out to find it.

Barr mailed the documents to a legal board office on Thursday,
June 6, 1996. But, despite the offer of a vaccine-damage test (for
a bargain price of less than sixty grand) they weren't greeted with
any dancing on desks. Class actions against drug companies had
always failed in Britain. And after the collapse, not only of the
DTP cases but also a massive suit over benzodiazepine tranquil-
izers (in which hundreds of claims from "victims" were found to
be bogus), the board's managers had begged the government for
reform, complaining of litigants "giving it a go."

"There is no incentive on the solicitor to act as a responsible filter for dubious cases," the board said in a thirty-six page report.
"This problem seems to be exacerbated by the fact that the appli-
cant is not funding the case him or herself and that the claim
may only arise due to the publicity."

Following a guarded response, however, the board caved in
after Barr pressed the argument that Ullstein's opinion showed
that a "prima facie case" existed. So, on Thursday, August 22,
1996, a twenty-nine-year-old board lawyer named Joanne Cowie
signed her name to a two-page "authority to do contract work,"

ordering a "preliminary report from Dr Andrew Wakefield," and approving the following grant:

> To facilitate the setting up of the clinical and scientific study proposed by Dr A J Wakefield in respect of 10 assisted persons at a maximum cost of £55,000.

"If the tests are positive, then I am reasonably confident that the Legal Aid Office will allow us to have further children tested," Barr wrote to Wakefield later, setting out the doctor's duties. "I have mentioned to you before that the prime objective is to produce unassailable evidence in court so as to convince a court that these vaccines are dangerous."

Barr was delighted. He'd tell anyone who asked that he'd got a hospital testing his clients. But, although Wakefield's personal fees were confidential between them, a month after Cowie's approval of the deal a check came through as a first installment, which set off a crisis in the Royal Free medical school that would rumble on, in secret, for months.

The dean, Arie Zuckerman, spotted straight off that the payment raised issues of propriety. In more than thirty years in academic research, he'd never encountered such a source of finance. In principle, it wasn't far from a lung disease study sponsored by a tobacco manufacturer. To him, the idea of Barr's role in the science was deeply, and obviously, contentious.

"The dilemma which the School faces is whether it is ethical for lawyers to fund a particular piece of research where a specific action in law is contemplated," he wrote to Michael Pegg, a burly consultant in anesthesia and chair of the hospital's ethics committee, in a "strictly private and confidential" exchange.

Pegg's reply did nothing to calm nerves. The ethicist knew something was wrong. "I have reviewed all submissions made by Mr Wakefield to the ethics committee in the last two years," he wrote back. "None of the stated sources of funding include the legal aid board."

> If you have evidence that Mr Wakefield has made a false statement to the ethics committee then I would be obliged if you would formally lay that evidence before this committee.

But Zuckerman blinked. He later said he was overworked. Personally, I think he was spellbound. Either way, two days later, he wrote back to Pegg, with underlining, saying his inquiry had been "misunderstood."

> There is <u>absolutely no suggestion of any misconduct</u> by Dr Andrew Wakefield.

So, instead of the school taking the money, the dean suggested it be transferred to a "special trustees" fund, managed by the hospital's chief executive, Martin Else. And all Else said he wanted, in a "private and confidential" request, was "written confirmation that there is no conflict of interest"—a Get Out of Jail Free card in the event of controversy—which Wakefield was glad to supply.

> I am writing to confirm that there is no conflict of interest in relation to the Legal Aid funding for our clinical study . . . which has been sponsored by the Legal Aid Board.

So what happened was this: the money from Barr for the clinical and scientific study was paid to the medical school, diverted to the hospital's special trustees fund, where, rinsed of its origins, it was then laundered back to pay for Wakefield's research, carried out in the medical school.

Who would know? Not the *Lancet*'s editors, peer reviewers, or readers. And not the millions embroiled in what would become a global alarm over the safety of vaccination. Who would guess at the deal—or the money-go-round—any more than they would guess about the rest I would reveal behind that history-making twelve-child study?

"I remember noting at the time that the funding acknowledgment wasn't there," Barr tells me of the paper, before refusing further comment. "But it didn't seem to be a big deal."

- - - - - - - - - - - - - - - - - - - -

TEN

Trouble in the Labs

On the last Monday morning of February 1997, a taxi pulled away from the Royal Free Hospital. It turned onto Pond Street, in front of the building, dense with patient transport and visitors looking to park, turned again, and gathered speed, heading south. It was a mild, rainy day, the wettest since November, and a grimy ceiling of sky shrouded the capital like a duvet abandoned to a dog.

The sole passenger was male. He was well built, with black hair, pricey clothing, and a somber expression. White, aged forty, from the Bay Area of California, he was an engineer and entrepreneur, owning an electropolishing business, specializing in stainless steel and aluminum. He was wealthy, shrewd, with an engineer's precision. I'll call him "Mr. Eleven."

His destination was the renowned Chester Beatty Laboratories: a unit of the Institute of Cancer Research, rated, in partnership with its neighboring hospital, the Marsden, as one of the top four such centers in the world. Once endowed by a New Yorker, whom they called "the King of Copper," and based in a narrow, brick building on Fulham Road, Chelsea, it was a place where puzzles of biology had been solved: as blue chip a center of scientific inquiry as the Hampstead medical school was gray.

Mr. Eleven's fingers gripped a plastic pot. He nursed it like it bottled his life. As the taxi negotiated six miles of central London, through Paddington, Hyde Park, and South Kensington, he sensed a gentle movement of liquid within the vessel, rocking as the car turned or braked.

Meanwhile, back at Hampstead, his son, Child Eleven, had returned to Malcolm Ward after undergoing ileocolonoscopy. He was five years old, and labeled autistic. But like many children with evidence of developmental issues, a more precise diagnosis seemed elusive. Unlike Child Two, or Child Four, he was smart. And one day, when I meet him, he'd just seem like a shy, geeky teenager, if somewhat socially gauche.

"My son can be quite rude," his father tells me, when we meet at a restaurant south of Los Angeles, when Child Eleven had turned sixteen. "He reads technical journals, and will lob off an email to a professor, and talk down to them in a condescending manner. And he is right."

For reasons unknown—his father suspected vaccines—his early years had been more worrying. He hadn't started speaking by the age of two, suffered from apparent malabsorption and immunity issues, experienced delays in cognitive development, and his behavior was obsessive and repetitive. "Everything was off," Mr. Eleven tells me. Then he corrects himself. "Twenty percent of everything was off."

Unusually, it was the father who led the family quest for reasons and remedies for the issues. Mr. Eleven believed there could be "two hundred different types of autism," blaming vaccines, heavy metals, pesticides, fluoridation, and viruses. "You name it," he says. The trip to London was but the latest of countless initiatives by which he sought to diagnose and adjust his son, like a technician at a panel of dials.

Early on, he learned about "oxidative stress," read countless books and papers on causes and treatment, and spent huge sums on blood tests and supplements, such as B_{12}, folic acid, and gluta-thione. "I can tell you one thing: my son's brain is healing," he says. "I've got specific tests, very specific tests, that I'm targeting on him, looking for what I would consider his dysregulation, or his deficiency."

Mr. Eleven knew nothing of the *Lancet* paper, which would be published twelve months after his journey across London. He'd simply heard from an immunologist in South Carolina—a pipe-smoking eccentric named Hugh Fudenberg—that the Royal Free had a test for vaccine damage.

"We would greatly appreciate the opportunity to bring our child to London as soon as possible to undergo testing at your facilities," Mr. Eleven had written to Wakefield as the twelve-child study neared completion. "We are convinced that his medical condition can be successfully treated and he will recover from this ordeal if identification of the virus and the extent to which the infection has spread is better understood."

Six weeks later, he was riding in the taxi, clutching the pot—inside which, drifting in formalin preservative, lay bowel tissue snipped from his son.

"I was in the room with my wife," he tells me. "They took the biopsy material, cut it in half, put the piece in a jar, in a special con-tainer. I ran out the hospital, hopped in a cab I had waiting. I was down this place within a half hour."

The mission, he explains, was the immunologist's idea. Fuden-berg, sixty-nine, recommended a second opinion. For all Wake-field's confidence that measles virus persisted to cause inflamma-tory bowel disease, any literature search on the US National Library of Medicine's PubMed database yielded a less hopeful consensus. Notwithstanding Wakefield's optimistic submission to the Legal Aid Board, study after study had tried to replicate his virology. But time and again, they failed.

The trail had begun nearly four years before, after the paper in *J Med Virol*. As the Holy Grail of gastroenterology, the cause of Crohn's disease couldn't be left to one institution. So, from April 1993, the race was on to reproduce the Royal Free's results.

First to hit the track was a Japanese group, led by Masahiro Iizuka, at Akita University, six hundred miles north of Tokyo. In a letter to *The Lancet* in January 1995 (three months before Wakefield's question-marked paper), they reported on tissues from fifteen Crohn's patients, using a different method to those reported from Hampstead. Deploying the molecular amplification technology of the polymerase chain reaction (the famed "PCR" genetic fingerprinting that catches rapists and serial killers who licked postage stamps years before), they hunted for sequences from four of six genes that code the virus's nucleus, capsule, and protrusions.

The researchers told the journal, "We found none."

Then a US group at the University of Connecticut broke cover. In the same month that Ms. Two phoned Wakefield at his desk, the journal *Gastroenterology* printed a nine-page study—Ying Liu et al.—that, as part of a bigger project, had tried to replicate a Wakefield method. In tissues from sixteen patients, they looked for measles proteins using immunohistochemistry (one of the three techniques in *J Med Virol*) with which Wakefield had reported thirteen of fifteen samples positive.

The immunohistochemistry was a staining technique. It was microscopic, not molecular. Specially made antibodies were meant to stick to their target protein, and a fluorescence, usually brown, signaled a match. Liu's people got their antibody from the Royal Free lab. But, where Wakefield reported success, the

Connecticut team failed, concluding that the antibody seemed to locate, and latch onto, normal components of human cells.

"Therefore our results," they wrote, "do not confirm the data of Wakefield et al. regarding the presence of measles virus."

Fudenberg could easily access this stuff. To any immunologist, the implication from Connecticut was that results from the Royal Free may have arisen from a cross-reaction: where an antibody mistakes "self" for "other." It was no big surprise. In biology, shit happens. Targets aren't always unique.

But Wakefield, as ever, remained cool under fire. Shrugging off his critics' work as "flawed" and "ill considered," he suggested they'd looked in the wrong place for the virus, or that it was present in tissues in such miniscule quantities that their methods—but not his—couldn't find it. He'd seen the bug himself, under a microscope, he insisted. Measles infection was both "persistent" and "confirmed."

Notwithstanding his rejoinders, the literature didn't lighten. In February 1996—the month he formally signed up to his deal with Richard Barr, and a year before Child Eleven was brought to London for scoping—Yoichi Haga and others at Japan's Hirosaki University published a six-page study in *Gut*. Claiming remarkably sensitive PCR amplification—which they reckoned could detect a *single* measles virion—they targeted the same gene sequence as in Wakefield's in situ hybridization, as he described it in *J Med Virol*. But where he reported success in ten out of ten, they failed in all of fifteen.

"The aetiology of Crohn's disease remains unknown," they noted, "although evidence for a viral cause has long been sought."

It was Fudenberg's idea to check all this out before getting in any deeper with Wakefield. Hence the taxi ride with gut tissue in a pot to test for the presence of the virus.

Mr. Eleven had gone to London, not to validate a hypothesis, or join a lawsuit. And San Francisco had better hospitals than

Hampstead. "I just wanted a simple little blurb, positive or negative," he tells me. "I didn't ask for a big report."

Child Eleven had been admitted to Malcolm Ward the day before, after arriving at the airport with his parents. Like the rest of the twelve, he was bowel prepped overnight and trolleyed to the endoscopy suite Monday morning. His mother and father had watched on the video monitor as the instrument pressed forward: rectum; sigmoid colon; descending, transverse, and ascending colon; cecum; valve; ileum . . .

And *behold*.

Amid glistening pink mucosa, the parents saw the patches: the protruding pale nodules, the ugly swollen glands, the ileal lymphoid nodular hyperplasia.

Was this confirmation of the measles hypothesis, which, unknown to Mr. Eleven, had been proposed to the legal board in the scientific side of the study? The glands, he was told, were reacting to an infection, which Wakefield felt confident was the virus. This would be the topic of the second—scientific—paper to be submitted to *The Lancet* (and rejected).

But even as Child Eleven was wheeled back to the ward, more controversy brewed over the measles idea—and not thousands of miles from Hampstead. As the American father headed for the Chelsea lab, Nick Chadwick, the "coordinating investigator-molecular studies," worked on PCR tests on gut, blood, and spinal fluid from the *Lancet* twelve, and others.

Chadwick—a quiet, waifish young scientist—had himself been diagnosed with Crohn's disease. He'd come to the Royal Free as a Wakefield disciple, and for a year had toiled as a lowly lab technician before enrolling in a PhD program. At first he investigated, and tried to replicate, the good news of *J Med Virol*.

He was a well-regarded, dogged, and meticulous investigator, able to handle the endless hours of repeating the same assays and the interpersonals of laboratory life. One joy of the hospital was seeing research in context: the patients, like Child Eleven, for whom it mattered. In Chadwick's case, he was a patient himself, receiving care from Wakefield's mentor, Roy Pounder.

Working in room 324 on the hospital's tenth floor, Chadwick was one of a team of usually four researchers, lab-coated at a pair of parallel, double-sided benches, split by bottle- and box-cluttered shelves. At right angles to the workstations were plate glass windows, with stunning views across a slice of north London.

His project had started with evaluating techniques for amplifying measles RNA. This led to a twelve-page paper, with Wakefield the last author, in a cousin publication to *J Med Virol*, the *Journal of Virological Methods*. Then he applied the most sensitive and specific to Crohn's tissues—and, *whoaah*, his working life soured.

The tests were negative, like those from Japan and Connecticut. He could find the virus—but only in spiked control tissues, plus occasional rogue contaminants. And when he reported his findings to his PhD joint supervisor—Wakefield—that supervisor was none too thrilled.

"He tended to believe, you know, positive data that fitted in with his hypothesis," Chadwick tells me, "and then disregard negative data."

Here was the downside of research in the hospital: direction by medics, not scientists. "Andy never actually did any of the techniques himself, from scratch," Chadwick remembers. "He would spend a lot of time looking at tissue sections, and looking at the results. And, like most lab leaders' jobs are, to raise money for the group, and to try to interpret results, and write up papers. But in terms of hands-on stuff, he never put a lab coat on really, as far as I can remember."

That February, Chadwick began testing the samples, as the legal board submission—of which he knew nothing—had prescribed the previous June. He looked for measles (as well as mumps and rubella) in biological materials from twenty-two kids, including Child Eleven, plus an additional six control patients for comparison.

"And are these children," I ask him in a television interview, "the same children that went on to be published in *The Lancet*, leading to the MMR scare?"

"Yeah, that's right," he replies.

"Did you find measles virus in those children?"

"No. No single case did I find any measles virus in those children."

"You looked at some cerebrospinal fluid, by lumbar puncture?"

"That's right."

"Did you find any measles virus in those?"

"No."

"So you found no measles virus in the children who were presented to the public, at the very foundation of the MMR scare—where Dr. Wakefield's theory was that it was measles virus itself that was responsible for a bowel disease, and then leading on to some kinds of autism—and you found no measles virus?"

"That's correct."

Unlike the material in Mr. Eleven's pot—fixed in formalin for hospital pathology—the bowel tissues Chadwick tested were frozen in nitrogen within five minutes of being taken from the patient. But, despite this advantage, and his status in the protocol as the "coordinating investigator," his data wouldn't be published, or supplied to the legal board in Wakefield's report on the study.

I only learned of these data from Chadwick's other supervisor: a respected molecular biologist, Ian Bruce. At the time, he was a professor at the University of Greenwich, southeast London, and he vouched for the power of the young scientist's methods. "Nick had developed the best test that could ever be carried out at that time for testing for measles virus in those samples."

Wakefield didn't think so. He believed that Chadwick's PCR wasn't sufficiently "sensitive." The methods had "major limitations," he'd argue. The results were "false negatives," he said.

But, what people couldn't understand was how Wakefield could find a virus with microscopic-level stains, and yet molecular methods—surely vastly more sensitive—so consistently drew a blank. Indeed, when I've presented his proposition, talking to biology undergraduates, they laugh. They think it's a joke.

Mr. Eleven didn't know about the conflict with Chadwick. But he knew that Wakefield wasn't happy about an external cross-check on the virology. After delivering the pot to the Chelsea lab—into the care of a senior virologist named Robin Weiss—and returning with his wife and son to California, the father waited on the findings. And waited.

"They wouldn't release the results to me," he tells me, still baffled. "In all honesty, I don't know why."

He waited and waited. He wrote letters. No luck. And as 1997 rolled through summer and fall, Wakefield always seemed busy. Behind the scenes, that June, he filed a first version of the *Lancet* paper, with the second, scientific, study claiming to find measles virus. In August, he stoked the media through statements to *Pulse*. In September, he met with managers to discuss the press conference. Then, two weeks later, he flew to Virginia, to speak at an anti-vaccine convention.

At home in California, Mr. Eleven struggled. He took advice from London lawyers. He warned he might sue. Then, long after the information could have made any difference—because a storm of provoked media was off and running—the Chester Beatty virologist issued a report giving his findings on the tissue from the boy.

This time yet another technology was employed—to see if the virus could be grown in human cells. And, no, it couldn't be grown. The "most likely reason," said the report, which the father shows me, "is that the child's biopsies do not contain measles."

- - - - - - - - - - - - - - - - - - - -

ELEVEN

Spartanburg Science

The medical school's command center nestled in the basement, accessed via a slope at the side of the concrete castle, then through glass doors, and down a wide, shiny corridor that ran east–west through the building. To the right was a suite, shared by the dean and the school secretary. Then deeper inside, past Student Planning, lay the office of the man in charge of money.

Just five days after the event in the Atrium, Wakefield arrived here for a meeting. This was Tuesday, March 3, 1998, and in the country beyond Hampstead, his profile now loomed like a white-coat leper messiah. Should anyone have missed his Thursday performance, the school had issued a statement on Saturday morning, recirculating data on the twelve *Lancet* kids, citing apparent backing from America.

> Parents reported the onset of behavioural symptoms in their children following either MMR vaccination (8 cases) or a likely measles infection (1 child previously vaccinated with MMR). Behavioural changes included repetitive behaviour, disinterest in play or head banging. This same temporal association with MMR has been observed by workers in the United States.

Through the weekend, the nation's local press joined the fray: the *South Wales Evening Post*, the *Belfast News Letter*, the *Northern Echo*, *The Herald* (Glasgow) . . . and London titles hadn't yet quit. The *Evening Standard* revealed a shortage of single vaccines. The *Independent* showcased the man. "If I am wrong I will be a bad person," it quoted him saying. "But I have to address the questions my patients put to me."

The Tuesday meeting had been scheduled before the press conference, and followed months of planning. Behind Wakefield's public image as a dispassionate researcher lay not only his deal with the lawyer Richard Barr but yet greater ambitions for a more personal success, which that day he would discuss with management. Forget Burrill B. Crohn, or Warren and Marshall. He'd be the greatest gastroenterologist who ever lived.

In his own mind, in those early months of 1998, he'd not only solved the riddle of Crohn's disease but had found in the children a new inflammatory bowel disorder, unrecognized by medicine. For now. It was part of the new syndrome with regressive autism: just like he'd told the Legal Aid Board about before any of the children were scoped. No matter his lab and its molecular tests, he was confident that the villain was measles virus, especially the strains in vaccines. Now, from this meeting, he hoped to scramble even higher: to barely imaginable peaks of achievement.

Two business associates came with him that day. Both were venture capital entrepreneurs. One was a professional investor named Alex Korda, who'd spent two decades in biotech start-ups. The other: Robert Sleat, with a similar background, and a PhD in environmental microbiology. Sleat was also father of one of the twelve *Lancet* children and had first met Wakefield at an autism meeting with the sentinel case's mother, Ms. Two.

They descended to the basement to meet with the finance officer and deputy secretary: Cengiz Tarhan, aged thirty-nine. Turkish by origin, with a wry sense of humor, he had a passion for classic rock and fast cars. The previous Thursday, he'd gone upstairs with the school secretary, Bryan Blatch, and heard Wakefield's call for MMR to be suspended in favor of single shots.

Tarhan (who later declines to speak to me) knew all about the Research Assessment Exercise and the money the *Lancet* paper might bring. But he was also responsible for a school company, Freemedic, which aimed to exploit any inventions or discoveries by staff that might be spun off to make a profit. That Tuesday's meeting was to explore one such venture that Wakefield had been touting for months.

This wouldn't be the first time that Tarhan engaged with the protégé of the powerful Roy Pounder. For all Wakefield's public image as an idealistic scientist, he'd long craved commercial success. Indeed, practically since the time he returned to Britain from Canada, he'd been filing for patents, launching business schemes, and shooting his cuffs over deals.

Tarhan didn't need to pull cardboard files from his cabinets. Wakefield's record as an entrepreneur was memorable. First came a company called Endogen Research, with the postal address of a store in Bath, Somerset, two and a half miles from Heathfield. Through this, for three years from August 1991, he'd negotiated with the school to develop monoclonal antibodies. Then came Inceltec, in September 1993, and Histogene, in December 1994. Nothing of any remained.

What lingered, however, was an impression of ambition going somewhat beyond expertise. One patent application was for PCR "primers": short strings of nucleic acid used to frame genetic sequences targeted for molecular amplification. My favorite is what I call "Wakefield's Box," an "apparatus and process for performing a chemical reaction," with a microwave element, turntable, and fan—like a well-known kitchen appliance.

Bold, certainly. Innovative, perhaps. But the objective never appeared selfless. After one venture, Tarhan warned him that "individual interests" must be secondary to the school's. In another, Wakefield talked of being "suitably incentivized by the allocation of Equity." And in a third, managers were stunned to learn of a £24 million "appeal" intended to fundraise from the question-marked paper, and elevate Wakefield to the rank of professor.

Tarhan's bosses balked at that. Such an appeal would clash with the school's own plans. And the intended self-promotion was intolerable. "It is not for you to determine whether or not a professorial title is conferred upon you," the secretary, Blatch, slapped him down.

Then came ideas about Crohn's and autism, producing flurries of business paperwork. Just two days after Child Two was scoped (and while the eight-year-old and his mother were still on Malcolm Ward), Wakefield broached a breathtaking scheme. Aimed at diagnosing measles virus in inflammatory bowel disease, he estimated an annual cash flow of up to £385 million (about £710 million or US $880 million at the time I write this)—from Britain and the United States alone.

"In view of the unique services offered by the Company and its technology," he wrote in an eleven-page "Inventor/School/Investor Meeting" document that I obtain (replete with bold emphases) "the assay can command **premium prices**."

No wonder the excitement when he thought Child Two had Crohn's. Wakefield had already filed a patent. Lodged in his own name, from his home address, his claims were frankly astonishing. Not only did he profess to have discovered a means of diagnosing the disease (as well as ulcerative colitis) by detecting measles virus in bowel tissue and blood, he also registered a "medicament for treating these diseases" and, even more remarkably, "a measles vaccine comprising a system which expresses part or all of the measles virus genome."

So that was Crohn's. Then came autism: with a patent so secret that even John Walker-Smith later said he knew nothing about it.

Almost nine months *before* the twelve-child paper was unveiled, with parents urged to shun the three-in-one, Wakefield had registered an even more ambitious moneymaker, claiming to have discovered a miracle drug, with a sensational three-in-one action.

It could be adapted as a "vaccine for the elimination of MMR and measles virus," as a "therapy" for Crohn's and other inflammatory bowel diseases (IBD), and as a treatment for what he called "regressive behavioural disease" (in other words, a remedy for autism). It could be administered by injection, pills, or suppositories. It was "remarkably free" of side effects.

"I have now discovered a combined vaccine/therapeutic agent which is not only probably safer to administer to neonates and others by way of vaccination," he claimed in a document I later reveal on page 1 of the *Sunday Times*, "but which also can be used to treat IBD whether as a complete cure or to alleviate symptoms."

It was this venture that he brought, with Korda and Sleat, to discuss with Tarhan that Tuesday. With Freemedic money they wanted to start a company, to be called Immunospecifics Biotechnologies. With the Royal Free's backing, they hoped to raise £2.1 million to develop diagnostic tests, therapies, and vaccines.

Tarhan listened and, three days later, received a draft prospectus. Notwithstanding the negative results from Wakefield's lab, it claimed that a Japanese collaborator, Hisashi Kawashima at Tokyo Children's Hospital, had found measles where Nick Chadwick failed.

Nine "objectives" were listed in the sixteen-page prospectus. Three were process issues, such as raising cash and finding partners. One was to commercialize "immunotherapeutics and vaccines," while the others were *measles, measles, measles*. There was a "measles specific" treatment for inflammatory bowel disease;

the same breakthrough for "developmental disorders"; plans to "purify" the products for regulatory approval; likewise for a "measles specific clinical diagnostic"; and plans to "establish the potential" for a vaccine.

Big ideas? Could there be many bigger? Just five days before, as Wakefield gazed into the glare of television lights, and voiced his torment over the "moral issue" of vaccine safety, he'd not only his secret deal with Barr in the background—to attack the triple MMR, but not single measles shots—but he'd also dreamt of his own product (including his own *single vaccine*), which, if credible at all, could only succeed if public confidence in the three-in-one was damaged.

Tarhan couldn't judge the science in front of him. The technology was something called "transfer factor": an extract of lymphocytes (a type of white blood cell) first raised by a few scientists in the 1950s as a would-be game changer in medicine. Drawing on an ancient bright idea—that you can take stuff from one person's body and stick it in another's—it aimed to pass clinical benefits from donors to recipients for everything from Alzheimer's to AIDS.

Even to the accountant, this seemed a tall order. Still, the project appeared reputable enough. His visitors were pitching a three-sided pact: firstly themselves, then Freemedic, and finally an entity in Spartanburg, South Carolina, called the NeuroImmuno Therapeutics Research Foundation.

It sounded tempting. Wakefield was nothing if not plausible. But, when Tarhan's secretary sent the proposal down the corridor, the dean's response was blunt and negative. "I have considerable research experience with transfer factor and viral infection," he'd told Tarhan, in a previous letter. "I would *not* support the investment."

Wise move. The impressively named therapeutics foundation was the vehicle of the pipe-smoking immunologist, Hugh Fudenberg, who advised Mr. Eleven. His résumé was, to say the least, colorful. Before relocating to Spartanburg, he'd been a professor at the University of California, San Francisco, where he succumbed to funding from the tobacco industry to probe the genetics of emphysema. He'd been sued by the Food and Drug Administration for prescribing hazardous treatments, suspended by his medical board for controlled-drug misconduct, and now ran a consultancy, charging eye-watering fees, to parents of autistic children.

He was also the first to report a proposed link between the MMR vaccine and autism. Although Wakefield would seize the crown as the "father of the anti-vaccine movement," and people talked of his twelve-child study as the first of its kind, Fudenberg had beat him to it. Indeed, it was this man's paper that the Royal Free's Saturday press release meant by "workers in the United States" who made the "same temporal association." ·

First presented in June 1995 at a conference in Bologna, Italy, Fudenberg's paper was published nine months later on five pages of a fringe journal called *Biotherapy*, which was soon to be discontinued by its publishers. He reported on forty autistic kids, fifteen of whom, he wrote, developed their "symptoms" within a week of MMR vaccination. Three had high fevers and convulsions within a day, he said, while the rest experienced a gradual onset of issues (the most common natural history of autism) at between fifteen and eighteen months of age.

He called his paper a "pilot study" and named as the source of his forty children a New York neurologist named Mary Coleman, a specialist in developmental issues. But when I phone her, she calls him "dangerous and crazy," says she thought that "something has happened to him mentally," and that "there's something about this field that attracts quacks."

But, quack or not, Fudenberg attracted Wakefield. So I drive to South Carolina to meet him. He was old and infirm by the time I get there, grinning from a wheelchair in a denim beanie hat, thick brown jacket, and dark glasses. He calls Wakefield a "gentleman," says he'd stayed at his London home, and that he, Fudenberg, had turned him down.

"He wanted to go into business with me," he says, as we talk on his upstairs deck on a humid afternoon, eighty miles southwest of Charlotte.

"And what would that have done, that business?"

"Make a lot of money for him."

"But apart from making money, what would it have done?"

"Maybe gave him some fame perhaps. I don't know. If you're a big businessman, you get famous."

He says he refused to go along with Immunospecifics, because he didn't like Wakefield's values. "He wanted to prove he was right," he says. "That was his main motive. To prove he was right. He kept at it through thick and thin. He was also just *money* too much."

We talk about transfer factor, where documents I obtain showed that the immunologist had experienced regulatory difficulties. "Now, using this technology," I ask, "do you believe that autism can be cured?"

This was a leading question, to test his reaction. I'd assumed that his answer would be the stock-in-trade of pioneers, whether quacks or Nobel laureates. The smart response was, "We're getting good results."

Fudenberg's reply was, "Yes."

I didn't see that coming. But these were early days. "*Cured?*"

"Yes," he repeats his claim.

So this was the man, the grandfather of the crisis, at whose feet sat the doctor without patients. Fudenberg tells me that he manufactured his cure on what he called "a sheet, about three cells wide," which he rolled out on his kitchen table.

"And where does that come from?"

"From my bone marrow."

"From your own, personal, bone marrow?"

"Yeah."

Wakefield's secret science proposed a modified approach: turning the transfer factor into pills. And where the American's product went straight from donors to patients, Immunospecifics planned to interpose animals. According to the patent supplied to Tarhan, the extract would be made by injecting measles into mice, from which lymphocytes would be isolated, grown with human cells, and injected into pregnant goats.

The goats' colostrum, their first milk, would then be collected, freeze-dried, and, I speculate, sold under the "Royal Free" brand. It was, as one expert (a professor of immunology at the University of Cambridge) explained later, an evolution from Fudenberg's "merely eccentric" to Wakefield's "totally bizarre."

Tarhan, nevertheless, was presented with a prospectus giving a detailed share-out of the spoils. The "initial equity position," as it described the planned ownership, was set out in the following order: Sleat, Wakefield, Pounder, Korda, Fudenberg (who says he declined the invitation), the medical school, and a "charitable trust."

But why, one might ask (I know that I did), spend time and money on a cartoon company, unless you're as crazy as a Spartanburg coot? Then I remembered the lesson of an investigation I'd done in the late 1990s into the "world's first AIDS vaccine," AidsVax. A clique of ex-staffers from the US Centers for Disease Control and Prevention, in Atlanta, Georgia, had been inspired, I think, by Mel Brooks's film *The Producers*, premised on the idea that you could make more money from a Broadway flop than you might from a successful musical. The CDC guys got $12.6 million in federal grants for their company (named VaxGen), a big tank of gunk in South San Francisco, floated stock on the NASDAQ, and retired.

Here was the beauty of biotech start-ups, although I can't speak to anyone's intentions. If Immunospecifics bombed—as you'd have to think was possible—the owners might nevertheless pay themselves. On top of their share of the initial equity (which they might sell to the faithful before the bubble exploded), the prospectus listed Wakefield drawing £33,000 a year as part-time research director (while still working for Barr and the medical school); Sleat, full time, receiving twice that amount; Korda getting £20,000 as executive chairman; and Pounder £7,500 a year.

Boosted by the Royal Free, *The Lancet*, and the media, if they could raise the initial capital, they should do just fine. Good money, win or lose. "Few VCs [venture capitalists] have the technical knowledge to understand what the patent was about," one source who knew about this project speculates to me in an email. "And even if they did realise this, many would consider it was worthwhile to invest anyway. They would put money in, hype the company on an AIM [alternative investment market] based on the huge public attention, and run."

TWELVE

Asked and Answered

Three weeks after the meeting with Cengiz Tarhan, somebody nearly beat me to unmasking Wakefield's twelve-child study for the project it really was. Her name was Anne Ferguson, aged fifty-seven: scientist, clinician, wife and mother, professor of gastroenterology at Scotland's University of Edinburgh, a fellow of no fewer than five royal colleges and societies, and a front-rank expert on bowel disease.

This was Monday, March 23, 1998 (twenty-five days after the press conference in the Atrium) at a daylong scientific meeting. She was there. So was he. And she asked him a question so simple, and basic, that had he answered her truthfully, openly, and completely—behavior expected at a scientific meeting—the public alarm over MMR and autism might have ended, there and then.

The event was organized by the Medical Research Council, expressly to consider Wakefield's work. Contrary to his later claims of sinister plots, he'd been accorded respect and tolerance of a kind that few enjoyed in twentieth-century Britain. Including Ferguson, Wakefield, and a CDC staffer who'd flown in from Atlanta, fifty-seven people were present: immunologists, virologists, epidemiologists, gastroenterologists, pediatricians, statisticians, and more. Twenty were professors (including six men knighted to the glorious title "Professor Sir").

The location oozed with privilege and grandeur: the neoclassical headquarters of England's Royal College of Surgeons—like the gateway to Heathfield, only bigger. Rising five stories and finished in Portland limestone, with six fluted columns across a giant Ionic portico, it overlooked the grass and trees of Lincoln's Inn Fields: the biggest garden square in London.

Their eyes met that morning at an open rectangle of tables, laid out across a wood-paneled room. She: a tousle-haired Scot, a strong, solid woman, who'd climbed in the Himalayas, played international basketball, and published three hundred papers and book chapters. He: a trainee gut surgeon turned charismatic crusader, whose name would live forever in medical history—albeit not in the way he planned. Behind them, observers crowded a second rank of chairs. A mechanical projector fired slides.

After introductions and coffee, Wakefield took the spotlight. Now attention was where he liked it. "He was flying high," remembers David Salisbury, the Department of Health civil servant and pediatrician, who, seven years before, received the demand for money after two vaccine brands were withdrawn.

"It is a great pleasure to be here," Wakefield began, screening the first of more than forty transparencies summing up his work on Crohn's. "I hope that you will at least try to reserve judgment, right to the very end, because the data do look interesting."

The gathering heard him out. People took notes. But when he finished speaking, the virologists and immunologists battered him like a southern fried chicken. How could it be, they wondered, that he claimed to find the virus using the protein-targeting immunohistochemistry (which nobody present doubted was "relatively insensitive"), and yet highly sensitive molecular amplification, targeting nucleotides, had so often drawn a blank?

The day was chaired by an urbane professor of medical micro-biology, Sir John Pattison, editor of *Principles and Practice of Clini-cal Virology* and *A Practical Guide to Clinical Virology.* "Where is that genome which produces the specific protein," he asked, posing the enigma most succinctly, "if you cannot find the nucleic acid?"

For the knights, professors, and doctors around the tables, the popcorn moment came quickly. Wakefield's best evidence that measles caused Crohn's—and which he previously claimed "con-firmed" his *J Med Virol* findings—was contained in a manuscript that he'd supplied in advance. It was the latest in a series, going back several years, staining for proteins with special gold-labeled antibodies, which, when viewed through an electron microscope, he said, found "persistent infection" with the virus.

But, as Ferguson sat listening, David Goldblatt, a Great Or-mond Street immunologist, projected a slide of the manufactur-er's instructions for the antibodies Wakefield had used. Critically, they specified a set of *four* negative controls—for example, using a different version of the antibody in parallel—to guard against false-positive reactions.

"I do not want to give you *my* opinion," Goldblatt said. "I would rather just show you what the company from whom they bought the gold conjugates say about negative controls."

Wakefield was nailed. The slide spoke for itself. Likewise, the study he supplied. Of the manufacturer's *four* required negative controls, Goldblatt could find only *one* in Wakefield's work. "These are simple to perform," Goldblatt recited from the instructions, as if reading aloud from a cake-mix recipe, "and should *always* be included."

The moment was tense, especially in light of the findings from Connecticut, which had suggested that another aspect of Wake-field's methods was picking up a cross-reaction.

Then, after a half-hour lunch, the proceedings changed direc-tion, with a talk by Wakefield's sidekick, Scott Montgomery. He was then thirty-six, a sometimes-untidy-looking epidemiologist, who'd been one of the four authors of the question-marked paper that was the peg for the *Newsnight* report.

Montgomery's contribution covered the efforts to link the virus (both in vaccines and natural infection) with the later development of Crohn's. But his cookie crumbled badly as the statisticians present chewed it. And, by the time he finished screening his selection of transparencies, he was admitting that his data didn't merely *not support* the question-marked paper but a*ctually* suggested that the shots reported in that study were *protective* against the disease.

"Our work and other people's work," Montgomery conceded, "does not support that monovalent measles vaccination, at a typical age, is a risk."

Does *not* support? But wasn't the claim that measles vaccines were implicated in Crohn's disease fundamental to all that followed?

Three speakers declared themselves "confused."

Looking back on the transcript of that day's discussions—112 pages, sixty-five thousand words—it's hard for me not to feel disgust. Here was Wakefield and Montgomery, who, three years earlier, with the cheap-thrills *Lancet*, a money-grubbing medical school, and a box-of-rocks reporter from the BBC's *Newsnight*, dumped on the public that question-marked paper—putting Jackie Fletcher on television, leading to the phone call from Ms. Two to Hampstead—and now it was a steaming heap.

Like, nobody suspected that comparing incomparables would generate junk? I think not.

But Wakefield, as ever, remained calm and unflustered. "If we were born all-knowing we would not be sitting round this table," he said, shedding, like snakeskin, the paper that first brought him to public attention. "Clearly, hypotheses evolve."

Ferguson's expertise was so broad and deep that she made two dozen interventions that day. But none hit the nail like one that she asked before afternoon tea was served. Now the twelve-child paper was the topic of discussion, and she wondered the same as I would, years later.

Where did he get the children?

This was a critical issue. And yet nobody had asked it, as if manners wouldn't permit the inquiry. At face value, the paper reported on routine patients—a write-up from the casebook of a pediatric bowel clinic where parents had repeatedly made the same shocking claim: of an association between autism and the MMR shot, with behavioral symptoms coming on *within days*.

"I am going to be forthright," Ferguson began. "Since it looks as if nobody else is going to raise the issue of bias in generating this series of cases."

Selection bias. Publishing rules sought to catch that in formal instructions to researchers. In a ponderously titled document, *Uniform Requirements for Manuscripts Submitted to Biomedical Journals* (adopted by more than five hundred publications, including *The Lancet*), what authors must disclose was stipulated. The code's fifth edition, in force at the time, said a paper's opening "abstract" section should state the "selection of study subjects," with a later "methods" section spelling it out.

> Describe your selection of the observational or experimental
> subjects (patients or laboratory animals, including controls) clearly.

Ferguson had a personal reason to wonder. She'd appeared in the *Newsnight* package. She'd seen herself saying there were no correlations between the introduction of measles vaccine and "any shift in the pattern of Crohn's disease." She'd seen a group of parents performing stiffly for the camera. And she'd seen Jackie Fletcher, the woman in scarlet, who founded that group called JABS.

"Maybe that the time scale I have got, and the facts I have got are not correct, but at least my perception is as follows," she addressed Wakefield at the meeting. "That, about 1994, your group became concerned about measles vaccine as a hazard, and that coincided with the organization JABS being either created, or supported, or sponsored, or some interest in the idea."

She was digging the right ditch. JABS was founded in January 1994, with Fletcher's determination to sue. Her son had been vaccinated in November 1992, just two months after the publicity over the brand withdrawals. And after she shared *Newsnight*'s platform with Wakefield, she referred clients and contacts to him.

Ferguson continued, with regard to the Royal Free. "I understood that there was a lot of publicity on the telly and newspapers, on the internet, suggesting that, if someone had a child with autism and bowel symptoms, that this was the center in the world to find out about it. I mean, I think, is that not correct?"

It *was* correct. But it was incomplete. Not only was there JABS, there was the lawyer Richard Barr inviting clients to seek contact with Wakefield. And the result—unspotted before my investigation—was a cohort of complainants who'd gone to the hospital, with nearly all of them intent on suing. Ferguson was gnawing near the heart of the paper that, unknown to her, was contrived with a lawyer, who paid the first author at hourly rates, and was sponsored by the taxpayer, through the Legal Aid Board, to make a case against MMR.

Such were these features that John Walker-Smith (who refused to attend the Atrium press conference) became concerned over the project's integrity. "It is clear that the legal involvement by nearly all the parents will have an effect on the study as they have a vested interest," he wrote to Wakefield before the last of the twelve kids was scoped.

I obtain a copy of that letter (headed "Enterocolitis and Regressive Autism"), and I publish extracts in the *Sunday Times*, including the Australian's most pertinent observation:

> Never before in my career have I been confronted by litigant
> parents of research work in progress. I think this makes our work
> difficult, especially publication and presentation.

Yup: especially *publication* and *presentation*.

Ferguson knew nothing of that private correspondence. And she wasn't a journalist, or a lawyer. So instead of pushing harder on a door that should have opened, her question segued into clinical observations, like ulcers, swollen glands, and sore ears.

But Wakefield responded. At last, a reply. After the day's embarrassments over histopathology and hypotheses, Ferguson had *impugned* without *proof*.

"Thank you for being forthright," he said, reframing her concerns in terms she hadn't used. "I imagine you are suggesting we are a sort of dumping ground for disaffected parents? No, we are not."

She hadn't said anything about "dumping grounds" or "disaffected parents." But, having denied his own charge, Wakefield doubled down with an assertion he surely knew was untrue.

"And, indeed, these parents came to us de nouveau," he said, "without any connection through any other organization."

Had JABS's founder been present, she might have said otherwise. With the family from California a notable exception, those crucial parents—at the foundation of the health crisis—nearly all had links to her group.

Could Wakefield have forgotten Walker-Smith's letter? Or the case of Child Four, with the "most compelling" history, whose mother had written to him, citing Fletcher and litigation in the opening paragraph of her flower-patterned letter? Or Ms. Twelve, the mother who met him at a JABS meeting before she brought her son to Hampstead? Or, another case I learned of, where Kirsten Limb, Barr's "scientist" wrote to the Royal Free, pressing for the admission of a client.

I've plenty more. But life's too short. I've no doubt that Wakefield *knew*.

In the wood-paneled room, however, he saw off Ferguson. She simply didn't have enough facts.

"Latterly," he continued, "parents have heard about our work—through the media, or through other organizations—and have come to us."

Latterly? Surely what he meant was *from the outset*. Right from Child Two, his "sentinel case," they were coordinated, organized, *schemed*.

Go no further than Ms. Two herself, referred to him by Fletcher after the *Newsnight* broadcast. He sent her to Barts Hospital, where Walker-Smith saw her son and discounted inflammatory bowel disease. But then *six months later*—from a report of the mother's account—she joined Barr's books for the proposed class action. Then *four months after that*, at Wakefield's suggestion, the professor *invited* her to bring her son to Hampstead.

At the Royal College tables, Wakefield offered a final thought. He didn't want any persisting confusion. "All patients that we have reviewed so far," he told the gathering, "have come to us through their general practitioners, or pediatricians, by the standard route."

The standard route? It went like this: on learning of a promising child for his research, he'd phone the mother, or ask the mother to phone him, and then would call her general practitioner. This conduct, in itself, was all but unheard of. National Health Service consultants didn't solicit. But in those calls he might speculate that the kid (whom he'd never seen) might suffer from a potentially appalling inflammatory bowel disease, and offer the Royal Free's help.

That would do it. Imagine the parents' worry. A rubber-stamp referral was assured.

Who in that wood-paneled room would have guessed that in doctors' offices scattered across Britain, lay medical records that, thanks to an old-fashioned newspaper investigation, would one day be exposed to the light?

Regarding a seven-year-old boy, sixty miles northwest of Hampstead:

> Dr Wakefield, consultant gastroenterologist, Royal Free rang and gave a v lengthy and convincing case for [Child Five] to be referred to Professor John Walker-Smith.

For a four-year-old boy, sixty miles south of the hospital:

> Dr Wakefield—Royal Free. To discuss association measles + Autism + inflammatory bowel disease . . . If we feel relevant can refer for treatment to Professor Walker at the Royal Free for investigation.

And for an eight-year-old girl, 280 miles northeast:

> Mum taking her to Dr Wakefield, Royal Free Hospital for CT scans/ gut biopsies. ?Crohn's—will need ref letter—Dr W to phone me. Funded through legal aid.

Then there were the referral letters, sent to Wakefield or Walker-Smith. They also made clear what was happening.

> This 7¾ year autistic child's parents have been in contact with Dr Wakefield and have asked me to refer him.

> [This little girl's] mother has been to see me and said you need a referral letter from me in order to accept [her] into your investigation programme.

> Thank you for asking to see this young boy.

Who in that room would know how it worked? Probably not even Montgomery. This choreography of referral, like the money from Barr, would have revealed a secret purpose behind the twelve-child paper: to pressure the legal board to fund a lawsuit.

Wakefield shook off his pursuer. *Easy peasy.* Then, a few weeks later, did it again. A *Lancet* reader, a doctor named Andrew Rouse, wrote in about a Barr fact sheet, which he'd found posted online by a little group called the Society for the Autistically Handicapped, which I never heard of before or since. Rouse was concerned about possible litigation bias and that this wasn't addressed in the paper.

Again, Wakefield saw him off, deflecting the suggestion. "No conflict of interest exists," he wrote to *The Lancet*, hurling a fist of blinding dust at his pursuer. "AJW had never heard of the Society for the Autistically Handicapped and no fact sheet has been provided for them to distribute."

To that, he added a line that one day he'd claim was evidence of his innocence and honesty:

> Only one author (AJW) has agreed to help evaluate a small number of these children on behalf of the Legal Aid Board.

He would say this covered it: that he'd disclosed the position. And he threatened to sue *The Lancet* after it condemned his conflict, when I revealed it in the *Sunday Times*. But the journal hit back: that he'd framed his admission in the present tense—"*has* agreed"—three months after the event in the Atrium. That made his "help" appear to *follow* the paper, when it had started *two years before*.

Ferguson did her best. But she didn't stand a chance. She was schooled in doctorly discourse. To take on Wakefield, specific facts needed nailing: data, documents, *proof*. And, after hearing his reply—laying on *her* shoulders the guilt *he* should have felt—she meekly backed away. He was safe.

"I apologize," she said, as if *she'd* behaved badly. "I wasn't suggesting any impropriety."

Yet, she'd come *so close* to the heart of his strategy. The "finding" in the paper, linking autism with the vaccine, wasn't any kind of *finding* at all. It was the crucial component of his research's *methods*; not a *discovery*, but his means of execution. Parents' concern over vaccine damage was why they came to the hospital: some traveling hundreds (in one case, thousands) of miles. It was a preplanned *inclusion criterion*.

But moments after the apology, and barely seconds before the day's concluding tea break, his mask briefly slipped, and he evidenced the nature of a mind made up, unchanged since his first big idea. Turning from Ferguson to address the gathering, he made remarks that, to a scientist, were so revealing of character that, of all the day's discussions, it will be the moment that Pattison, presiding from the chair, recalls twenty years later, when I phone him.

"I have a different perspective, clearly, to most people in this room," Wakefield told them, as the event drew toward its close. "And it comes from, I expect, with actually having looked down the microscope, looked down the electron microscope, and seen these things, and done the work. And I stand by that absolutely. I still feel there is a link between measles virus and chronic intestinal inflammation in these situations. Now my job is to go away and try and convince you of that."

Then he added, "And that's what I'll do."

THIRTEEN

Turn of the Century

Doom-mongers forecast the end of the world. In the final twelve months of the twentieth century, talk was rife of a computer bug, "Y2K," which, at the stroke of midnight to welcome the year 2000, might make bank deposits vanish, aircraft plummet, and launch war between the United States and Russia. It was said that old programs clocking dates in double digits might run out of numbers, and go berserk.

At the Royal Free, however, the closing year of the second millennium kicked off looking sweet for Wakefield. By January 1999, his office had moved up eight floors to the tenth, lightening his life with luscious views across London. His mailbox was stuffed with referrals and queries, meaning plenty more kids to be scoped. And his once-parallel schemes in litigation, science, and business ventures converged like one of those night sky alignments of Jupiter, Venus, and Mars.

First up: his secret contract with the lawyer Richard Barr to produce evidence for the government's Legal Aid Board. Asking for its money two and a half years previously, he'd promised results with molecular amplification, "strain-specific" sequencing of measles virus, and Nick Chadwick as his coordinating investigator. But all that yielded nothing, so now, on Tuesday, January 26, 1999, he filed a report on the pilot study based on his staining tests.

Nobody cared. He could have filed his lunch. What would the board know of proteins and nucleotides? The storm created through *The Lancet* guaranteed that Barr's lawsuit would be funded by the taxpayer. Four national newspapers now backed the crusade. Some eighteen hundred families swelled Barr's contact lists. And the first "writs," as they were called, against vaccine manufacturers, had been stamped in red at the Royal Courts of Justice.

Wakefield's report to the board was a secret dossier claiming his discovery of the new gut-brain "syndrome," which he predicted before the first child was scoped. That ticked the box for Lord Justice Stuart-Smith's checklist item 1: a "specific clinical syndrome." And here, too, was a candidate for Wakefield's disease: a specific pathology (checklist item 2), which he named "autistic enterocolitis."

"Both those affected children funded by Legal Aid and, subsequently, a larger group of similarly affected children who were referred independently by their General Practitioners, have been investigated," he submitted, through Barr.

> The conclusion of this report is that in some children there is a strong likelihood of a causal relationship between measles virus and possibly some other component of the MMR vaccine and the new syndrome.

The bowel story was the same as he told it in *The Lancet*. The colitis and swollen glands—the ileal lymphoid hyperplasia—were a "consistent pattern of intestinal pathology," he told the board, that was "consistent" with the cause being a virus. But his "temporal link" (checklist item 3) had notably undergone evolution. Reporting not on twelve kids but now more than forty, that association had weakened from the fourteen-day *maximum* before behavioral symptoms to *four weeks, on average*, after the shot.

I think Barr must have watched that evolution too. He knew the importance of the timings. Before the paper's publication—even before the kids were scoped—the lawyer, with his wife-to-be and scientist, Kirsten Limb, had advised on the temporal link. For the board to cover the costs of parents hoping to sue, the pair stressed that it needed to be told of a "clear reaction," and a "close link up in time," preferably in a "number of days."

That didn't mean the couple told their clients *what to say*, only what *needed to be said*. "Let's get this straight," Barr insists, during my early inquiries, before he refuses further comment. "My role is to do the best for my clients. It always has been, and always will be. Clients came to me and told me what was happening to their children."

True. But in an outpouring of fact sheets and newsletters, the couple did a great deal of telling. Perhaps no wonder, with Limb believing that her daughter was a victim of medical negligence. Or maybe they were impassioned for a cause, or billings. Either way, they didn't merely brand doctors *wrong*, but implied that they were *dishonest*.

> We are concerned that risks associated with the actual illnesses may have been exaggerated, perhaps to frighten people into having their children vaccinated.

And:

> Even in the face of quite an obvious link between the vaccine and the injury, doctors are dismissive and say the cause was anything but the vaccine.

And:

We are troubled that there seems to be a certain amount of massaging of the figures.

Slippery suggestions. And fantastic advice for parents with broken hearts. In the decades to come, such poisonous acorns would mature into a dark ideology. Little was more potent in building a campaign than opponents branded fools and liars.

"She was very full of herself," one mother in the lawsuit tells me of Limb. "She talks for Britain, seldom letting up, and was full of the conspiracy stuff."

"I've got to be really honest with you, Brian," claims a former colleague of the pair, who helped to prepare the class action for court. "Going to work for them was like having to dunk my arm in a pot of boiling oil."

Barr and Limb told clients that Wakefield was a "paediatric gastroenterologist," which he wasn't; claimed that those who "in any way challenge" the safety of vaccines were "publicly discredited," which they weren't; and even admitted that they aimed to "raise a question-mark" over the "rationale" for immunization.

"Needless to say, both Kirsten and I are satisfied that the link between the vaccines and the injury to our individual clients is not a fanciful one, but one of direct causation," Barr had declared in a newsletter, even before the meeting with Augustus Ullstein two years before the *Lancet* paper.

At public expense, they'd made up their minds, and had no mind to keep it to themselves.

One angle, which they plied their clients with for years, insinuated profession-wide shenanigans. Comparing lay medical books created for family use, they noted that in the days before vaccines were available, doctors downplayed measles, mumps, and rubella, telling parents they were usually mild.

But in a marvelous contrast—spread across seven pages—fact sheets revealed that, after vaccines were licensed, "perception of the illnesses" apparently *changed*. Now doctors "inexplicably" stressed the *risks*.

"Something curious has happened to the 'official' perception of the childhood illnesses," they informed their clients, many of whom weren't sophisticated people. "They have all officially become more serious since vaccines were introduced."

With arguments *that* smart and a surge in client numbers, Barr and Limb moved to a bigger firm, with offices in London, with maybe less room to maneuver. But parents were free to tell it how they saw it—with Ms. Two, as usual, in the lead. "CYNICAL ATTEMPT TO DISGUISE THE TRUTH," she shouted in a statement from her group, Allergy-Induced Autism, over a government-funded research paper. "SCANDALOUS PUBLIC DUPE."

Ms. Two was a gem, a one-in-a-million. She delivered like a midwife on speed. In March 1999, she organized a conference, with Wakefield the star, drawing nearly four hundred, including the Australian professor, to the National Motorcycle Museum. And, all but incredibly, it was she who'd first suggested the mechanism of damage, the Stuart-Smith checklist item 4. She'd raised it in her phone call after the *Newsnight* broadcast, and it would survive to the end of Barr's lawsuit.

Her mechanism went back to the "opioid" idea that even made it into the *Lancet* paper. It was borrowed from an Estonian psychobiologist, Jaak Panksepp, who injected morphine into lab rats and guinea pigs. Then he watched them sink into stupor or go crazy. In a two-and-a-half-page paper published in July 1979, he hypothesized that "opioid peptides" (most notably found in wheat and dairy products) led to what he called "opioid excess." Moved over to children, this caused an "emotional disturbance"—which is what he believed autism to be.

"Think morphine or heroin and you'll get the basic drift," Ms. Two popularized this idea.

How many loaves of bread it might take to get wasted wasn't part of any Wakefield equation. But he seized on this mechanism—what I call the "stoned rodent model of childhood autism"—soon after he heard it from the mother. In his *Lancet* paper, he gave it two hundred words, with more in his secret report to the legal board.

"A coherent explanation for a link between the gut, persistent measles virus infection, autoimmunity and autism, is embodied in the 'opioid excess' hypothesis," he told the board. "The hypothesis proposes that early in life, opioid peptides—principally in ß-caesomorphine and ß-gliadorphin—derived from dietary casein and gliadin [a gluten component] respectively, enter the circulation through a damaged or leaky gut."

So, here was how MMR was meant to cause autism. Persistent measles virus led to bowel inflammation. Then an "excess" of peptides from food escaped into the bloodstream, traveled to the brain, and caused damage. As Ms. Two would file in court papers for her son:

> The presence of measles vaccine virus in the tissues of the gut
> causes immune dysregulation and/or autoimmune reactions which
> lead to the development of inflammatory bowel disease, which in
> turn initiates a biochemical cascade resulting in an excess of opiate
> peptides in the circulation damaging the brain so as to cause autism.

Speculative, yes. But it *was* referenced to an -ologist, a psychobiologist. And 1999 was a year of new ideas about immunization impacting the brain. In July, there was concern in the United States when the US Public Health Service and the American Academy of Pediatrics called for the retirement of a mercury-based preservative, thimerosal, then contained in many vaccines, in case of possible neurodevelopmental effects.

Thimerosal had been used for some seventy years to protect multidose vaccine vials from bacteria. The plan to phase it out echoed Britain's brand withdrawals—and triggered a similar reaction. When the government made a move to tighten vaccine safety, lawyers pounced, campaign groups formed, and a class action lawsuit was raised.

The "live virus" MMR never contained thimerosal. Yet here was power to Wakefield's elbow. At the time, however, his mind was still on measles and, after servicing Barr's lawsuit at hourly rates of pay, and poring over the stoned rodent model picked up from Ms. Two, his third priority for that good-looking year was business—a.k.a. making money.

His biotechnology company, Immunospecifics, was still in talks with the medical school, which by now had been swallowed by University College London—a blue-chip institution with more than sixteen thousand students, and seven thousand staff, in countless buildings. It was this that now owned his patent claims— for the tests, treatments, and single measles vaccines—which, although he lodged without his employer's permission, he devised while on its payroll.

And more news bubbled on the business front: another company was good to go. With his venture capital partners, Robert Sleat and Alex Korda, as well as Roy Pounder, the professor of gastroenterology, he was readying a scheme for a more ambitious enterprise, which they named Carmel Healthcare. It was to focus, first, on selling diagnostic kits based on the detection of measles virus.

I obtain the draft prospectus, the pitch to investors, stamped "Private and Confidential." It was brave.

> Carmel has positioned itself, uniquely, to be part of the solution to what is going to be one of the major healthcare problems of the new millennium.

> Carmel is a new biotechnology venture specialising in the development and commercialisation of measles specific clinical diagnostics.

In all the years of my investigation, I never worked out why finding measles virus would diagnose anything but measles. But the plan was to launch the venture—on Monday, January 17, in the new year, 2000—before Wakefield spoke at a conference. In advance of the event, he'd be media-coached, ready to sound an even louder alarm than two years earlier in the Atrium.

His team, he planned to say, had used molecular methods to find "unequivocal" evidence of vaccine-derived measles in the guts of autistic children. Ms. Two would be with him to give the parents' view, and the results, he would say, were to be published in *Nature*: one of the two top science journals in the world.

He saw this moment as a turning point—and a new feedback loop to himself. The London lawsuit, which rested on his advice, wasn't merely to pay him through fees agreed with Barr, but was to create the launch pad for Carmel. Citing "the UK Legal Aid Board" as a founding customer, its thirty-five-page prospectus argued that "autistic enterocolitis," shortened "AE," had the potential to make a fortune.

> It is estimated that the initial market for the diagnostic will be litigation driven testing of patients with AE from both the UK and the USA. It is estimated that by year 3, income from this testing could be about £3,300,000 rising to about £28,000,000. [About £48 million or US $59 million at the time I write.]

This was no charity venture. A big chunk would be his. Having created the evidence that lay behind the scare, with his secret legal deal, and his hold on the media, his share of the stock was to be 37 percent. Sleat, the father of a child among the twelve, would get the next slice—22.2 percent—with Korda, 18 percent; Pounder,

11.7 percent; and a fifth owner 11.1 percent. Wakefield would also bag a £30,000-a-year consultancy, with corresponding arrangements for the others.

Here was final victory over the naysayers. And, win or lose, the company would pay him. The only minor remaining challenge was to oil a squeaky wheel: a newly arrived head of medicine at Hampstead. It was one of those situations that, as often over the years, would call upon his charm, and *charisma*.

The new head, Mark Pepys, started work on October 1, 1999, settling into a new center at the rear of the building built expressly to house his team. Aged fifty-five, he was a slim-framed South African–born high achiever: professor of immunology, Cambridge double first, and a fellow of the Royal Society (the world's most elitist club of science, with a past president named Sir Isaac Newton). He was the school's biggest catch since 1959, when Sheila Sherlock, a liver specialist, arrived to become Britain's first female professor of medicine.

Pepys's specialty gave him insight into Wakefield's methodologies. He was a leader in the field of amyloidosis: a group of mysterious, rare conditions that could damage practically any organ through the buildup of rogue protein fibers. In the 1980s, he'd invented a diagnostic for the problems. And, in the following decade, he devised a screening system to identify potential therapies. So, while his quarry was elusive, Pepys cast his net wide in the clinical, cellular, and molecular.

He also drove red Jaguars, wasn't easily schmoozed, and arrived with a predisposition. "They made me an unrefusable offer," he tells me of the negotiations that brought him to Hampstead. "And I said, 'Here are twenty-five conditions under which I will come, and I want the dean to sign at numbers one to twenty-five—twenty-five signatures—for these things that I want.' And one of those was Wakefield out of the department when I take office. Because I knew he was a wanker and a fraud."

Here was a twist at the turn of the century that the doctor without patients couldn't control. The doctrine of "tenure" made dismissal tough, but Pepys wasn't only a formidable scientist. He was also an adept office politician. And when Wakefield asked permission to accept two consultancies—one with a drug company, Johnson & Johnson, and the other with a biotech start-up called Carmel—it didn't take the new head of medicine long to find out that "Carmel" was the name of Wakefield's wife.

"He said, 'But we've proved it, and we've got this *Nature* paper,'" Pepys tells me of their first meeting, in his office at Hampstead. "I said, 'Stop, what *Nature* paper? Is it accepted?' 'No.' 'Have you submitted it?' He said, 'No.' I said, 'Thank God for that. What were you proposing to submit?' He said, 'We've proved it, because we've got ten cases of this, and seven cases of that' . . . And I said, 'Do you not understand statistics 101, Mr. Wakefield?'"

Now it was Pepys who made the unrefusable offer. Wakefield could choose between paid leave of absence, to work for a year with his biotech business, or conduct a gold-standard test of his hypothesis. With University College London funding, help, and facilities, he could mount a molecular study—with definitive genetic sequencing—that would endorse, or refute, his ideas about measles virus. Once and for all. Without doubt. He should include at least 150 of the children he said he'd recruited, and his methods should be mirrored at two external sites, to ensure accuracy and publishing speed.

You would think any scientist would be delighted by such an offer: with time, support, and *money*. But Wakefield balked. He didn't seem keen. Response from him came there none.

Meanwhile, Pepys learned of an extraordinary negotiation in which the school's commercial arm, Freemedic, sought options to profit should the business venture succeed, but to deny any involvement if it didn't. "They may choose never to exercise such options," Cengiz Tarhan, the finance officer, wrote to Wakefield in November 1999. "Therefore neither Freemedic nor the School are in any way involved with Carmel until such options are formally exercised and shares are taken up."

So Pepys bypassed the school and had Wakefield summoned downtown and, in administrative parlance, *upstairs.* They traveled, with Pounder, to Bloomsbury, three miles south, where, at the university's headquarters, guarded by stone lions, a soft-spoken silver fox and theoretical physicist repeated Pepys's offer. His name was Chris Llewellyn Smith, formerly director-general of the CERN particle collider in Geneva, Switzerland, also a fellow of the Royal Society, and the occupant of an office about half the size of a football field, as the college's provost and president.

Seated at a hefty conference table, Llewellyn Smith asked Wakefield to conduct the research that frightened young families deserved. He also asked him to stop making public statements until he'd published the results of his findings. Not only would the university support the project, on those terms, but, if he agreed, it would *give him* his patents for the tests, vaccines, and products to exploit as he pleased through Carmel.

"We urge you not to publish prematurely observations that you may have or be making in this field," Llewellyn Smith wrote to him afterward, in a two-page letter that Wakefield received on Monday, December 13. "Good scientific practice now demands that you and others seek to confirm or refute, reliably and above all reproducibly, the possible causal relationships between MMR vaccination and autism / 'autistic enterocolitis' / inflammatory bowel disease that you have postulated."

And that's how things stood at the concrete castle as the twentieth century slipped toward closure. As fears of Y2K did the rounds in table talk, lights burned late in the head of medicine's office as Pepys mulled the likely response. In Pepys's opinion, Wakefield was a fantasist. He was unlikely to agree to proper science.

But then, just eleven days before the first light of January, Wakefield fired back a response. "Further to our meeting and the Provost's letter," it said, in part, "I am prepared to comply with the request."

FOURTEEN

On Capitol Hill

John O'Leary had the gift of the gab. In room 2154 of the Rayburn House Office Building, 350 yards from the US Capitol, he seemed to speak with such authority—*independent* authority—it felt like game, set, and match for Wakefield.

"I can confirm," O'Leary declared, in a soft Irish lilt, "that his hypothesis is correct."

As viewed from the front of the high-ceilinged committee room, O'Leary sat toward the left of a narrow strip of tables, which were draped in white linen, as if for dinner. Bald, but for a monkish dark fringe behind his scalp, and obese beyond the threshold of clinical concern, he bulged in a navy suit, white shirt, and gray tie. He peered through wire-framed glasses.

He was aged thirty-six, an associate professor of histopathology, and spoke toward an ornately carved two-deck platform, from which a dozen or so lawmakers gazed back. Here was a defining moment in the emerging controversy outside Britain over the safety of immunization.

"*Ninety-six percent* of the children's biopsies that he sent to my laboratory," O'Leary continued, "children with autistic enterocolitis, harbor measles virus genomes."

This was Thursday, April 6, 2000. In the morning. Nearly four years before my first report. O'Leary had been invited to give evidence as an expert. His testimony was the day's big event. Ms. Two had flown in to watch proceedings from a side room, and Lorraine Fraser, the *Mail on Sunday* medical correspondent, monitored the proceedings from her office in London for a major write-up that weekend:

Exclusive: The damning evidence that the medical establishment has chosen to ignore

O'Leary had come to the tables twenty minutes before, after nearly two hours of listening. First were statements from the politicians at the front, then a panel of six parents assembled along the tables: all to address the House Committee on Government Reform, with Congressman Dan Burton in the chair.

Burton was a Republican, representing a patch of the state of Indiana, and convened that hearing—an intense five hours—in pursuit of a personal quest. He was convinced that his much-loved grandson, Christian, was a victim of vaccine damage.

"I can't believe that that's just a coincidence that the shot is given," Burton had said, as the parents yielded the tables to a medical panel of O'Leary and five others, "and within just a matter of a few days, instead of being the normal child that we played with, and talked, and everything else, he was running around banging his head against the wall, flailing his arms."

Burton named the next six witnesses. Then they stood, shoulder to shoulder, right arms raised, to take the oath on the accuracy and completeness of their evidence. The congressman quizzed them at the rapid-patter speed of TV warnings about drug side effects. "Do you solemnly swear to tell the whole truth and nothing but the truth, so help you God?"

O'Leary confirmed that he did.

Behind him sat well-dressed women and men: a half dozen rows, mostly the day's contributors. And, to his right, sat Wakefield, importing his crusade to his next big market: the USA. With a press conference that morning alongside anti-vaccine campaigners, and live coverage by the public affairs network C-SPAN, today was his chance to plant his message, and lay the groundwork for his business schemes.

I'd rarely seen him so sharply turned out as he appeared, far left, at those tables. His hair, trimmed and thinned, spoke of money well spent, and his complexion bore a smoothness that, for a man of forty-three, might suggest a light touch of cosmetics. He wore a formal black suit with the faintest of pinstripes, black shirt, and rectangle-pattern tie.

He'd spoken before O'Leary: talking through slides screened on a monitor mounted high on a wall. "Nothing in this testimony should be construed as anti-vaccine," he began. "I advocate the safest vaccination strategies."

Then he cruised through his evidence for thirteen minutes—effortless, articulate, elegant, plausible—like a hang glider riding a thermal. "Autistic enterocolitis" was a "real syndrome," he said, with a "remarkably consistent" bowel disease and "regression." He said the swollen glands were "the important image." He screened before-and-after pictures of the blond-haired Child Two. He spoke of opioid peptides "impacting on the brain," made a distinction between *regressive* and *classical* autism, and gave the lawmakers a summary of the first sixty children to pass through Malcolm Ward.

"The great majority had autism," he said, fingering a pencil. "But there was a spectrum of neuropsychiatric problem, including Asperger's syndrome, and attention deficit disorder."

Given the evolution of developmental diagnoses, this was a worthy contrast to highlight. "Asperger Syndrome," as it was then called in Europe under the World Health Organization's International Classification of Diseases—or "Asperger's Disorder" in the American Psychiatric Society's manual—took a less troubling slot than autism on the spectrum.

But central to the case he set out that morning was, as ever, his big idea. Measles. And here, two and a half minutes before O'Leary began, he gave the hearing what resembled a confession. "We had failed completely to identify this virus by molecular amplification technology," he admitted—meaning Nick Chadwick's PCR tests, promised to the Legal Aid Board at the start of the deal with Richard Barr.

The technology of which he spoke, the polymerase chain reaction, was an immensely powerful tool. Long a lab workhorse throughout the scientific world, it split the double helix of DNA to allow the specific amplification of any target sequence. In quick, repeated cycles of heating and cooling in a test tube, the double-stranded DNA came apart, unzipped, into something like broken-runged ladders. Then a miracle enzyme danced the snapped rungs, joining on fresh nucleotides, replacing what was missing, to create *two* double strands of identical DNA where previously there had only been one.

Wakefield's buddy, measles, was coded in RNA, and required a prior step ("reverse transcription") to convert it to DNA. But with PCR methods, it could be doubled just the same: exponentially increasing until it was present in such numbers that sequences of the famed building blocks of life—adenine, thymine, cytosine, and guanine—were sufficient to be detected, read, and checked again with nucleotide sequencing techniques.

TGACTCG TTCCAGCCAT CAATCATTAG TCATAAAATT AATGCCCAAT . . .

But the young scientist, Chadwick, had found nothing in the samples, whether from autistic or Crohn's disease patients. And although Wakefield had supervised him (even coauthoring a paper validating the test), the former surgeon reached a different conclusion. The lab's failure, he argued, was in the technology itself. The PCR wasn't *sensitive* enough. He'd reported measles proteins using *microscopic* staining, and insisted that the *molecular* method was unable to find the genome (which determines the proteins' component amino acids, without which the virus didn't exist).

"In my laboratory we had a reaction that was sensitive to about ten thousand copies," he told the committee, before O'Leary's turn came, referring to virions one would expect by the million. "Anything less we couldn't find."

Now for the Irishman, seated to Wakefield's left. They'd known each other, and worked together, for two years. On the advice of Robert Sleat, the venture capitalist and *Lancet* parent, the doctor without patients had flown to New York—billing the legal board for the cost of his trip—to propose a research collaboration. At the time, O'Leary was a visiting professor at Cornell University, but had since returned to Ireland to supervise a lab at the Coombe Women's Hospital, Dublin.

"May I inform you that I am a pathologist and a molecular biologist," O'Leary proclaimed in oddly stilted vocabulary. "These studies were undertaken following an approach made to me by Dr. Andrew Wakefield, who has just submitted independent testimony."

Then he explained his success where Chadwick had failed, peppering his talk with technobabble, and speaking of a novel piece of kit. His lab had a revolutionary detection system, he said. He called it "TaqMan PCR."

"I have worked in this technology for the last six years," he explained, glancing back and forth between Burton and the video monitor. "It's approximately a thousand times more sensitive."

Unlike what he called "standard" or "solution phase" methods (with which researchers like Chadwick relied on reactions in conventional test tubes), what he called "TaqMan"—more usefully referred to by its supporting equipment, the ABI Prism 7700—was automated, with bells and whistles. Laser beams scanned trays in a closed machine and, when amplifying the target during heating and cooling, it didn't merely give a signal if a gene segment was *present* but, by counting the cycles before this signal was elicited, it also quantified *how much* was there.

With this neat device—about the size and general finish of a big Xerox copier—O'Leary said he'd tested gut samples from forty children. They included twenty-five kids with "autistic enterocolitis," and fifteen developmentally "normal" patients as negative controls for comparison.

Now came the big moment in room 2154. O'Leary gave headline results. He'd found measles gene sequences in inflammatory bowel disease, he said, and, especially, in Wakefield's enterocolitis.

"Twenty-four out of twenty-five children—that's *ninety-six percent* of the children's biopsies that he sent to my laboratory, blinded—children with autistic enterocolitis—harbor measles virus genomes," he declared. "One of fifteen—*six point six percent*—of control children harbored measles virus genome. And I think it doesn't take great statistical analysis to work out that there is a significant difference between twenty-four out of twenty-five, and one out of fifteen. Next slide."

It was like the bloody glove scene from the trial of O. J. Simpson. The very air seemed to drain from the room. "In terms of the association that Andrew Wakefield alluded to, I can confirm that his hypothesis is correct."

Here was vindication. And O'Leary had more: to showcase the *independence* of his data. He had slides of black material, spidery, looking evil, which he explained was the virus in tissue. He said his lab had "strict anti-contamination measures" to "outrule" false-positive results. And he confirmed his discoveries, he said, with "fluorescent-based sequencing"—outputting the strings of As, Gs, Cs, and Ts—to definitively fingerprint the bug.

In fifteen minutes, he stressed sequencing seven times. He called it the "gold standard" confirmation. In a written report to the committee, he even identified his equipment: an ABI Prism 310 capillary sequencer—a different piece of kit to the 7700—which checked results, nucleotide by nucleotide.

"We can sequence measles virus isolates from these children," he said, as a brown-haired woman in a blue dress, behind him, twisted her head from side to side. "And, of course, we can sequence it, and we can say that this is measles virus RNA present in the biopsies of these children."

What more needed saying? Wakefield was endorsed. The professor appeared to have the proof. As Fraser reported in the *Mail on Sunday* that weekend:

> The potential importance of Professor O'Leary's results will not be lost on solicitors for some 200 children—large numbers of them autistic—who are already suing the makers of MMR.

But not everyone in room 2154 was convinced. Four places to O'Leary's left at the white-clothed tables, sat another professor, who'd also flown from Europe to address the committee on vaccines. His name was Brent Taylor: a white-haired, stubble-cheeked, New Zealand–born pediatrician, who not only worked at the Royal Free medical school, but had published on MMR in *The Lancet*. He'd looked for, and didn't find, any "step-up" in autism cases corresponding with the triple shot's introduction.

O'Leary's results were as yet unpublished, and Taylor was one of a handful of observers in the room who didn't assume they were correct. "This information does have to be verified by an independent laboratory," he told Burton, when his turn came to contribute to the discussion.

The implication provoked fury from the Irish pathologist, who demanded permission to speak again. "What I present is evidence, direct evidence," he stormed. "It was done at a separate laboratory from Dr. Wakefield's. If Professor Taylor has a beef with me, he should say that. But my work is *completely independent*. I stand over it. I've come here to tell the truth. There is nothing for me to be gained in not telling the truth."

His resentment was understandable. He was confident of his findings. Certainly I can't challenge them. But in his oath to the committee, he swore to tell the *whole* truth. And I wonder if he protested too much.

He didn't say, for example, that, on Wakefield's recommendation, he too had a deal with Barr. Only a week before the hearing, as I discover later, O'Leary had renamed a Dublin-registered company, "Unigenetics," (of which Wakefield himself would become a director) to receive payments from the London class action. More than one hundred children, whose parents were suing over MMR, would be tested with his 7700 machine. And his company's bill, picked up by the taxpayer, would be nearly eight hundred thousand British pounds.

Could these interests have impacted his possible independence? And those interests *still* weren't the whole story. After gaining publicity, he would charge parents for tests, and his relationship with the man to his right, Wakefield, was yet more complicating than that. Company records, I find, from four months before the hearing, show O'Leary joining Immunospecifics as a shareholder. And the "Private and Confidential" draft prospectus for Carmel—which, until the head of medicine, Mark Pepys, intervened, had been planned for launch three months before the hearing—named a "Professor John O'Leary" as its fifth listed owner, with 11.1 percent of the stock.

"The company will have its technical base in the Department of Pathology, Coombe Women's Hospital, Dublin," the prospectus said, identifying the ABI Prism 7700, which O'Leary had praised on C-SPAN live, like he was selling committee members a Mercedes. "One of the founders of the business, Professor John O'Leary, has taken the concept of quantitative PCR much further."

Ironically, Congressman Burton was a hawk on conflicts. And the discussion that had prompted the pathologist's outburst had thrown this up as a topic. The committee's ranking Democrat— Henry Waxman of California—had urged that O'Leary's research be reviewed by federal agencies. But this suggestion was taken badly by the chair.

"We have been checking into all the financial records of the people at FDA, HHS, and CDC," Burton hit back. "And we are finding that some of those people, even on the advisory panels, do have some possible financial conflicts."

Evidently, he hadn't checked the records of his witnesses. Yet the congressman looked to the tables. "Who funded your study, Dr. Wakefield?" he asked.

"We did," Wakefield replied, after two seconds' thought. "We have a small charitable contribution."

"A charitable organization did, I see."

"But we found it a little difficult to get funding."

O'Leary wasn't asked. Burton's question was theater. Taylor acknowledged he was funded by the government.

I was surprised by O'Leary's stress on his independence. Yet something he *did* tell the committee that morning was, to me, if not to them, more revealing. There appeared to be an anomaly, a contradiction in the science, grating on his associate's evidence. Wakefield had said—as he often would—that Chadwick's PCR was *insufficiently sensitive.* So it was, at least, logical that if O'Leary possessed a more sensitive gadget, it might find the virus. *Made sense.*

"TaqMan PCR is a thousand times more sensitive," O'Leary said, "than standard solution phase."

The machine's manufacturer doesn't support this, when I ask. But five times in his fifteen-minute talk to the committee, O'Leary also spoke of running "standard" PCR on the selfsame tissues from London. He even put up a slide with distinctive gel bands that were then staples of Chadwick-style work. And using this, he told Burton, "all children with autistic enterocolitis" *also came up positive for measles.*

"By solution phase PCR, by what we call fairly standard laboratory protocols," he explained, "we can detect the measles virus in gut biopsies from these children, and the negative controls are appropriately negative."

But, if that was right, I wonder, who needed the 7700? It might be nifty, but was it *essential*? And if standard, chopped liver, meat-and-potatoes PCR could detect measles genes in bowel samples from the children, why couldn't Chadwick find it?

It was a riddle that nagged with the Crohn's work, too, where Wakefield's staining for proteins had been challenged. Why couldn't the Japanese teams, at Akita and Hirosaki Universities, find the virus using PCR? And why, most pointedly, had there been a research letter in *The Lancet* on Saturday, February 28, 1998—just five pages back from the twelve-child paper—in which scientists at the British government's flagship public health labs had likewise announced they'd failed?

O'Leary tested samples from Crohn's patients, too, reporting measles in three out of four. "That's an interesting biological fact," he told Burton.

We'll meet this pathologist again.

FIFTEEN

Letting Go

They'd had enough. Wakefield had to go. Only the means of his dispatch was undetermined. Within days of reports from Washington, DC, his managers, back at University College London, began debating the process to effect it.

Mark Pepys, the head of medicine, first got pertinent news at eight twenty-seven on the evening of April 5, 2000, thirteen hours ahead of Congressman Burton's meeting in Rayburn Committee Room 2154. "Mark," read the cover sheet of a three-page fax:

> I attach the cast list for a Press Conference scheduled for 6 April
> before the Congress hearing. You will see that Andrew Wakefield
> will be taking part.

The source was David Salisbury, the civil servant and pediatrician who first encountered Wakefield after the brand withdrawals. He was assisting Democrats at the hearing. He'd now had more than seven years of the gastroenterologist, spent his working life dealing with a raging vaccine crisis, and knew that its architect, whom he'd grown to pity, had been asked to refrain from public statements.

Parents' confidence in MMR was now sliding in Britain like a truck losing grip on the slope of an icy hill: a slow-slip skid to misfortune. From a peak of 91.8 percent before *Newsnight*'s package, the proportion of kids vaccinated with the three-in-one by the age of two had now slipped to 87.6. Outbreaks of disease crept inevitably closer as the cohort of susceptibles grew.

Wakefield had agreed to run a gold-standard study to endorse, or refute, his hypothesis. But he'd still not submitted any protocol to Pepys, and had ignored a reminder from the provost and president. "Three months have elapsed since I wrote to you," Chris Llewellyn Smith had pointed out on March 16. "I would now ask you to send me, if possible within the next week, a progress report on the study proposed."

Wakefield's reply wasn't a good omen. Any "further communications" on this issue, he wrote, should be made through his union, the Association of University Teachers.

Pepys was right. Wakefield wasn't going to do it. He'd turn down a scientist's gift of a lifetime.

So, now a staff file was pulled for a big-shouldered powerdresser by the name of Sarah Brant. She was University College London's human resources director, leading a department of fifty at its Bloomsbury headquarters, and was assigned to the task of getting him out of the institution as quickly as possible, at the lowest cost, and with the least adverse publicity.

To Pepys, Wakefield was a waste of space. Not just a doctor without patients, but a teacher without students; not a scientist, but a zealot and opportunist. "He does no clinical work, and to my knowledge he does no teaching," Pepys wrote to Brant and colleagues, in a memo I obtain. "My view is that his activities bring our institution into severe disrepute."

Eyeballs scanned his more obvious research, and what they saw left managers' jaws swinging. While newspapers lauded him like Galileo reborn, and mothers of children with developmental issues sometimes sobbed just to meet him, such papers that could be checked without access to his data (unlike the twelve-child *Lancet* report) were examined and told the tale.

Most technically complex was Kawashima et al. It was published in a low-rank journal, *Digestive Diseases and Sciences*, with Wakefield's name following five Japanese physicians', in the same month as the congressional committee hearings. First-authored by the Tokyo pediatrician Hisashi Kawashima, and cited in the prospectus for Immunospecifics, it didn't merely report measles genes in children's blood but claimed that the sequences of As, Gs, Cs, and Ts were "consistent" with *vaccine strain*.

"Nine children with autistic enterocolitis—proved by ileocolonoscopy and histology—were all UK cases," the paper said. "All had ileal lymphoid nodular hyperplasia and nonspecific colitis."

Those patients reported positive included Child Two, whose case had been filed as the leading example in Richard Barr's class action. And, to Wakefield's supporters, the seven-page paper was explosively close to conclusive. "Dr Kawashima from Japan has confirmed that the virus found comes from the MMR vaccine," was how a former *USA Today* columnist reported it. "Sounds like a smoking gun to me!"

But specialist scrutiny revealed peculiarities that a virologist could find with a wet finger. Not only did Kawashima use the same technology as Chadwick (contradicting the argument that it wasn't sensitive enough), but the sequences were, indeed, smoking guns. First, they didn't match any vaccine used in Britain. Second, they didn't match themselves.

A measles virus genome is crammed with nearly sixteen thousand nucleotides, which (when converted from native RNA to DNA) could be run out in As, Gs, Cs, and Ts. To demonstrate that strains were consistent with vaccines, Kawashima had printed portions of those he found—sometimes including *twice from the same patient.* But when scientists compared the repeated sequences, they discovered that nucleotides *changed.* An A became a C, a G became a T, a T became a G, and so forth.

"Anomalies of this nature," said an expert review, "are usually produced by cross-contamination."

Two reports were also looked at that Wakefield had published with his sidekick, Scott Montgomery. This was the epidemiologist who not only coauthored the question-marked paper but joined him with the knights, professors, and doctors at the Royal College of Surgeons event. Like Kawashima et al., the texts and tables could be checked without data. And in these, once again, contamination was detected—but with origins that could only be human.

These texts were published across three columns of the *Lancet*'s letters section and five pages of an Israeli journal. Both contained a diagram ("Temporal trends for autism") with two steep lines, from bottom left to top right, superimposing two graphs previously published by others on data from California and London. The texts claimed that the graphs showed how autism took off, *ten years apart*, "coinciding with the introduction of MMR."

But the graphs were misaligned. MMR was licensed in the United States *seventeen years* before it was in Britain. Moreover, the California data was misrepresented. And, most importantly from the point of view of Wakefield's managers, the graph from California had been doctored.

Like the question-marked paper, the diagram tried to make a point by comparing data collected by others. But the two rising lines only looked comparable because a word, "enrolled," had been deleted from a caption for the California figures, and the surrounding space closed up. This transformed the graph from what it really was—the ages of children receiving support at state service centers (good news)—to the purported incidence of autism (bad news).

Number of [Enrolled] *Persons with Autism*

Who was responsible? It was impossible to say, but Wakefield continued to circulate it to parents, even after he'd been challenged over its truth.

By the time Wakefield's staff file hit Brant's desk in Bloomsbury, such anomalies were common-room banter. And later, another scientist, Tom MacDonald, professor of immunology and dean of research at Barts and the London School of Medicine, spotted another astonishing discrepancy. Two photographs, published in the *American Journal of Gastroenterology*, were labeled as comparing the "normal" small intestine at the terminal ileum of a purported MMR-affected child, with "severe" ileal lymphoid hyperplasia in another. But somebody had left date stamps visible on the images, revealing that the pictures were taken less than two minutes apart, and so could only have come from the same patient.

I admit I found Wakefield incapable of embarrassment. To me, he'd got no conscience. But his response to the university's requests to do his job and prove claims that, by now, were terrorizing a generation, went beyond such errors (or whatever they were) into a blank refusal to answer the question with the gold-standard study—claiming this would infringe his "academic freedom."

Months passed. Then came a last straw: a blunt confirmation, in September 2000, that he wouldn't mount the project he'd agreed to. He wrote to Llewellyn Smith:

> It is the unanimous decision of my collaborators and co-workers
> that it is only appropriate that *we* define our research objectives, we
> enact the studies as appropriately reviewed and approved, and we

decide as and when we deem the work suitable for submission for peer review.

Two months later, he defied the request that he stop making public statements and appeared on the CBS network's *60 Minutes* program: his biggest chance yet for publicity.

Five weeks after that, Brant swiveled to her screen and wrote a paper of her own: three pages:

Mr Andrew Wakefield—mutual termination of employment

A plan was constructed to ensure that the university's senior managers were on board to weather the inevitable storm. The *Mail on Sunday*'s Lorraine Fraser had now moved to the *Sunday Telegraph*, and she was sure to spin the story his way. So on the document's third page was a list of seven names, seven job titles, with seven dotted lines: as if for a failed state dictator's execution.

From the president and provost to the vice-provost (administration) and the director of planning and management accounts, between November 2000 and January 2001, Brant's document went back and forth between Hampstead and Bloomsbury, until every dotted line was signed.

The plan was final. But execution would take forever. Such was job security in academia at the time that it would take nearly another year to complete. External lawyers were hired. Accountants went to work examining his spending. He'd be asked to explain long absences in the United States. And even his letterhead—the printed paper he wrote on—was studied for irregular claims.

Wakefield's correspondence had long provoked mirth. Now it was eyed as evidence. A typical doctor or scientist, like almost any office staff, would sign work letters above a short designation. Simon Murch, for example, who scoped most of the *Lancet* kids, used "Dr. Simon Murch, Senior Lecturer." But Wakefield communicated—even within the school—with a grandiose panoply of *self.*

He was only a mid-rank lab researcher, after all. But, not content with the dignity of this station in life, he'd fashioned a personal letterhead. After the name of the school, the university, the department, and the "Centre for Gastroenterology," he added:

> Inflammatory Bowel Disease Study Group
> Director A. J. Wakefield MB BS, FRCS

Fair enough, I suppose. Ink on paper. But, as if this wasn't enough to announce him to recipients, below his signature were typed thirty-two further words, that, if he needed them at all, would have filled five lines, but were configured to occupy a more impressive six lines, like scrambled eggs on an admiral's cap.

> A J Wakefield FRCS
> Reader in Experimental Gastroenterology in the
> Departments of Medicine and Histopathology
> Hon. Consultant in Experimental Gastroenterology to the Royal Free
> Hampstead NHS Trust
> Director, Inflammatory Bowel Disease Study Group

Murch could have padded his dignity too. But here were shades of Wakefield delusion. Brant wrote to him pointing out that he left the histopathology department in March 1998, and so should stop describing himself thus. He'd not been entitled to "FRCS" since July 1996, when, according to the Royal College of Surgeons, he'd resigned by withholding his fees. The "Hon. Consultant" was a courtesy title, of little significance outside the building. And the last line (repeated from the top of the page) had been dealt with during his bid for a professorship, when the school secretary, Bryan Blatch, had told him:

The Inflammatory Bowel Disease Study Group is not a department of the School, and I have no recollection of the title Director being conferred upon you.

Low self-esteem? Anything but. All the signs said Wakefield thought he was *special*.

And on it went, into 2001, when he revealed how special that was. Instead of agreeing to prove his career-defining claims, he coauthored another paper with his favored sidekick that was so wildly wrong that when I came to study it—pulling the source materials from the British Library's vaults—I found anomalies line by line.

It was nominally published in February 2001, in a short-lived journal called *Adverse Drug Reactions and Toxicological Reviews*, with a circulation of just 350. Wakefield had it press-released the month before, however, through a not-for-profit entity called Visceral that he'd set up to raise money outside the medical school.

Fraser, at the *Telegraph*, was primed in advance.

Shame on officials who say MMR is safe

As was another acolyte, at the *Daily Mail*:

MMR: A marvel or a menace?

But Britain's worried parents didn't have a clue about the junk that lay behind such headlines. The new paper appeared to be an independent review of science, running to nineteen pages. Coauthored by Montgomery (who, legal records indicate, would be paid nearly £90,000 to support Barr's lawsuit), it was grandly titled "Measles, Mumps, Rubella Vaccine: Through A Glass, Darkly."

Indeed.

The official position is that MMR vaccine is safe; this paper examines the evidence.

Except that it didn't. It was a campaigning pamphlet, framed to make a case. Claiming to review prelicensing safety studies—conducted between the 1960s and the 1980s—the authors made it look like researchers had long known that combining three vaccines was risky.

A government safety watchdog denounced Wakefield and Montgomery in a fifteen-page press-released analysis. But "Glass, Darkly" could be tackled with a more telling method, which I would bring to bear long after. The paper was dominated by a table, filling a page, purporting to summarize six studies. And, after ordering a stack of musty volumes to be trucked to London by the library, I find *none* were accurately reported.

In a two-thousand-word email to Montgomery, I point this out, with a line-by-line comparison, for example:

> (b) With regard to the second paper (Stokes, 1971) you say in the table that 228 cases, including 77 from the United States, were compared with 106 unvaccinated controls, and that the length of follow-up was 28 days. This is wrong. The paper reported on 685 children, including 228 in the United States, compared with 281 controls, and the length of follow-up was six to nine weeks.

Another:

> (d) With regard to the fourth paper (Schwarz et al., 1975), you say in the table that the study had no relevant outcome. This is wrong. The study had the very relevant outcome that MMR was found to have a similar adverse event profile to monovalent measles vaccine.

Montgomery replied from Sweden's Karolinska Institute, where he'd worked since leaving Hampstead. He addressed other issues but, despite being named as an author on both, declined to comment on the "Glass, Darkly" paper or the doctored caption from California. "It would be inappropriate for me to speculate or comment on specific aspects of the work that I was not involved in and were not my responsibility," he wrote.

It seemed that Wakefield believed rules didn't apply to him: in research, or anything else. As health agencies raged against damage from "Glass, Darkly," professors at Hampstead complained of his unexplained absences, of him making job offers without authority, and of his registering patents in the Royal Free's name without managers' knowledge or permission.

For his part, in the war of words during that bitter year of conflict, Wakefield threatened to report Pepys to the UK doctors' regulator, the General Medical Council, and took advice on suing a professor for libel. Then, in a curt email to Brant in July 2001, he revealed a persona behind the charisma:

> Under no circumstances delete my name from the payroll or I will take legal action immediately. I hope I make myself clear.

A brief moment of pause came in September 2001, when, on Tuesday the eleventh, London's sky fell silent, and it would be weeks before attention broke away from New York and the attack on the World Trade Center. But the skirmishes with Wakefield then resumed with a "Settlement Agreement," under which he would resign from the school. In exchange for £10, he'd be assigned his patents for tests, treatments, and vaccines—a sum Pepys thought was excessive.

Wakefield signed the document—twenty-five pages, witnessed by his wife—on November 14, ending his career in academia. After tax and deductions, his payoff was £109,625 (about £178,000 or US $223,000 at the time I write this) plus a bloodless reference from the school. "As a team leader, he has shown the ability to engage the enthusiasm of his co-workers," this said, in part. "He has published work in journals such as *Gastroenterology* and the *Lancet* and has been in demand as a speaker."

The school agreed to say nothing about the reason for his departure: his refusal to set up the study. But straightway he fed the journalist Fraser, donning an identity that was to serve him well, as he set out to make his fortune in America.

> Andrew Wakefield, a consultant gastroenterologist whose research has linked the vaccine to autism and bowel disease in children, said last night that he had been asked to resign because of his work.

She quoted him saying, "I have been asked to go because my research results are unpopular."

- - - - - - - - - - - - - - - - - - -

SIXTEEN

The Bridge

It was a wet afternoon back in Washington, DC, from which the first public appearance of a renewed Andrew Wakefield was reported by people who were there. This was five months after he cleared his office in Hampstead, and now, with no employer except Richard Barr, he was at last free to speak his mind.

"We are in the midst of an international epidemic," he was quoted as saying at a rally on the grass of the National Mall, on a rainy, windy, and unseasonably cold Sunday toward the end of April 2002. "Those responsible for investigating and dealing with this epidemic have failed. Among the reasons for this failure is the fact that they are faced with the prospect that they themselves may be responsible."

That was some allegation. His epidemic was vaccine damage. And he was making the case that the people who should tackle it didn't because they thought they might have caused it.

"Therefore," he continued, "in their efforts to exonerate themselves, they are an impediment to progress."

Printed and read aloud, his words had a cadence that invoked a stentorian oratory. Maybe a speech by the war leader Sir Winston Churchill, transposed to the United States in some feature film fantasy as an artistically licensed crowd pleaser. The great man standing proud, within sight of a monument, with a ring of stars and stripes, crackling on a hill, under a gusting drizzle of rain.

"I believe that public health officials know there is a problem. They are, however, willing to deny the problem and accept the loss of an unknown number of children on the basis that the success of public health policy—mandatory vaccination—by necessity involves sacrifice."

It was a noxious charge: of conspiracy and cover-up by those he felt had slighted him. They were people like David Salisbury, the civil servant and pediatrician, whom he asked for money ten years before. And although Wakefield never submitted a written proposal for any funding, he'd never forgotten that insult. He accused Salisbury of slander, in a letter copied to Barr, and would still rail against him decades later.

Now he didn't just *assume* MMR caused autism (a claim he made squarely in his patent applications), but went way beyond even the newsletters and fact sheets from Barr and Kirsten Limb. The law firm couple's output was salted with insinuation, but their chief expert (whose deal remained undisclosed) now summoned visions of evil.

"Neither I, nor my colleagues, subscribe to the belief that any child is expendable," he declaimed, in a transcript ascribed to the Washington event. "History has encountered and dealt with such beliefs."

This wasn't bombast. This was a state of mind. But that miserable afternoon, when a few score parents had gathered near Fourth Street to listen to speeches and a Louisiana rock band, it wasn't clear if they got much benefit. The weather was appalling: 51.8°F, with rain, at 4:00 p.m. And even hot gumbo and a boy with Asperger's singing "America the Beautiful" couldn't lift a desultory mood.

Mobilized by a campaign group called Autism Unlocked, they'd mostly come to the capital for another congressional hearing. And, to be frank, I'm not convinced that Wakefield was even there, and that his words weren't delivered as a message. Yet his accusations rang out, echoed to hundreds of thousands—via another man, listed to speak.

His name was Lenny Schafer, from Sacramento, California, and it was he who built the bridge that Wakefield would cross, trafficking his epidemics of fear, guilt, and disease, from Britain to America, and then the world.

It had happened before with vaccine scares: made in England, marketed in the United States, and from there to everywhere on the globe. That was the story with John Wilson's DTP panic. And even he wasn't the first on the path. In October 1879, an English businessman-crusader named William Tebb had crossed the Atlantic to give the keynote address to the inaugural meeting, on New York City's East Side, of the Anti-Vaccination League of America.

"The statistics showed that 25,000 children were slaughtered every year by being vaccinated," Tebb declared, urging a campaign against smallpox immunization, as reported next day in the *New York Times*.

Already in his fifties, Schafer wasn't an orator, or even much of a campaigner. But he'd got what it took for his role. As an angry young man in Detroit, Michigan, he'd been a left-wing activist, dabbling as a publisher in the "alternative press," and later, in middle age, he faced up to autism: through an adopted son named Izak. That led him to a community: a local parents' group called Families for Early Autism Treatment, or FEAT.

Densely mustached and with a quirky sense of fun, Schafer pooled his assets in 1997 in a pioneering internet bulletin. Just six years after the World Wide Web went live, he began culling reports on autism issues, which he forwarded to a mailing list of parents. In the first six months, that list grew to one hundred. Then, as the web became part of daily life, by the time of the National Mall rally he claimed ten thousand subscribers to what he named the *FEAT Daily Newsletter*.

Alongside Izak, here was his pride, reaching out into America from a cramped condominium on Sacramento's Old Placerville Road. "Every parent who takes on this cause brings with them their light of hope to the rest of us," he wrote, referring to the struggle of supporting children with developmental issues. "This is my little light, and I'm going to let it shine."

The newsletter—which he later renamed after himself—was as crude as it proved to be effective. Aided from the living rooms of a handful of parents, he searched for and collected media stories on autism, copying them into plain text files. Overruling formalities of copyright law, he republished these squirrelings for free, to subscribers, in what he called a "news clipping service."

In the early years, he was guided by FEAT's core interests, passing along reports on, say, restraints in residential homes and surveys on mental illness. But as Wakefield's campaign took hold in Britain—the world's most competitive newspaper market—Schafer harvested the ever more strident coverage and, by the logic of his process, delivered it to the most susceptible: mothers and fathers like himself.

Study Links Measles Virus to New Form of Bowel Disease

Scientists: MMR Vaccine Should Not Have Been Licensed

Were All Of These Children Killed By The Triple MMR?

Just think of that drumbeat, banging around your inbox, from a trusted, not-for-profit source. "It is important to point out that we do not write this news, we only deliver it," he assured his subscribers. "And this editorial policy gives us as much room for partisan spin as your newspaper route delivery person."

He republished results from the defective Kawashima paper. He scooped endorsements of the much-covered but wrong "Glass, Darkly." And story after story—ignored by US media—was imported and relayed to families touched by autism, until the noise from across the Atlantic grew so loud that, ten weeks before the Washington rally, he proclaimed a "Wakefield Fest."

"We are having so much coverage over the MMR issue," Schafer explained, "because currently the British public is obsessed."

The Fest was triggered by a paper from John O'Leary in a short-lived journal, *Molecular Pathology*. Using his ABI Prism 7700 machine for gene amplification, the Dublin professor, who'd appeared in Washington two years before, claimed what sounded like more proof over measles. The guts of seventy-five of ninety-one children—diagnosed with a combination of autistic disorders, enterocolitis, and the swellings in the ileum—were positive for the virus, he reported. That compared with only five of seventy control patients. His data "confirm an association," he said.

This was bound to attract big coverage in Britain. The "MMR debate" was now a national recreation. Everyone from the prime minister to celebrity chefs were stroking their oars in the controversy.

Wakefield—a coauthor of O'Leary's paper—had an extra advantage with media. His entity, Visceral, that he'd set up to fundraise, had a chair whose sister-in-law (a woman named Sarah Barclay) was a BBC television reporter. And, though she assures me that her managers *knew* of her relationship, she presented an hour-long fest of her own for the BBC-1 channel's investigative *Panorama*.

"We have found measles virus," the Irishman told her on camera. "And the next thing people want to know is, you know, what's the sequence strain?"

With American media, O'Leary's paper went nowhere. But Schafer published a link to a BBC webstream, allowing him to focus the output from London to where it might most hit home. He'd a hard-core audience of mothers and fathers, many of whom must have wondered, while skimming his clippings, "Is this saying we injured our own child?"

Likewise, the newsletter ran Wakefield's Mall epistle: with its grandiose phrasing picked up as a meme and republished at countless websites. "You, the parents and children, are the source of the inspiration and strength for our endeavors," his tones rang out online. "Our quest for truth through science—a science that is compassionate, uncompromising, and uncompromised."

Nothing would compare with Schafer's little light for building Wakefield's bridge into America. But he wasn't alone. There was also the Republican congressman Dan Burton, with his hearings on Capitol Hill. Certain as he was that his grandson was vaccine damaged, he ran a string of show trials, year after year, at which Wakefield—"All the way from merry old England"—was feted like Shakespeare on wheels.

After his 2000 appearance, with O'Leary at his side, he'd returned a year later to the witness tables—with him dressed this time in a loose cream suit—and said much the same as before. The syndrome. The bowel disease. The persistent measles virus (which he said had been sequenced to the vaccine strain). "Bear in mind that we are dealing with regressive autism," he stressed, "not of classical autism, where the child is not right from the beginning."

But, as he learned from the Royal Free's head of medicine, Mark Pepys, charisma wouldn't smooth all paths. Further down the table, and crowned with frizzy hair, sat America's top expert on gut-brain interactions: the "father of neurogastroenterology," he'd been called. His name was Michael Gershon, chairman of the department of anatomy and cell biology at Columbia University, New York.

Gershon told Burton that if measles made the gut wall leaky, as proposed, it should be leaky in both directions. *And it wasn't.* If opioid peptides escaped from the gut into the bloodstream, so would many similar-sized peptides. *And they didn't.* For the components of foodstuffs to do the harm Wakefield said, they would need to evade the liver—and Gershon believed that they couldn't—and would then require a "miracle" to occur: the protective blood-brain barrier opening, "like the Red Sea did for Moses."

Wakefield never responded to these big-picture points: then or, to my knowledge, ever after. But what he did take up at his next appointment with Burton were things Gershon had said about O'Leary. These would rankle and fester until the hearings resumed, two months after the rally on the National Mall. And then, revealing a less beguiling nature, the fugitive from Britain lashed out with a venom that made the words reported from him in Schafer's newsletter read like a Buddhist meditation.

After Gershon's Moses miracle simile, the professor had recounted information he'd picked up from a preeminent scientist. His name was Michael Oldstone, the world's go-to guru on measles virus, at the Scripps Research Institute in San Diego, California, the world's top-ranked research institution. Wakefield had hoped to collaborate with Oldstone, until Pepys found out and suggested to the Scripps man that he check O'Leary's lab. So blind, coded specimens were dispatched to Ireland and, as Gershon relayed it in his testimony to Burton, the results came back crawling with anomalies. Some samples sent twice, with deliberately different codes, he said, were reported as both positive and negative.

The most likely explanation was lab contamination. The fragile, light-as-air, will-o'-the-wisp RNA virus could hang in a room for hours, attach to coat sleeves, or be blown by a door, to turn up where it shouldn't in a lab. Or, the 7700 might be wrongly configured, or run without a required raft of safeguards. Another possibility was some form of misconduct by a person, or persons, with access. But, in any event, the Scripps institute scientist opted for no further involvement with the Irishman.

"Oldstone has concluded that the record of performance would not be acceptable for certifying a clinical laboratory," Gershon told Burton's committee.

Wakefield was outraged. He was planning more papers, and the tests from Dublin were vital to Barr's lawsuit, now edging toward show time in London. The virus had been sequenced as vaccine strain, he insisted, and, *if there was* contamination, it had occurred at Scripps, not O'Leary's lab at the Coombe.

"I would like to put the record straight," Wakefield declared from the table in the Rayburn committee room. "Dr Gershon's behavior was a disgrace."

Here surely were matters for scientific debate. But Wakefield also lashed out, in a five-page letter, with all the grace of his departure from Hampstead. Gershon, he informed Burton, wasn't just guilty of "obvious errors" but of "unprofessional behaviour," "false testimony," "demonstrably false assertions," "shoddy science," "lack of integrity," "what amounts to perjury," and "malicious disinformation" that may add up to what he called "defamation."

For Oldstone's part, Wakefield wrote that the measles expert was culpable of "obvious errors," "sloppy practice," and, if he was aware of the "substance" of Gershon's testimony, he "may be considered to have perjured himself."

No more Mr. Nice Guy from merry old England. And he hadn't yet finished his rejoinders. Now back at the table in June 2002, he filed a dramatic statement for the congressional record that hinted at what was crossing the bridge. Had the Columbia scientist appeared for a second time, he wrote, "I am sure he would have enlightened the committee, somewhat belatedly, as to any proprietary rights his wife might have in the Merck chickenpox vaccine."

His wife's rights in a vaccine? Inquiries found *none.* But here, un-spotted by the listening lawmakers, lurked a disturbing, mirror-ing phenomenon. It was *Wakefield* who had rights—in his pro-posed *measles vaccine*—not only as the purported inventor of the product, but with all entitlements handed over by University Col-lege London, five months before Burton's hearing.

Was this some kind of psychological projection, I wonder? If so, it wasn't one-off. Back in London, with his sidekick, Scott Montgomery, and Ms. Two, he'd done something similar. They'd been invited by the Medical Research Council to a workshop on autism. But just days before, all three pulled out, saying they'd learned that some participants were being paid to advise drug companies in a lawsuit.

The lawsuit was Barr's. But the target participants were on the *other* side. And had Wakefield attended, it might have come out that he'd the same conflict as them. Nevertheless, he wrote to the workshop's organizers:

> While we have no doubt that these individuals have declared their obvious conflict of interest, declaration of such a conflict in an area that is as charged and sensitive to public scrutiny as this one may be interpreted as being merely cosmetic. Such a conflict is irreconcil-able and should have precluded them from acting in both roles.

Acting in both roles? A curious reflection. And, even before his conflict regarding the twelve-child paper and his performance in the Atrium to launch a public health crisis, Wakefield's deal with Barr—to create bespoke evidence—went way beyond acting as an expert.

To be fair to Burton, he couldn't have known. And he, too, had made up his mind. He couldn't have run his committee with more partisan glee if the topic was Democratic Party finance. So he posted Wakefield's letter on the congressional website and likened its author to a titan of medicine.

"I believe other scientists who have differed with the prevailing opinions have suffered similar castigation as you have," Burton announced when Wakefield finished giving evidence to the committee. "You may rest assured that eventually the truth will out. Louis Pasteur found that out, after seventeen years, when he was knighted. So eventually the truth will come out, and those who criticize, and continue to denigrate what you have done, will be eating a heck of a lot of humble pie."

Here was a bridge-builder as keen as Schafer. But, back in London with Barr's class action, the other end of that bridge was on fire.

- - - - - - - - - - - - - - - - - - - -

SEVENTEEN

Unblinded

Were it a few years later, there might have been video. Someone might have pulled out their iPhone or Android and captured the behaviors—reactions, expressions—when, at last, the music stopped. The scene: the *unblinding*, the moment of truth, when, as far as Richard Barr's lawsuit was concerned, all would be revealed.

Well, *enough*.

A year before, the BBC had filmed a precursor. They were present at the scoping of a sixteen-year-old boy whom Wakefield had cited to the congressman, Dan Burton, as a case of vaccine damage. But the green-aproned endoscopist, Simon Murch, gazed at the monitor in the Royal Free's endoscopy suite and pronounced nothing diagnostic of any condition.

In the BBC video (broadcast on the *Panorama* investigative program reported by the sister-in-law of the chair of Wakefield's Visceral entity), the mood was caught in a four-second clip. Here was Wakefield, peering over the endoscopist's shoulder, with a demeanor resembling the way I think he must have felt as the unblinding ground painfully forward. His right hand rises and covers his eyes, like he's suffering from migraine, or jet lag. His palm slides to his cheeks, then the back of his neck. His head twists left, with his right elbow rising. He fingers the collar of his shirt.

The unblinding took place over two spring days in 2003: April 27 and 28. The location was a window-walled seminar room, in a low-rise, oddly shaped Venture Centre on the edge of campus at the University of Warwick, in the rolling green midlands of England. The host: Micropathology, a contract diagnostic and research company, which shared a front desk, coffee shop, and bathrooms with maybe twenty small businesses like itself.

Eyewitness reports said that Richard Barr was present, with his scientist and wife, Kirsten Limb, plus a huddle of retained experts and aides. Their purpose: to decode the final laboratory results on both measles virus and opioid peptides.

For the first time ever, the Wakefield hypothesis of viral causation, and the stoned rodent model of childhood autism, would be checked against data from controlled, blinded studies. So the status of the children from whom samples were taken—whether autistic cases or neurotypical controls—wasn't known to researchers in advance.

Here was the climax to a project unheard of in the annals of forensic medicine. Working under Limb, the agricultural graduate, the lawyers had hired a nurse to travel around Britain, collecting blood and urine from client children and others, then delivering it to Micropathology. In turn, the research company dispatched it to labs, including to the pathologist, John O'Leary, at the Coombe Women's Hospital, Dublin.

"Our nurse, Sarah Dodd, is working hard to try to collect as many samples in the quickest possible time," Barr explained to clients in a "strictly confidential" newsletter from his office, where the bottles and boxes were kept. "She has managed to collect blood and urine samples from a total of approximately 100 children so far. This includes 'control' children (age- and sex-matched children who have not been affected by the MMR vaccine)."

No question about it, this was a race against time. A decade had elapsed since the case of Richard Lancaster: the Norfolk schoolboy who, after MMR, developed mumps-meningitis, and on whose mother's house purchase Barr did the paperwork.

Court deadlines loomed: the evidence on autism must be ready for exchange with the drug company defendants no later than the fourth of July.

The once small-town solicitor now ran with the big dogs. By the time Nurse Dodd set off on her rounds, Barr worked for a law firm with a backroom team of dozens. There were week-long meetings with experts from America, conferences with Queen's Counsel in book-lined chambers, foreign expeditions to keep abreast of the science, and nights at swanky hotels.

"The ironic thing is they were always going on about how 'you know we've hardly got any money compared with the other side,'" a veterinary vaccine specialist by the name of John March, who attended the unblinding, tells me. "And I'm thinking, judging by the amount you're paying out, the other side must be living like millionaires."

Some surely were. Pretrial court hearings were like parties of middle school geography teachers pitched against the Roman army. Alongside Barr's team of about eight—to the judge's right—would be three dozen from the defendants, to his left. The opposition was the same as it was all along: Big Pharma in all its might. Headquartered in Lyon, France, was Aventis Pasteur (later Sanofi Pasteur). From the United States: Merck Inc. of New Jersey. And, from Britain, what was then called SmithKline Beecham (later GlaxoSmithKline, or GSK).

Until now, Barr and Limb had traded on arguments over the ever more elaborate hypothesis-upon-hypothesis that Wakefield had glued together. Born of his inspirational moment in Toronto—speculating on the cause of Crohn's disease—it had embraced measles virus after he read an encyclopedia. Then he'd picked up the psychobiologist's opioids conjecture in the post-*Newsnight* call from Ms. Two.

With minimal forays into other possibilities (such as that measles might damage neural structures directly), they lined up their ducks with the same ol' same ol': MMR → persistent measles virus → enterocolitis → leaky gut → opioid excess in blood to the brain → regressive autism.

Bada bing, bada boom.

"I was convinced that one day all of this would come out," says March, an expert on rinderpest virus, the cattle equivalent and ancestor of measles. "Basically what you had was two legal people running a five or six million pound research program. And that would be unprecedented. If you went to the Medical Research Council and said you were going to have your entire research budget for this year run by a lawyer and a legal assistant, they would just be incredulous. But that really is what happened."

The pair worked all hours. But whether or not MMR did or didn't cause autism, their case was in chaos from the outset.

"I cannot overemphasise the fact that to embark on the litigation in this state would be catastrophic," wrote a Queen's Counsel advocate, Jeremy Stuart-Smith (son of the judge, Sir Murray, of the DTP checklist). He'd been hired to work alongside Augustus Ullstein and gave this advice in twenty-two secret pages, two months *after* the first writ was served.

Despite such warnings, little improved, while fees and costs sprouted like bamboo. So tough was the challenge that, in July 2000, Barr's team even proposed (the judge called it "daft") that autism be indefinitely "left to one side" and a trial proceed purely on the claim that MMR caused "autistic enterocolitis."

And yet, to me incredibly, this alleged new bowel disease was often "subclinical," they submitted in court, meaning the sufferer didn't even know they had it. "The fact that the infection may not cause clinical symptoms," insisted a statement filed from Barr's team, "is not an indication that it does not exist."

Even six months before the showdown at Warwick, Queen's Counsel remained unconvinced. After an intermediate opinion from Stuart-Smith Junior that without better evidence the claims would "fail," three QCs (Barr hired another, Simeon Maskrey) reported to the Legal Aid Board on the strength of the case over autistic spectrum disorders, or ASD.

> We are still not able to say, on the balance of probability, the vaccine has caused ASD.

The *balance of probability*. Nowhere near scientific proof. And yet, beyond the lawsuit, in both Britain and the United States, fear and guilt over the shot was causing turmoil in families—and outbreaks of disease were crackling. Even the mayor of London, a man named Ken Livingstone, urged parents to shun MMR. "There is no way I would inflict that risk on a child," he opined on a radio show. "Why whack them all into a child at the same time?"

But behind the veil of Barr's multiparty suit—which maxed out with compensation claims for sixteen hundred children—his QCs still struggled with the logic. Wakefield's attempts to satisfy the Stuart-Smith checklist offered little explanation as to why the triple product, over which they were suing, was less safe than single shots. At the heart of the action remained the big idea, shining as brightly as any time in his life.

As one of two judges in the proceedings noted:

> The mechanisms all take their point of departure from the demonstrated persistence of measles virus in the body of children with regressive autism.

Wakefield himself couldn't solve the riddle. He wasn't a virologist, immunologist, epidemiologist, or any kind of -ologist to render his opinion admissible on such matters in court. And, when interviewed in writing by Britain's national Science Museum (for an exhibition in London at the time of the unblinding), he admitted that he didn't know.

> SCIENCE MUSEUM: Andrew Wakefield has suggested separating the jabs by one year to be on the safe side, and that's what most doctors offering single jabs are sticking to. What's his reasoning?
> WAKEFIELD: It's purely empirical—we have no idea. It's the public health people's job to look into that.

And so, back to Warwick: with the coded results from Nurse Dodd's gatherings of blood and urine. "It was all blinded beforehand," recalls March, a clean-cut molecular biologist, virologist, and former Harvard Medical School fellow. "And you had one of the people there give results, and say, '*That* was an autistic child, *that* was a control.'"

The action opened like an Oscars-night envelope, and closed like a Las Vegas daybreak. "Once it started being written up on a board," March says, "it became blindingly obvious that, for every test that was done, there was no difference between autistics and controls—whether that was looking at urines, or looking at measles virus."

March was a great source. Relieved to talk. And he'd a close relative diagnosed with autism. "I've never actually seen this published—I don't know why—but, bizarrely enough," he tells me, "there were more of the *control* kids that apparently had measles virus in them than there were *autistic* kids."

I can vouch for such anomalies, using a spreadsheet I obtain of results from the Dublin lab. While Child Two's blood, for instance, was reported *negative* for measles, three control subjects—with the family name "Wakefield" and initials I recognize—were tabulated as infected with the virus.

March's commission was to prove *opioid excess*—measured by peptide levels in urine. He worked at the Moredun Research Institute, a center for the study of livestock diseases, south of Edinburgh, Scotland. And Barr and Limb hired him to use mass spectrometry—bombarding test samples with electrically charged particles to weigh their molecular components.

In a post-results interlude, March, with a colleague, stepped from the meeting room into a wide, carpeted corridor where, previously blinded to their own test results, they contemplated the implications of the data. To them, "opioid excess" looked dead in the water. Measles: just as bad.

"And I went back in, and they just continued as if nothing had happened," he remembers. "I kind of said: 'I'm sorry, I don't understand. *There is no case.*' And they looked at me: 'What do you mean?' I said, 'Well, obviously there's no case here.'"

He says he was asked to sign a confidentiality agreement. The data would never be published. "It was almost like it had become a religion. And if you got a result that you didn't like, you ignored that result and carried on."

No surprise there. That was the logic of litigation. The goal wasn't truth. It was to win—or, at least, maximize billing to legal aid. And, understandably for a lawyer, Barr kept his nerve, even after the unblinding opened eyes. A peptides meeting was promptly convened in Norfolk (flying four academics from the United States to huddle with March), at which "opioid excess" was unsentimentally dumped for a new "opioid suppression hypothesis."

Defending the big idea was less straightforward. Persistent measles was integral to the argument. So, after doubts were raised over the Dublin lab, Barr had commissioned a backup. Based at Barts and the London Hospital (into which John Walker-Smith's old workplace was merged), a team with many years of PCR experience was hired to duplicate O'Leary's tests.

Their machine was the same as his: an ABI Prism 7700. Their "primers" (short strings of engineered nucleotides to seek and bookend gene sequences for amplification) were identical to those at the Coombe. Their "probe" (a different string, meant to bind to the target, so as to trigger a fluorescent signal upon detecting the virus) was, similarly, a perfect match. Everything was set for the Irish pathologist's findings to get impeccable backup confirmation.

The London work went well. Except for one snag: the English lab couldn't find the virus. Well, they *could* find the virus, in positive controls, and a few samples preprocessed in Dublin. But where blood for the tests came directly from Warwick—and never crossed the choppy Irish Sea to the Coombe—they found nothing. *Nada. Zilch.*

"The lack of positive results in RNA extracted in our laboratory," wrote Finbarr Cotter, the lab chief and professor of hematology, in a report filed on behalf of Barr's clients, "leads us to conclude that these samples had no detectable measles virus at the level of detection in our laboratory."

Reports were now exchanged with the defendants' advisers (twenty-eight from Barr's team; thirty-two from the drug companies). Both sides now saw each other's hands. The companies' experts—mostly leaders in their fields—were uniformly excoriating of each and every aspect of the MMR-autism allegations. But leading counsel for the children—the three QCs—also bumped rocks close to home.

Wakefield's report ran to two dense volumes, totaling 198 pages. To my count, the word "consistent" appeared fifty-nine times, and there were five boilerplate statements on causality. "It is my opinion that, on the balance of probability," he affirmed for Child Two, and four more of eight test cases, "the disease was caused by, or at least contributed to by, MMR."

That was his conclusion. It could hardly be otherwise. But, in volume 1, paragraph 1.1, of his epic analysis, he rushed over an extraordinary admission.

I will not be relying on the data of Kawashima et al. I have been told that according to Dr Kawashima, the data are not available for further scrutiny.

This was the Japanese pediatrician who claimed to find gene sequences "consistent" with vaccine strain measles: the so-called "smoking gun." But Wakefield's "coordinating investigator-molecular studies," Nick Chadwick, had warned him of issues at the time. Kawashima had reported sequences from autistic children's blood cells that precisely matched tissues from a patient in London with the fatal SSPE brain disease. They'd been sent from Hampstead as positive controls to evaluate the Tokyo doctor's PCR.

This neatly chimed with Chadwick's inability to find any measles himself. He was sure the Japanese had reported false positives, and he later made this clear in a statement. "Each of the SSPE positive controls I had been using had quite specific changes in its sequence and so it was easy to determine when a sample had been contaminated from this source," he wrote. "I mentioned this to Dr Wakefield, but he did not seem to take any particular notice."

Barr's three Queen's Counsel absorbed Kawashima as they pored over reports from both sides. Then, on Friday, August 8, 2003, they put Barr's lawsuit out of its misery. "Upon the assumption that no further test results would be admitted in evidence by the judge," they concluded in a secret 218-page opinion, "we consider that the claimants would not prove that the vaccine has caused, or is capable of causing, ASD."

So that was that. Applicable law kicked in. The legal board stopped the money. And while its decision would be appealed to an independent review panel, to the High Court (twice), and to the Court of Appeal, it would never be overturned. And on Wednesday, October 1, 2003, the board, now renamed the Legal Services

Commission, or LSC, issued a statement from its chief executive, with a small-print footnote harking back to the board's fatal mistake, years before, when it approved Wakefield's "clinical and scientific study."

> This was the first case in which research had been funded by legal aid. In retrospect, it was not effective or appropriate for the LSC to fund research. The courts are not the place to prove new medical truths.

Ms. Two, Ms. Four, and hundreds of other parents were shattered when the news came through. Troublemakers blamed an establishment conspiracy—so blighted had spirits become. Some vowed to fight on and refused to sign papers withdrawing their claims for damages. But the game was up. The music had stopped. And almost none of them ever knew why.

Undoubtedly many had been "giving it a go"—joining a lawsuit they'd heard of through the media—just in case it might pay out. That was the history of the board's class actions over pharmaceuticals, as it had noted nearly twenty years before. Lawyers had dangled the prospects of up to £3 million in compensation per autistic child. Who wouldn't put their name down for that?

But even those who never blamed MMR before Wakefield were nevertheless mostly families supporting members with real issues and uncertain futures to consider. Some of Barr's young clients might have thrived on mere tolerance. But, at the unfunny end of the autistic spectrum were challenges for parents 24/7. And what would happen when those parents were gone? Many had waited for five, or more, years dreaming of help that now wouldn't come.

They'd been spared the hell of litigation stress: night terrors for those who might face legal bills. But they suffered a peculiar agony. The things that we dwell on become the shape of our minds, and many who'd been goaded to seek comfort blaming others had grown bitter and suspicious in their waiting. I'd find them, bewildered, fingering torn manila envelopes stuffed with press clippings, newsletters, and fact sheets.

The rest was just money. Lots of money. "We were always being told, throughout this, that there are these 'indications' from this, that, and the other piece of evidence," a lanky, donnish type named Colin Stutt, the legal board's head of funding policy, tells me. "'We need to do just a bit more, and then we'll be okay. And we'll be home on proving that causative link—if you'll just give us a bit more money.'"

That money mostly went into the pockets of a small group of lawyers, doctors, "experts," and their staff. On Barr's side, the final bill was £26.2 million (about £41 million or US $51 million at the time I write this). And Wakefield's allocation was £435,643 (about £677,000 or US $846,000 now), plus £3,910 in expenses. That was roughly eight times his annual medical school salary. He claimed, but was refused, much more.

Barr and Limb did well. They retreated to Norfolk and a barn-style thatched house, built in 1593, with seventeen acres of land. And after "spectacular results" with Limb's daughter, Bryony, Barr became a board member of the Society of Homeopaths, while his wife set up shop as a "CEASE" homeopath: a program targeting autism, devised by a Dutchman, offering practitioners certification in treating developmental issues after three to five days' training.

"I have some idea of what the anonymous sculptor of the Venus De Milo must have felt," Barr chuckled in a column for a lawyers' magazine, likening the lawsuit, on which he spent a decade, to an exercise in chiseling and polishing. "He had chipped away for years, slowly transforming a piece of the best available marble into a work of unimaginable beauty."

Lawyers tell me that the drug companies, between them, spent roughly the same as Barr's side on the action: offset against tax, investor value (mostly pension funds), and perhaps a little medical research. So, the gross cost of his Venus totaled about £52 million—convertible to approximately eighty million at the time I write, or one hundred million US dollars.

A fortune down the toilet? Campaigners thought not. Parents throughout the world had heard the message. In the United States, a deluge of new claims were pending, with lawyers now recruiting thousands of families as Lenny Schafer's newsletters and Dan Burton's committee hearings imported the alarm from Britain.

Again, the culprit: measles in MMR. Again: the Dublin lab. Again, a feeling tone of mistrust and resentment, as hearts, already broken, were poisoned.

And still, behind it all lurked that twelve-child paper, with its fourteen days from shot to symptoms, lymphoid hyperplasia, and nonspecific colitis—of which much remained to be revealed.

EXPOSED

- - - - - - - - - - - - - - - - - - - -

EIGHTEEN

Assignment

As with many a media project in the golden age of ink on paper, what became my investigation of that twelve-child study started with a three-course lunch.

My host was Paul Nuki, a pugnacious former reporter, who'd just been promoted editor of the *Sunday Times* "Focus" section, and was looking for big, space-filling stories. He was a lean-forward kind of guy: a surfer and rock climber, lean and wiry, with the demeanor of a pool player. He was the son of a doctor (a rheumatologist) and the father of one girl and three boys.

We dined on the terrace of a white-tablecloth restaurant, next to London's iconic Tower Bridge. To my right, Nuki's left, chugged Thames river barges and sightseeing cruisers, trailing sun-sparkling waves and squealing gulls. This was Tuesday, September 16, 2003: a classic, cloudless, English summer day.

Nuki, thirty-nine, first proposed an inquiry into Heinz tomato ketchup. He was convinced that its color and texture were too uniform to be consistent with a natural product. I wasn't so sure. I thought his premise was sketchy. In any event, he didn't really need me. I had a big-time award citation as probably the only British journalist who "polices the drugs companies," and to the best of my knowledge, H. J. Heinz didn't make medicinal claims for its sauce.

My favorite pharma investigations began in 1986: first exposing a biochemist who faked safety studies of a new generation of contraceptive pill. He was contracted to the Schering AG company of Berlin, and I tracked him from Deakin University, in Geelong, Australia, via a conference hotel in Chicago, Illinois, to a rented villa in Marbella, Spain, where he opened the front door, and practically fainted.

I remember his wife, a family doctor, goading me. "But what can you *prove*," she sneered. "What can you *prove*?"

Her husband drank himself to death after we published.

A good story. Page 1. And I fared even better with a man who was already dead. That was Henry Wellcome, the Wisconsin-born salesman, whose last will and testament, signed in February 1932, bequeathed a part drug company, part grant-giving charity with all manner of money-go-rounds. One skeleton in its closet, which I dragged into view, was a blockbuster combination antibiotic behind a tsunami of deaths and injuries. His empire was broken up after we ran five pages, spawning a richer, revamped Wellcome Trust: a giant biomedical research benefactor of vast international repute.

Wellcome's product was called Septrin, or Septra—identical to another, Bactrim, from the Swiss pharmaceutical behemoth Hoffmann-La Roche—which bolted two drugs together, one from each company, in rough proportion to their manufacturer's capital. But when I called a researcher involved in the recipe, he slammed down the phone. So I *knew*. After we published, I got hundreds of letters and emails, saw the government curtail the product's use in Britain, and acquired the memory of a mother describing the sound of life-support equipment when her eighteen-year-old daughter died.

Nuki liked that kind of stuff. It was a *Sunday Times* specialty: fusing public and human interest. Years before, the newspaper had branded itself with a campaign by the then editor, the legendary Harold Evans, over a notorious morning sickness drug, thalidomide. It was responsible for thousands of appalling birth defects, and he ran page after page for justice.

I guess I followed that tradition: from an eight-page magazine piece on the dark side of Viagra, to five on "an epidemic of medical fraud," which kicked off with a kidney specialist forging patients' signatures. But that kind of journalism was so, so expensive—with reporting not in hours, but over months, sometimes years—while my lunch friend wanted words within weeks.

As the waiter brought desserts, we kicked around ideas. I proposed the death of a government weapons expert. Then, eventually, we got to "MMR." In Britain, parents' confidence had now sunk to its lowest. Only 79.9 percent of kids were getting the shot. In parts of London, it was 58.8. Outbreaks of measles, with deaths, looked certain. So any new angle would get space.

I said, "Okay, Paul." But I wasn't busting for the gig. To be honest, I felt vaxxed out. First I'd done the investigation of DTP, inspired by the victory of the Irish mother. That took me almost a year. Then later came AidsVax, the no-hope AIDS vaccine, which produced an eight-pager in the *Sunday Times Magazine*, and dragged on long after that. I discovered that a staffer at the US Centers for Disease Control and Prevention who cheer-led for VaxGen and negotiated grants, had a secret deal to join its payroll.

I felt I'd done enough. And such work was life-crushing, to get on top of all the -ologies involved. Vaccines were a hugely multidisciplinary topic, and to go beyond the trivial platforming of experts—*he says this; she says that*—you'd be quicker becoming fluent in Russian. The temptation with medicine is like reading Shakespeare: you hope the tricky words will make sense from their context. But when I investigated DTP, I made a pact with myself: I wouldn't skip one "delation" or "Pale Hecate's off'rings." I was determined to know what they meant.

Medicine wasn't even my specialist beat. My first commitment was to social issues. My instincts were toward things like poverty, homelessness, prisons, disability: inequality in access to power. But when I reported on that stuff, my stories would appear between pages 3 and 9, whereas almost anything about doctors made the front. So after lunching with Nuki, instead of gleefully pouncing on the MMR controversy, I sent a few emails but otherwise did nothing, except spend the next few weeks writing a novel.

I wouldn't finish that novel for thirteen years. It seemed life had other ideas. Because, on a Sunday afternoon in late November, I was walking through London from Buckingham Palace to Trafalgar Square, when I came upon a little arts center that, for one day only, was previewing a TV show. It was described as a "docudrama," called *Hear the Silence*, in which Wakefield and a mother—both played by actors—battle a mustache-twirling medical establishment.

The on-screen mother was a fictional character. But it was based, I'd learn, on Ms. Two. And when the screening finished, she rose and gave a speech: a smartly presented woman, even more smartly mannered, with her Lancashire accent calling people to order in a confident, controlling style.

According to the drama, she was the first to contact Wakefield, dramatically rushing into the hospital. So, I phoned her the next day, and four days after that I traveled to her home: a small, yellow brick house on the edge of an unmemorable Cambridgeshire town (which I won't identify, so as to enhance her son's privacy) eighty-five miles north of London.

Ms. Two lived with her husband and two neurotypical children, twenty-two and twelve years old. Child Two, then fifteen, was away at a special school, but there were signs of his needs in a securely fenced yard, with a trampoline and unbreakable toys.

On the phone, I'd told her that my name was "Brian Lawrence," from the *Sunday Times*, to keep our chat free of inhibitions. I'd got clearance from Nuki and a *Times* lawyer to do this. It's common in investigative work. By now Google searches were up and away, and the last thing I wanted was for her to read my DTP story and get defensive when answering questions. "'Brian Lawrence' was actually Brian Deer," reported the *Washington Post*'s London bureau chief, Glenn Frankel, later, "a prize-winning investigative journalist."

By now, I'd read the twelve-child paper, and particularly noted its time link. The parents of eight kids were reported to blame MMR, with the first behavioral symptoms said to have followed the shot by no more than *fourteen days*. That was, I knew, the same time frame picked by John Wilson in the 1970s for his selection of suspected DTP victims.

It was also the time frame in a government report in my files, dated May 1981. In a bid to sort cases of brain illness after the whooping cough element of DTP, a chapter on "causality" segregated times of onset based on the Great Ormond Street neurologist's paper. When "spasms and behavioural disturbances" occurred "more than 14 days" after the shot, a link was considered to be "more unlikely than likely." But when the problems were reported within *two weeks*, it was deemed "more likely than unlikely" to be the cause.

Seated in Ms. Two's living room with my microcassette recorder, I ask, like I had with Ireland's Margaret Best, about the day of her son's vaccination. And although Child Two received it in November 1989—before any controversy in Britain over MMR—

his mother says she was so concerned about its possible side effects that she'd raised this with both the doctor and a nurse.

"I remember going out and actually spoke to the doctor," she says. "Because I was saying about this vaccine, saying I'm concerned about this vaccine."

Smart lady. She explains her prescience by remembering her father: a family doctor in Preston. One of her "jobs," she tells me, as I sip warm tea, was to "tidy up the drugs room," and one day, she says, she found unused cartons of thalidomide.

"I remember saying 'These boxes here haven't moved,'" she tells me. "'There's no stock control here. Why aren't you using these boxes, Dad?'"

She says he replied with words that lay behind her later caution over MMR. "And he sat me down, and said, 'That's actually something called *thalidomide*.' And he said, 'And I will not use it.' And I said, 'Why not?' And he said, 'Well, because it hasn't been tested properly.'"

With my tape gently turning, I ask what followed, on the day her son got his shot. "I suppose, you leave the surgery, you go shopping, or something?" I suggest. "What happened then?"

"No, I was at work, actually," she replies. "I was at work. So I didn't go shopping. I came back, and the nanny looked after him. *Uhhm* . . ."

On the transcript of this, I would note, "Pauses, sounds confused." Then she takes off on a riff about her position with a travel agent, which she'd earlier mentioned, in passing. "Sorry, I just, we just talked about the job that I was doing. I'm a bit tired this morning," she explains.

Tired or not, she talks and talks, continuing without interruption.

I was still working in the IT department, because, and I moved over, I actually moved over, so when he at that age, I'm just—it's not particularly crucial is it—but I was still in the IT department. I was doing this management facility, my own department job when I left, when I left, because actually I was, what happened . . .

And on she goes, some 370 muddled words: all about a travel company in London. It's pretty confusing, and I struggle to restore order, zeroing in on the first behavioral symptoms experienced by her son, who she'd confirmed was among Wakefield's dozen.

She says, "What happened was he started not sleeping at night. He'd scream all night, and he started head-banging, which he'd never done before."

"When did that begin, do you think?"

"That began after a couple of months, a few months afterward, but it was still, it was concerning me enough, I remember going back . . ."

"Sorry," I interrupt. "I don't want to be, like, massively pernickety, but was it a *few* months, or a *couple* of months?"

"It was more like a *few* months because he'd had this, kind of, you know, slide down. He wasn't right. He wasn't right, before he started."

"So, not quicker than *two* months. But not longer than how many months? What are we talking about here?"

"From memory, about six months, I think."

From time to time, she got up and made phone calls. One was to Richard Barr, and another to Jackie Fletcher of JABS. And when I got back to London, I spent a day or two trying to make sense of my recordings.

Ms. Two's father had died when she was aged eleven. So her memory of tidying up thalidomide in the drugs room seemed to me somewhat improbable. This might, I thought, be an error of recall, so many years after the events. Or, she might be grandstanding for a *Sunday Times* reporter. Or, her late father, James Lunn (secretary of the Preston medicoethics committee) should have been arraigned by the General Medical Council for allowing a child access to drugs.

She'd had remarkable foresight to question MMR's safety and was considerate of her nanny's schedule. But although she claimed she didn't know which child in the *Lancet* paper was hers, I noted the disparity between her *"about six months"* and Wakefield's *fourteen days*.

Of course, I didn't know then that, seven years before, she'd twice been logged as telling doctors at Hampstead that her son started head-banging *two weeks* following the shot. So days after the interview, I meet with John Walker-Smith and share with him my confusion.

"There is no case in the paper that is consistent with the case history [she] has given me," I tell him. "There just isn't one."

The Australian professor doesn't seem surprised. "Well, that could be true," he replies, matter-of-factly. Not only was he the last author of the twelve-child report, but he'd seen this boy many times. He says he didn't think that parents should talk about such things. It was a "confidential matter," he stresses.

"Well, so either what she is telling me is not accurate," I persist, "or the paper's not accurate."

"Well, I can't really comment," he says.

That was enough for me. There was something going on here. If the paper's senior author couldn't offer a better answer, I suspected the disparity was real. And if that child's case was wrong, what else might be wrong in that five-page, four-thousand-word paper?

I was kind of tempted to give it a spin. But how could I investigate a clinical case series? Here was medical information of the highest security: anonymized patients, child patients, developmentally challenged patients. The chances of discovering who their parents were, and when their kids showed the first signs of autism, were probably about as good as winning a lottery for which I'd not bought a ticket.

But then, even before I'd reported back to Nuki, my attention to this matter was sharpened. We got a complaint from Ms. Two that was so over-the-top that, in my opinion, its unstated, but transparent, objective was to get Mr. Lawrence taken off his story.

"I remain deeply shocked that such a journalist who, in my opinion is neither well informed nor particularly intelligent, should be let loose as a representative of a newspaper with the reputation of the Sunday Times," she wrote, in a three-page email headed "Serious Concerns re Sunday Times journalist," to the newspaper's editor, John Witherow. "The questioning began with a launch into the exact nature of what happened on the day my younger son had received his MMR vaccine down to questions about where I worked, what the surgery was like, what time of day it would have been."

And in case *that* didn't do it, her charges went further. I only vouch for the bit about my bladder.

> Surprised and shocked by the tone . . . stopped little short of interrogation . . . repeatedly displayed arrogance . . . did not appear to know . . . consistently revealed a dangerous bigotry and clear ignorance . . . exceptionally insulting . . . complete waste of my time . . . methods seemed more akin to the gutter press . . . his whole appearance was shoddy and shifty . . . kept turning the same tape over every time it ran out . . . he paid many trips to the toilet saying that only just drinking tea again was affecting his bladder yet prior to that he had said he was a regular tea drinker.

The next day, Nuki got a phone call from Wakefield's publicist, a man named Abel Hadden. And later, I got a warning from a lawyer called Clifford Miller (who would one day resurface representing Wakefield) hilariously trying to gag me. In a dense two-pager, littered with comedy legalese, he claimed that what he called the "gratuitous license" granted me to record the interview was "void ab initio," demanded that I "deliver up" my recordings within twenty-eight days, and told me that the use of "the words spoken" by Ms. Two would infringe his client's "copyright literary work."

Call me suspicious. But, after her letter, I figured she had something to hide.

- - - - - - - - - - - - - - - - - - - -

NINETEEN

Cracking the Coombe

With Richard Barr's lawsuit crashed and burned, I assumed I was alone in the wreckage. Other journalists who'd spent any time on Wakefield had mostly either offered themselves as his mouthpiece or platformed a crossfire of "experts." Nobody, it appeared, was out looking for a story: old-style newspaper reporting.

But, just five weeks after my visit with Ms. Two, came an investigation about which I knew nothing. At the Coombe Women's Hospital, on the south side of Dublin, a lawyer and two scientists, retained to advise the drug companies, arrived at the front desk for a showdown with John O'Leary and his miracle measles-finding machine.

"The Coombe," as locals called it, was in a rough part of town. With Holles Street to the east, and the Rotunda north of the Liffey, it was one of the Irish capital's three maternity units. Not renowned for molecular biology. Ringed by thin-walled terraced cottages and gang-friendly public housing, it wasn't really the kind of place you'd want to walk past at night, much less take your scientific riddles.

"This isn't the Great Ormond Street of Dublin, trust me," says a friend whose brother was born at the Coombe, and who knew the neighborhood well. "They've spruced it up a bit lately, so it's not as much of a shithole as it used to be. An awful place, it is."

It was, nevertheless, a place where fear of vaccines was reborn for the twenty-first century. Second only to the twelve-child *Lancet* paper, O'Leary's cherished machine ("a thousand times more sensitive") was as integral to the delivery of Barr's Venus De Milo as any midwife or obstetrician on the hospital's wards to the latest baby Patrick or Mary.

The visitors were led by Gillian Aderonke Dada. She was both a lawyer and a medical doctor. Aged forty, and praised as "confident" and "inspiring," she worked for a heavyweight firm of commercial solicitors—which had earlier been retained in the DTP trials—that day representing the three vaccine manufacturers: SmithKline Beecham, Aventis Pasteur, and Merck.

The class action was dead. But a string of hopeless appeals kept its sweating corpse technically breathing. So the companies exploited this ventilated state, with their eyes on the United States. Spurred by Dan Burton's congressional hearings, Lenny Schafer's republishing of British media reports, and Wakefield's appearance on CBS's *60 Minutes*, thousands of parents were being recruited, coast-to-coast, for a yet bigger lawsuit on the way.

This was where the story gets briefly complex, as I am obliged to pursue Wakefield, Barr, Kirsten Limb, and Ms. Two to the molecular level of evidence. When I learned of it later, it would prove the biggest challenge in mastering all those interminable -ologies behind which sheltered the real people and specific facts.

So while I plodded forward with my inquiries in London, waiting with Dada in the Coombe's reception area were two top biomedical detectives. One was Malcolm Guiver, head of molecular diagnostics at the British government's public health laboratories in Manchester. The other: Stephen Bustin, reader (later professor) in molecular science at London's Queen Mary school of medicine. Both were specialists in the polymerase chain reaction and had worked for years with the same equipment as O'Leary's, the ABI Prism 7700.

Compared with later devices for amplifying DNA, the 7700 was a heavy metal beast. Although only ninety-four centimeters (twenty-seven inches) wide, it weighed 130 kilograms (286 pounds) with an attached Apple desktop computer. Finished in the color of aircraft interiors, its front sloped to a bevel above a row of ventilator slats that ran nearly the length of the machine. Wrapping its right front corner was a plastic, lift-up window, behind which a boxlike, heatproof cover shielded its exquisitely delicate reactions.

The manufacturer's manuals were a walk in the park. I've owned washing machines with more baffling instructions. O'Leary's operatives lifted the window and raised the cover, exposing a "plate" of ninety-six tiny wells, which rested on a heating "block." Into these they popped "runs" of sealed plastic tubes containing bowel tissue, blood, or cerebrospinal fluid, each in a solution of chemical reagents. Around these in the runs were placed various control tubes for comparison: some negative, containing, for example, distilled water; some positive, spiked with measles.

Technicians set the computer. And off it all went: automated molecular amplification.

If any samples in the tubes contained what O'Leary hoped to find (single strands of measles virus RNA), the machine allowed these to be converted into DNA: first a single strand, complementary to the RNA, then the full and famous double helix. Rapidly heating the tubes made this come apart, like the ladder unzipping, after which an enzyme, called the "Taq polymerase," went to work with a miracle of life.

Taq rebuilt the ladder's rungs by creating fresh nucleotides of adenine, thymine, cytosine, or guanine—A, T, C, or G—to create partners for the separated strands. Then the machine cooled the tubes, and the ladders reformed: only now there were twice as many. Thus each single RNA strand became one, then two complementary DNA strands, which exponentially doubled, and doubled with each cycle, until billions of copies were present.

Each tube was laser-monitored, second by second, and with the 7700 counting the cycles, it graphed how much (if any) of the target was present at each cycle, so as to calculate how much was there in the first place.

Quick. Easy. Lab staff liked to think so. But therein lay traps for the unwary. Although Wakefield's Carmel business planned to advertise to investors that its 7700 would diagnose both Crohn's disease and "autistic enterocolitis," its manufacturer said such use was improper. The machine's operating manuals, technical guides, and brochures expressly warned, in bold, standalone statements:

For Research Use Only. Not for use in diagnostic procedures.

One reason for this was that, when working with such sensitive molecular technologies, if something could go wrong, it would. Despite a digital stream spewing data from the machine, which the Apple mashed together into real-time line graphs, you never stepped in the same river twice. Behind all the gadgetry lay biological phenomena: calling for art and integrity from researchers and technicians, working more like violinists than mechanics.

Hence Dr. Dada, and her two detectives. They'd come to collect the music. Unlike a violin, every performance was recorded, digitally archived, and disclosable to the lawsuit's defendants. O'Leary had supplied the court with "experimental reports," giving results on many samples from the Royal Free, well by well. But the Apple also logged a great deal more—some *four thousand data points* on each tube's progress—which the drug companies wanted. Very much.

Guiver, forty-six, with black hair and chiseled jaw, was a catch for more than his looks. With a PhD degree in molecular virology, his lab was among the first to get a 7700. And he'd filed a forty-nine-page analysis, based on reports from the lab, evaluating the Coombe's performance. He alleged "wholly inappropriate" and "entirely unreliable" methods, "lack of judgment," "inadequate controls," and complained of "spurious false positives" from the machine.

Big Pharma had paid for his professional opinions. But he wasn't alone in his critique. There was a second analysis from a Dutch adviser, Bertus Rima, professor of molecular biology at the Queen's University, Northern Ireland. He'd spent thirty years studying measles. And a third from a virology professor, Peter Simmonds, of Edinburgh, Scotland, who in the past decade had grabbed the cape as Britain's most cited microbiologist.

Rima and Simmonds took the same view.

Meaningless . . . suspicious . . . no validity . . . dubious practice . . .

Wholly unacceptable . . . results invalid . . . unreliable . . . contradictory . . . untenable

It would take me weeks to get my head round judgments like these. But one simple issue, very easy to grasp, concerned the machine's most basic operation. If you wanted, you could run it for as long as you liked. But if the lasers didn't quickly detect a signal from the tubes—essentially after no more than about thirty-five cycles—then you needed to accept that your target wasn't there, or tweak your preparations, and start over. Because by then the process would be running out of reagents—the juice—and the hiss from billions of random amplified molecules could, metaphorically, drown any tune.

Every source concurred. Even on YouTube. But, to be safe, I ask the manufacturer. Later owned by a multinational, Thermo Fisher Scientific, the 7700 became a legacy product of its Life Sciences Group, whose vice-president for research and development, Vinod Mirchandani, briefs me from San Francisco. "We've learnt that, if you go beyond thirty-five," he tells me, "and you're starting to see some small signal, most likely they're not the real thing."

He says that robust results are found sooner in the cycles: when the graphs on the Apple plot strongly rising lines, before these plateau as the process falters. In later cycles, he explains, on behalf of the machine's makers, you can "get a lot of noise" and "false positives."

But the Irish pathologist and his team saw things differently in their enthusiasm for measles virus. Reports from the Apple that they filed in the lawsuit revealed that samples taken at Hampstead—including from Child Two—were often tested in runs of up to *forty-five* cycles. And, in one case, *fifty* heatings and coolings. Rima even said that Barr's firm had told him that they planned to retest samples unblinded at Warwick with a, frankly ludicrous, *seventy*.

Meanwhile, Bustin came at O'Leary by another route, after experiencing a personal epiphany. Aged forty-nine, with a cheeky manner and a PhD in molecular genetics, he was England's Dr. PCR Geek. He wrote about it, taught it, probably dreamed in thermocycles. And within days of being hired to evaluate O'Leary's methods, Bustin found himself wondering . . . and wondering.

He'd been studying an Apple graphic of a 7700 plate generated from a disclosure in the lawsuit. Of the ninety-six wells, fifty-one were shown in use: labeled from A1 to E3. They'd been loaded in duplicate (two per child or type of control), which was common in this kind of work.

But he'd learned at school that fifty-one was an *odd* number. It looked to him like E4 had gone missing.

Right or wrong, he was keen to learn more. This anomaly might be a clue. What appeared to be absent was a "no template" control—meaning a tube of reagents, with Taq and other stuff, but *no biological sample*. No measles. If a tube in that well had tested *positive* for measles, it would suggest contamination: the scourge of PCR. And if that was the case, he speculated, but the well reported *empty*, then maybe someone had airbrushed the result.

For six months Dada had been pressing for this visit. But after her experts' analyses were disclosed to Barr's people, dealings with the Coombe became fraught. First O'Leary was in Australia and couldn't be contacted. Then none of fifty-nine dates from Dada were convenient. It would take £20,000 and up to five weeks to prepare for guests. The 7700 broke down.

But now here she was with her molecular detectives, being ushered toward the back of the building. O'Leary's lab was bright and modern, with plenty of kit—and anomalies screwed to the walls. Above doors to side rooms, the visitors spotted a pair of signs that set the scientists murmuring with the lawyer. One read "Plasmid Room," and the other "PCR Set-Up": the first generally meaning where positive control materials were prepared, the second where amplifications were run.

"The doors of these side rooms were single swing doors," Dada explained later in a statement, filed at the Royal Courts of Justice, in London. "I did not see any facilities for changing coats and/or shoes."

Happily, Barr was her best witness to this. He'd also flown to Dublin for the visit. And he'd brought a camera, which he offered the visitors. But O'Leary wouldn't allow any pictures. Nor, Dada said, would he release any data that hadn't already been disclosed to her clients.

It soon became clear that legal force would be needed. And the drug companies could afford to get it. Weeks later, after O'Leary refused to consent, a London judge issued a request to the Dublin courts to compel the pathologist to comply. This man who'd bragged in Washington of his "independent" achievements—on matters potentially critical to the safety of millions of children—had become uncommonly shy.

The visit that Monday was productive, however. Although the visitors spent most of it in a conference room, waiting, Dada, Guiver, Barr, and an O'Leary associate witnessed Bustin pull a rabbit from a hat. With them huddled around his laptop, the PCR geek displayed a report on a sample of blood from a *non-autistic* child included in the Warwick unblinding.

The report was *negative* for measles virus: good if you aimed to show that the vaccine caused autism. But Bustin also displayed the underlying raw data, from a small amount that O'Leary had disclosed. It was derived from the *same child—same well*; *same tube*—and was reported to be *positive*.

Oops.

"Richard Barr acknowledged that this was an important scientific issue," Dada drily recounted in her statement.

So here was another anomaly, spotted by the geek. And more would be alleged in court. "He is beginning to find a mismatch," counsel for SmithKline Beecham told the judge in London, weeks later. "These findings are raising very serious concerns."

Guiver, Bustin, Rima, and Simmonds all agreed that much was wrong. Along with excess cycling likely producing false positives— precisely the phenomenon the manufacturer warned me of— they thought the lab was awash with measles. "The overall impression is one of inadequate care, slipshod compliance with protocols, and a lack of basic understanding," Bustin argued.

Contamination, they believed, might have occurred at any stage. It might have arisen at Hampstead, even with Wakefield himself, who personally delivered samples to Dublin. It might be related to the plasmid room, and the drafty swing doors. Maybe the reagents, careless fingers, or pipettes. Rima recounted how, in his own laboratory, traces of mumps RNA (another paramyxovirus) had lingered on a bench for *nine years*.

A bigger shock, however, was proposed in court: that the experimental reports, submitted in Barr's lawsuit, didn't give the true results from the machine.

I can't say. But, if the visitors guessed right, the upshot was surely serious. O'Leary's claimed findings were pivotal to Barr's lawsuit. They were the peg for the BBC's *Panorama* program. They were the basis for the pathologist's endorsement of Wakefield in front of the congressional committee. They were the occasion for Schafer's "Wakefield Fest," importing the claims into the United States. And they'd convinced countless parents of children with developmental issues that a cause, MMR, had been found.

In reply, O'Leary was certain all was well: his lab hadn't failed in any way. Its findings backed claims by parents like Ms. Two. The Coombe was clean of stray measles. "Appropriate environmental and laboratory set-up controls" were maintained, he insisted, in a report. Results of testing had shown "clearly and unequivocally" that no contamination had occurred.

Better than that: he'd the means to prove these assertions—as he'd explained to the Washington lawmakers. What he'd called the "gold standard" was DNA sequencing: running out all the strings of As, Gs, Cs, and Ts after PCR amplification. This couldn't merely confirm whether the virus was present, but "outrule" false positives, detect contamination, and definitively fingerprint the measles viral strains: as found wild in nature, brewed for vaccines, or reared in labs for experiments.

Rima, the scientist, had read O'Leary's Washington speech. So Dada's team couldn't say they weren't warned. The pathologist even identified to Burton's committee his equipment: an ABI Prism 310 capillary sequencer (94 kg / 210 lbs.). It sifted nucleotides, one by one.

And this technology, with his 7700, wasn't only the kind of kit that caught serial killers from a smudge of spit or strand of hair.

It was what Wakefield had promised to the Legal Aid Board in the summer of 1996. "Strain-specific" sequencing was a key element of the research he was contracted to perform in his vaccine damage test, now more than seven years before.

But O'Leary never delivered. Sequencing wasn't done—as I later find in papers from the lawsuit. Just as Wakefield had refused to mount a definitive study, when the claims for Barr's test cases were filed in court the same phrases were deployed, again and again, with regard to the pathologist's gold standard.

For samples from a thirteen-year-old boy with autism:

It is denied that sequencing is necessary

For those from a second boy, aged fifteen:

Sequencing is unnecessary

And, of course, for those from Child Two, the sentinel case:

It is denied that sequencing is necessary

For these children, the claim was that the vaccine virus in MMR was the ultimate culprit for their autism. But doctors and scientists, supervised by lawyers, able and equipped to fingerprint the suspect—and so maybe save humanity from a repeat offender— had considered this, and chosen not to do it.

TWENTY

The Spoiler

The editor-in-chief of *The Lancet*, Richard Horton, stared at me like one of us had broken wind, and he feared the finger of suspicion. Seated to the side of a long, polished table, his face was stone, eyes narrowed, lips stretched, as I outlined the first findings of my inquiries. During eight years at the top of the world's number two general medical journal, his bravest gamble had been the doctor without patients. Yet, here was I, a newspaper reporter, showing him how dumb that was.

"Dapper" is a word I've seen used to describe Horton. "*Adjective: neat and spruce in dress and bearing; trim.*" In his case, "*Pleased with themselves.*" Still only forty-two at the date of our meeting—which came twelve weeks after my conversation with Ms. Two, and six weeks after Gillian Dada went to Dublin—he'd seized the journal's chair after two years in New York, seeing off more experienced contenders. I'd heard whispers that he was shrewd to the point of cunning. But he'd still much to learn, as we'd see.

Still unaware of the events at the Coombe, I stood at the table's head, in the *Lancet*'s conference room, with my right fist clutching a Magic Marker. Horton sat diagonally to my right, occasionally scribbling, while five of his senior staff, mostly to my left, leaned forward in their chairs, doing the same. At the far end lounged my witness—a member of Parliament named Evan Harris—who I hoped would protect me from any complaints to my editors, of which investigative reporters get a lot.

"And then there's this," I say, sketching a row of squares on a flipchart pad mounted on an easel behind me. "Here's the case series of twelve, extended to *thirty* kids seen at the Royal Free. So, here it's got the first twelve from the paper, and then it runs on with another eighteen. Okay? Now look at this."

In my investigation so far, I'd found a couple of "abstracts" that threw open a window on the pilot study. They were near-identical texts, about three hundred words each, that Wakefield had filed for gastroenterology conferences in the north of England and New Orleans, Louisiana. They were mere snippets of information about the Royal Free research but gave headline data on more of the patients admitted to Malcolm Ward for scoping.

I move along the squares, marking *eight* of the twelve from the paper's Table 2: those whose parents had apparently blamed the three-in-one shot for their child's "developmental regression."

Eight of twelve. So, two out of three.

"But, according to the abstracts," I continue, "out of the next *eighteen* cases, only the parents of *three* more children—only *one in six*—named MMR. So why would that be? Why would there be this cluster, right there at the start, and then it fades?"

By then, I knew the answer: the Legal Aid Board contract. What Wakefield couldn't have expected in 1996, was that a soon-incoming government would introduce a Freedom of Information Act. So I'd made an application, got a briefing from the board—by then renamed the Legal Services Commission—and eventually obtain the two-page document commissioning the "clinical and scientific study," stating the amount of money involved.

At the time I meet Horton, that deal was still secret. Even Wakefield's coauthors didn't know of it. And, although the Scottish professor, Anne Ferguson, nearly rumbled him at the Royal College of Surgeons meeting six years before, he'd even covered his tracks in the lawsuit. "This study received criticism from several quarters," he noted in his report to the court, citing among that criticism the complaint that the children studied were "a highly selected population."

Indeed, they were. But he'd an answer for that to make the kids seem like routine patients.

> This is a specious argument. Children with gastrointestinal symptoms present to paediatric gastroenterologists. Patients with inflammatory joint pain are referred to a rheumatologist, patients with optic neuritis (inflammation of the optic nerve) come under the care of neurologists. Patients are self-selecting by virtue of their symptoms and disease—this is the nature of medicine.

In fact, the cluster was of children brought by parents intent on complaining about the vaccine. So the paper, and the panic that Wakefield unleashed, had guaranteed public money for the lawsuit (and himself) while, contrary to the rules of biomedical publishing, obscuring the source of his subjects.

There was plenty more at *The Lancet*. The meeting lasted five hours, with plates of sandwiches brought in for lunch. The next big thing—in some ways the biggest—was the matter of who protected those children from exploitation as they were forced through the hospital, some kicking and screaming, for the battery of sedations, scopings, scans, spinal taps, blood draws, and barium drinks. The paper said the "investigations were approved" by the hospital's ethics committee. At the table, I tell Horton this is false.

I could see him struggling to suppress a reaction. Not only was he a licensed medical practitioner, but for years he'd virtue-signaled on just such matters. He was the inaugural past president of the World Association of Medical Editors, a coauthor of the *Uniform Requirements for Manuscripts Submitted to Biomedical*

Journals, and a founding member of the Committee on Publication Ethics. He was Dr. Squeaky Clean on propriety.

And he wasn't the only one—in that room or beyond—to be perplexed that day by my findings. This was Wednesday, February 18, 2004—four days before my story (what little I had at the time) was scheduled for page 1 treatment. As I spoke at the *Lancet*'s offices—two miles south of Hampstead—two miles south of those, at Wakefield's publicist's in Mayfair, three of my colleagues were interviewing the man.

By now he was living in Austin, Texas. And after refusing, through his publicist Abel Hadden, to speak to me, he'd flown to London on the condition that I shouldn't be present when he was questioned for the story. Rather, he saw a chance to work his charisma on journalists who lacked my grasp of the facts.

Our side, however, was led by the paper's third-in-command: an eerily calm executive, Robert "Whispering Bob" Tyrer, who'd spent years wrangling tricky situations. And with him was Paul Nuki, the "Focus" editor—who, I thought, raised the killer issue in a question that morning that captured the character of our subject.

"I'm saying to you," Nuki put it, "that the fact that you were an agent, being paid to work for Barr and his clients, was something that should have been disclosed."

"I don't agree," Wakefield replied.

"*You don't agree?*"

"I don't agree."

And there he was. Rules didn't apply to him. Not even rules to protect the integrity of potentially life-impacting medical research. The world, he believed, was however he said that it was, just because he said it was so. The kids were referred "solely on clinical need," he claimed. The investigations were approved by the hospital's ethics committee. *There were no conflicts of interest.*

"I acted with due propriety in every case," he told Tyrer and Nuki. "I have no regrets."

But the *Uniform Requirements* were clear on this point. Both third-party funding and expert witness work must be acknowledged as conflicts of interest:

> Financial relationships with industry (for example, through employment, consultancies, stock ownership, honoraria, expert testimony), either directly or through immediate family, are usually considered to be the most important conflicts of interest.

In the past, he'd scrupulously adhered to the principles. In his first *Lancet* study—photographing blood vessels—he stated that he was a Wellcome Research Fellow, and that a coauthor was "supported by a grant from the Crohn's in Childhood Research Appeal." In *J Med Virol*, he again cited Wellcome, plus two foundations. And in his question-marked study, he declared a coauthor as supported by two charities and Merck.

His MMR coauthors and associates were stunned when they learned of what we'd got. John Walker-Smith declared himself "astounded" to hear of the legal board contract. "There was no awareness of any legal involvement when we saw these children," he tells me, when I phone him at home (referring to the board under its new identity as a "services commission").

"You must have known that in August 1996, the Legal Services Commission entered into a contract," I put it to him.

"Absolutely not."

"For fifty-five thousand pounds."

"Absolutely not."

"And that the preliminary report was submitted to the Legal Services Commission in January 1999."

"Absolutely not."

The Irish pathologist, John O'Leary, professed himself similarly "shocked." Simon Murch, the endoscopist, reacted, "We are pretty angry." And another of the paper's authors, who asked not to be named, said he was "very, very" angry.

"I would never have put my name to the study if I had known there was this conflict of interest," he fumed. "And had I not done so, it would never have got published."

That Wednesday, the two meetings—me at *The Lancet*, and Tyrer and Nuki in Mayfair—went forward in parallel. Then it was my turn to be stunned. When I finished my presentation, I expected a response. Something like, "We need time to investigate." But Horton refused to comment and, moments later, told me that Wakefield had entered the building.

On the phone before the meeting, and again before it started, the chief editor had agreed that our discussion would be private. He even offered to sign an undertaking. "You don't need to worry," he told me. "We are all, you know, very experienced here in dealing with confidential material."

But what I didn't know, because I hadn't researched him, was that Horton had history with Wakefield. Before joining *The Lancet*, he'd spent two years at Hampstead, where they'd worked alongside each other. And, just eight months before I stepped into that conference room, the editor revealed himself smitten.

"He is a committed, engaging, and charismatic clinician and scientist," Horton simpered in a book. "I do not regret publishing the original Wakefield paper. Progress in medicine depends on the free expression of new ideas. In science, it was only this commitment to free expression that shook free the tight grip of religion on the way human beings understood their world."

Now it seemed that Horton wanted a tight grip himself: over a story that threatened his image. Within hours of the meeting, he put together a team of doctors to investigate and report on my discoveries. He picked Wakefield, Walker-Smith, Murch, and another coauthor, Mike Thompson, who scoped two or three of the kids.

Naturally these four wouldn't work unsupervised. That wouldn't do for *The Lancet*. There would also be a hepatologist named Humphrey Hodgson, who'd taken over from Arie Zuckerman as the Royal Free's vice-dean. Plus Abel Hadden, Wakefield's personal publicist, at whose offices Tyrer and Nuki had quizzed him.

"Is it customary," Horton would be asked later, when a panel of the UK's General Medical Council was convened to reinvestigate my first findings, "for an investigation of possible serious research misconduct to be carried out by the people who have been so accused of the misconduct?"

"It is customary for the institution to lead an investigation and to gather the data which will inevitably involve those who took part in the investigation," Horton replied. "It is then the responsibility of the institution to make sure that there is some kind of separation between its interpretation of those findings and those who are involved in the investigation who are being in some sense accused of a set of allegations, and once that interpretation by the institution has taken place and has been conveyed to whoever has brought the allegations to them then we can go forward. So there certainly should be some separation, which is why in the first instance I wanted to get the reaction from Dr Wakefield, Professor Walker-Smith, and Dr Murch, but after that my duty was to go to the head of the institution, the vice-dean, in this case Professor Hodgson."

They did a great job: exonerating each other on each and every matter they examined. But there was no "separation" and no "independent inquiry"—as the medical school later confirmed. The day after the meeting—Thursday—Horton moved to the hospital, where Walker-Smith, now retired, returned to work with Thompson, rooting through the children's records. They concluded that all was well, noting they found referral letters, so purportedly disproving my submission of Wednesday that families were marshaled for complaints.

Murch, meanwhile, dug into institutional review files and dismissed any ethical error. He was himself a member of the ethics committee, and even fished out a code number, 172/96, as proof that it authorized the research. "I can confirm that the patients presented in the *Lancet* study were investigated in accordance with the ethics committee approval," he ruled on behalf of Horton's team.

Wakefield wasn't allowed onto Royal Free premises. But from his family's house at Taylor Avenue, he supplied the children's names (which the hospital, medical school, and other authors didn't have) and drafted a claim that his work for the legal board was for an "entirely separate study." Whether parents made a link with MMR, he said, had "no bearing whatsoever" on their inclusion.

But a mass of documents told a different story. Starting with the children's records. None of the twelve lived in London (the nearest's home was sixty miles away), and files were thick with signs of orchestration, as local doctors rubber-stamped requests from parents (sourced to Jackie Fletcher, Richard Barr, and, in one case, Ms. Two), with Wakefield phoning to ensure cooperation.

Four children were sent to Walker-Smith's bowel clinic with referral letters not even mentioning bowel symptoms. The Australian proactively solicited two kids. Two more were referred to Wakefield, a laboratory researcher. One boy's notes contained a legal aid letter. And there were plenty of giveaway phrases.

This 7¾ year autistic child's parents have been in contact with Dr. Wakefield and have asked me to refer him

[This little girl's] mother has been to see me and said you need a referral letter from me in order to accept [her] into your investigation programme

Thank you for asking to see this young boy

Simply reading the records would have captured those clues. But Walker-Smith declared nothing amiss. Meanwhile, the claimed approval from the ethics committee concerned a different vaccine, a different number of children, and a different developmental diagnosis. Murch would eventually admit (three years later) that his statement for Horton was untrue. And Wakefield, of course, had privately told managers (when Barr's check came through) that the study was "sponsored" by the board.

But Horton's investigators confirmed their innocence. So *The Lancet* rejected nearly all of my findings. It did so, moreover, in a sneaky maneuver to try to pull the sting of my story. In those days, the standard PR advice for slipping out bad news was to release it as a "spoiler," on a Friday afternoon, inconvenient for newspapers' schedules. And (while ignoring emails and phone calls from me) that's what Dr. Squeaky Clean did.

Vice-dean Hodgson knew of this ruse to frustrate me and forewarned his colleagues in an email. "No doubt one—but I believe only one—motive," he wrote, "is to safeguard the *Lancet*'s reputation by getting the riposte in first, and 'spoiling' the story."

But if that was the aim, it proved a disaster. Horton's maneuvers sparked a media firestorm. Given his coauthorship of the *Uniform Requirements*, one thing he *couldn't* deny was Wakefield's conflict of interest. We even had the figure for the legal board money—not much compared with his personal fees, I'd later learn—for his "clinical and scientific study." The very word "clinical" was enough to nail it down: from both Latin and Greek for *at the bedside*.

"This funding source should, we judge, have been disclosed to the editors of the journal," Horton admitted that Friday afternoon in a three-page public statement. "We believe that our conflict of interest guidelines at the time should have triggered such a disclosure."

He refused to tell journalists where he'd gotten the information. But that only made the press more curious. Within minutes of him releasing a sheaf of denials that anything else was amiss with the research, Britain's news industry pounced. A half hour later, the BBC snapped a report. The member of Parliament, Evan Harris, appeared on screens. And every editor in the business could now predict the front page of the country's market-leading Sunday paper.

Horton battled for control. But given the nation's plummeting vaccination levels, even the fifty-five grand was incendiary information: revealing that the study was carried out to an agenda and wasn't independent research. "If we had known the conflict of interest Dr. Wakefield had in this work, I think that would have strongly affected the peer reviewers about the credibility," the editor admitted under questioning that evening. "In my judgment it would have been rejected."

Next morning, our rivals were running my story, albeit gutted to a fragment by Horton.

MMR Doctor in £55,000 Fund Row

'Tainted Research' of Doc Behind MMR Alert

Scientist's Two Roles in Study May Conflict

Damn, I thought. I've lost my scoop. But I was as wrong about that as was Horton. Tyrer and Nuki had seen such things before and knew how to handle a spoiler.

"Full details are disclosed today," Tyrer hammered onto his keyboard that Saturday morning, "of the four-month *Sunday Times* investigation that has uncovered a medical scandal at the heart of the worldwide scare."

With Sunday's *Independent* splashing with "'Misconduct' inquiry for doctor in MMR scare," and the *Observer* and *Telegraph* likewise going big, we hit the streets with a simple message.

Revealed: MMR research scandal

Plus a two-page "Focus" in narrative prose.

MMR: THE TRUTH BEHIND THE CRISIS

We'd only got the guy for the fifty-five grand, the deal with Barr, and the fact that children were recruited to make a case. Not the huge sums of money that I didn't yet know of, or the secret business schemes, the patents, the measles vaccine, the Dublin lab—and things yet to come that would finish Wakefield in medicine for good. But that February weekend, Britain shared a Guinness Moment: *Wakefield—lawyers—ahh!*

Right through the next week, the fire blazed on. The *Daily Mail* hit back, claiming their hero had been "smeared." The prime minister backed us on breakfast TV. Wakefield threatened to sue.

Then ten of his twelve coauthors—including Walker-Smith and Murch—stepped in with a statement, issued by the journal on the evening of Monday, May 3. Sensationally, they repudiated the paper's conclusions, retracting its twenty-five-word "Interpretation" section: where they'd claimed that the children's "developmental regression" was "associated in time" with the vaccine.

Doctors disown Wakefield Study

Research scientists retract link with autism

Docs dramatic U-turn

Which is where I'd have been happy to leave the story and write not another word about vaccines. Later, we'd learn that, in those frantic days, immunization rates in Britain reversed and began to climb.

We'd gotten a result. *Job done.*

But, if the "Interpretation" was wrong, I wondered, how could that happen? And it threw me back onto the logic of Ireland's judges in the case of *Best v. Wellcome*. The paper was so meticulous, and so defended by Wakefield, that if the conclusions weren't accurate (as also suggested by my interview with Ms. Two) then surely one, or more, of the authors must have known this at the time the paper was written?

- - - - - - - - - - - - - - - - - -

TWENTY-ONE

Texas

Anybody else might have said, "I'm sorry." They might have apologized for not making the position *more clear* about the deal with the lawyer and the source of the children. They might have said they misunderstood *The Lancet*'s rules for authors. Or blame the media for confusion. *Whatever.* They'd regret any mistakes, but profess good faith. And my attention might then have moved on.

But that wasn't Wakefield. He was untroubled by regret. He raged like an indignant shoplifter. Still concealing the turkey under his coat—the enormous hourly payments he received through Richard Barr—he stormed that there was "no conflict of interest at any time"; that the fifty-five grand went to the hospital for a "quite separate study"; that my "allegations" were "grossly defamatory"; and that I "conflated" them to help his enemies.

"My family and I have suffered many setbacks as a direct consequence of this work," he lamented, casting himself as the aggrieved.

By now he was settled in Austin, Texas, ready to start all over. People didn't know why the English lawsuit collapsed or that he'd refused to mount a definitive study to validate, or refute, his hypothesis. So instead of being greeted with anger or suspicion, thanks to Dan Burton, Lenny Schafer, and others, he was welcomed by those whose help he would need as if Lady Liberty herself ought to kneel.

"It takes a man of great courage and integrity to stand up against overwhelming pressure from his scientific colleagues and refuse to say what is false when he knows what is true," was the view, for example, of Barbara Fisher, founder of the confusingly named National Vaccine Information Center, based a half hour's drive from Washington, DC.

Fisher was the Jackie Fletcher of US activists: the anti-vaccinators' woman in scarlet. With the startled demeanor of a Tupperware host, she'd embarked on her mission in 1982 after NBC broadcast a rehash of the DTP claims from the Great Ormond Street neurologist, John Wilson. These were screened in a feature called *Vaccine Roulette* (which relied on research later gutted by Lord Justice Stuart-Smith), and she deduced that her son, Chris, was vaccine damaged.

Wakefield's arrival stateside thrilled Fisher's group. But he was grabbed by a yet fresher sponsor. This was a tough-dealing lawyer named Elizabeth Birt, who was to become the brains behind a string of anti-vaccine groups (Advocates for Children's Health Affected by Mercury Poisoning, the National Autism Association, SafeMinds) and would mastermind his crusade's migration.

He'd caught her attention with the twelve-child paper, which she read soon after publication. Her backstory was that some time following her first son Matthew's MMR, she'd noticed in him symptoms of autism. According to a New York journalist, David Kirby, she studied *The Lancet*, thinking, "My God, this sounds like Matt," and the next day went to war on her pediatrician.

A year later, she met Wakefield at a conference near Chicago, run by a group called Cure Autism Now. She was then forty-three (four weeks his senior), with pencil-sharp features and golden hair. And she lived with Matthew, age five, his two younger siblings, and a husband, Maurice, in one of the Windy City's rich northern suburbs.

I've seen Wakefield perform at events like that one. In those days, he fronted as a scientist and clinician, as young mothers raced to take down his words. But this time he went further than a technical talk (*lymphoid hyperplasia . . . non-specific colitis . . .*) and invited Birt and Matthew to his hotel room, where he examined the boy, felt the kid's abdomen, and told her: "I think we could help him."

Three months later, Matthew was at Hampstead, being trolleyed from Malcolm Ward for scoping. "I took my son to London," Birt recalled in an online post, "and found out at the Royal Free Hospital that he was and is very sick. He had a fecal impaction the size of a melon and had colitis."

According to Kirby (who worked with Birt on a book), on the evening of the day after Matthew was scoped, Wakefield joined her for dinner. And judging by Illinois state records that I find, she flew home to Chicago convinced. Just three weeks later, she incorporated a foundation—Medical Interventions for Autism, she called it—which would raise for his projects, as well as him personally, many hundreds of thousands of dollars.

Birt also fixed his US resident's visa and toiled to plot his future. Plan A was to join an enterprise in central Florida: the International Child Development Resource Center, founded by a physician and autistic boy's father named James Jeffrey Bradstreet.

"The British doctor forced out of his job because of his studies on the childhood MMR jab and autism," crowed Lorraine Fraser in the *Telegraph*, back in London, "has been appointed the head of a multi-million dollar research programme in America."

As "research director" at Bradstreet's operation, Wakefield was meant to head a "research campus," leading a team of molecular pathologists, immunologists, and biochemists, in a renewed effort to prove his hypothesis.

It sounded great. A fresh start in the sun, where he was careful to protect his interests. "All intellectual property owned personally by AJW," he cautioned Bradstreet in a memo I obtain, "will remain property of AJW and subject to his control."

But, like so many of his dreams and schemes over the years since that now-distant night in the Toronto bar, his latest cried out for scrutiny. So, within weeks of his denials of what I knew to be true, I made a few further inquiries. After rooting among records at the London Patent Office, searching for Nick Chadwick (who was named on virology papers) and retrieving Hugh Fudenberg's Spartanburg study, I trawl the web for the Florida center.

> Welcome to a place where you and your family can find answers and hope for your child. . . . A place where the most advanced research in developmental disorders is a daily event.

By now, I'd more resources to support my reporting through a contract for a TV film. So after interviewing Fudenberg in South Carolina, I drive south with my producer and crew to Florida, where we find Bradstreet's international center. It was a humdrum doctors' office in a suburban shopping mall, in the sleepy town of Melbourne on the state's east coast, with a reception crammed with racks of quack remedies.

There were pricey pots of products to "enhance cognitive abilities," such as "*Learner's Edge®*," "*ChildEssence®*," and "*ImmunoKids®*,"—all formulated by Bradstreet (who later shot himself dead, after a raid by federal agents). There was secretin, "a natural body hormone" (usually from pigs), and "*Sea Buddies© Concentrate!© Focus Formula*" to provision travelers on the desperate quest.

Bradstreet's website, meanwhile, splashed promotions for events—some touting Ms. Two as one of the "world's leading specialists"—charging hundreds of dollars to attend.

Be among the first to hear about this comprehensive integrated new treatment program from Drs. Bradstreet, Kartzinel & Wakefield.

At the Melbourne office, I ask to speak with the latter. But, if he'd ever been there, he was gone. And while personal embarrassment wasn't part of his repertoire, he seemed anxious to put this chapter behind him. His lawyers write to me that his connection was purely "honorary," and from which, they say, he "never derived income."

Florida flopped. But Birt wasn't discouraged—even when her husband filed for divorce. According to Kirby, he accused his wife of "harboring more love and affection for Andy Wakefield." And, according to a source who emailed me later, she "basically turned her life over to him." Apparently, one day he phoned her in her car, said that measles virus had been found in her son's spinal fluid, and she was never the same again.

"She began a long spiral down after that," my source tells me, "into some terrible things and some really dark places."

Texas followed. The show moved on to a business in Austin, the state capital. Plying his famed charisma and a new identity as a martyr, Wakefield inspired other parents to help Birt fund a clinic and a proposed "hub" for a "virtual university." Leasing a basement suite in a three-story brick office building, he was thus installed as executive director of the Thoughtful House Center for Children.

The name was borrowed from a tiny stone cottage on the property of his latest benefactor: a woman named Troylyn Ball. She was a real estate agent, wealthy, owning horses, and who, like Birt, would do anything for answers.

"It just seemed like, 'You know what? Here's a smart doctor who *knows*, who's got a *vision*,'" Ball said, years later on YouTube. "I couldn't solve the problem, but I could pull together a bunch of people who could try to solve the problem."

For Troylyn and her husband, Charlie Ball (also a realtor), that "problem" touched two of their sons. Marshall, seventeen, and Colton, two years younger, were affected by profound developmental issues, which first manifested as seizure disorders. The original Thoughtful House was Marshall's retreat on his parents' seven-acre ranch.

Both boys had strengths. But Marshall was a celebrity, having three times been featured on the talk show *Oprah* as an author and spiritual guide. Although he never spoke, and was severely challenged, it was said he relayed messages from God. With his right elbow cupped by a relative or family friend, it was reported that he channeled divinely inspired poetry by erratically stabbing letters on a board.

> Even though my individuality finds sweet
> Knowing perfection I listen for the
> Answers to wishes from above. I listen to
> Good thoughts like something cloudy over
> mountain tops . . .

His mother was proud of his communication skills. "If you held up two objects and asked 'where's the cup?'" she'd say, "he would lean forward and touch it with his forehead."

According to a writer for the *Dallas Observer*, Brad Tyer, Troylyn (who was three years younger than Wakefield) was "an attractive blonde with an open smile and the look and bearing of a woman long familiar with horses."

She also struggled with misplaced guilt. "There's a lot of this looking at yourself and saying, 'What did I do wrong?'" she'd say. "'What did I do wrong that caused my child to be born this way?' Or, 'What did I do wrong to deserve this; did I do something wrong?' You know? And it's very, very hard, especially as the mother. I think it's worse for the mother."

In time, Thoughtful House would boast a dozen staff—with two or three MDs leading a schedule of sessions, a therapist, nutritionist, researchers, and administrators. A fine product of a mother's determination. Although Wakefield wasn't licensed to practice medicine, his employment package—mostly funded through Birt—would top out at nearly twice that of a typical family doctor's. And he was also doing a land deal in London.

A board of directors brought advice and credibility to the business. From its first calendar year—2004—this included the chief executive of Dell Financial Services, a Venezuelan-born movie producer, a retired major general, a former Major League Baseball player, and a country singer with the Dixie Chicks band.

Such endorsements were priceless. But a "managing co-director" was next with what Wakefield most needed. This was a Manhattan socialite, Jane Johnson, thirty-eight: supermodel slim, exquisitely styled, whose family forbears once controlled Johnson & Johnson, the pharmaceuticals and healthcare colossus. Accounts kept by Birt showed that, in year one alone, Jane's personal foundation gave a whopping million dollars toward the efforts of the doctor without patients.

Johnson had a son with developmental issues, whose privacy she fiercely guarded. Pretty much all I know of him was from a Thoughtful House chat room, where she mentioned a gluten- and casein-free diet, nasal secretin, and an apparently failed therapy involving at least eighty "dives" in a pressurized oxygen tank.

Her road to Wakefield began three years earlier, when her journey of discovery led her to a conference run by an organization called the Autism Research Institute, based in San Diego, California.

The institute was founded in 1967 by a then thirty-nine-year-old psychologist named Bernard Rimland. Like Bradstreet, he had a son with autism. Challenging psychiatrists, Rimland made his mark early, helping to bury a theory of autism (almost as strange as the stoned rodent model) sometimes dubbed the "refrigerator mother." This held that the classic constellation of symptoms—in thinking, communication, and social interaction—was a legacy of cold, aloof parenting.

But by the time Johnson found him, Rimland—seventy-two—had long since left the reservation. With an impressive salt 'n' pepper beard and wise-man eyes, he presided over a network of some four hundred fringe practitioners (marketed to parents as "Defeat Autism Now!") whom, as a condition of him listing them on his institute's website, he required to sign up to a creed. This embraced a catalog of unproven speculations, including that vaccines caused autism.

To be fair, his efforts spoke to a reality for parents—as one mother captured it in a Thoughtful House chat room, with a snapshot of autism in her family:

> Constipation, severe self injurious behavior (biting himself, chewing fingernails/toenails, biting a hole out of chair and ultimately pulling out a tooth—only five years old), not sleeping well, not eating well, tantrums constantly, can't wear shoes now due to tight heel cords from toe-walking, doing SCD—no yogurt, running out of ideas. What in the world is going on with my baby?
>
> PS 1 husband paralyzed (quad due to surgery for a spinal tumor), 2 other kids to care for, 1 dog, 1 cat, 2 frogs, 2 fish, bills, clean house etc . . . How are you all doing it?

Up against all that, what mother or father wouldn't share Rimland's impatience? If not quick progress, then at least *something*. With autism as elusive to medical science as dark matter remained to gravitational physics, when the psychologist ran surveys, it seemed that, for some kids, anything, *anything*, worked. Vitamin A: he reported that parents told him 41 percent "got better." Beta blockers: 33 percent, "better." Transfer factor: 39 percent, "better." Giving up chocolate: 49 percent, "better."

His list went on, column after column.

Rimland learned of Wakefield in November 1996, more than a year before the twelve-child paper. On the twenty-ninth of that month (when only five of the dozen kids had so far been scoped), Rimland's fax machine in San Diego spat out a thirty-six-page "fact sheet" from a lawyer. It was from Richard Barr, with Kirsten Limb, explaining, "We are also working with Dr Andrew Wakefield."

In the next edition of the institute's newsletter—the *Autism Research Review International*—Rimland trumpeted "alarming" news on page 1:

Autism-vaccination link in the UK?

Still scrabbling for answers, Rimland never looked back. By the time Thoughtful House was shopping for furniture, he published a list of what he said was evidence that MMR caused autism. It comprised one review article, three reports by an ex-collaborator of the crazy professor, Hugh Fudenberg, and twelve authored by Wakefield.

To Johnson—who returned every year to Rimland's conferences—the project in Austin offered hope. But some parents, online or writing to me, voiced concerns over the center's priorities.

I heard of instances of kids being scoped (at a neighboring hospital) when their mothers said they'd no bowel symptoms. Others complained of what felt to them like pressure to agree to the procedure. One told me she wanted to enroll her son in an "equestrian program" advertised by Thoughtful House—but was informed that it was in a "package" with colonoscopy.

"The first thing I was struck with, other than the expense, was that they said they may determine that my son may need a scope," wrote another mother. "And if so, they required you to use their facilities, and most insurances do not cover it . . . my son has never had any bowel problems."

By now, Wakefield knew that I was back on his trail: not least because I'd written to say so. My TV contract was with the UK's Channel 4 network: a national broadcaster, with legal mandates for accuracy and fairness. By now, I had the patents, the business scheme documents, and a boxful of Bradstreet's remedies. I'd got Chadwick, Fudenberg, and the agony of a mother who blamed herself for letting her son have MMR. I'd got complaints alleging horrors involving children on Malcolm Ward. All I needed now was the man.

I trawled his schedule. Texas would be best. But it seemed there was nothing on the horizon. His next listed engagement was at the Indiana Convention Center in Indianapolis, where on Friday, October 22, 2004, he was to speak at a conference run by the Autism Society of America. So, when he descended from the podium to mingle with mothers, I walked right up and extended my hand for our prime-time 9:00 p.m. slot.

Anybody else might have responded, "Go away." But that wasn't the real Andrew Wakefield. He stepped sideways, struck our camera, slapping his paw over the lens, and took off, with me in pursuit. The chase went on . . . and on . . . and on. The conference center was vast. It was perfect. With him dressed in a cream jacket, one-strapping a black rucksack, he strode—escorted by a heavyset man—past mothers, past Rimland, and only eventually to safety, through a lockable glass door. Where I stopped.

"Parents have very serious questions to ask you," I called, as we'd careened down corridors, our cameraman dancing. "If you're confident about your work, sir, and the quality of the research, sir, and that your commercial ambitions will withstand public scrutiny, you will stand your ground, and answer these questions."

- - - - - - - - - - - - - - - - - - - -

TWENTY-TWO

Nothing As It Seems

It was a scorching summer morning in Washington, DC, when Wakefield announced his vindication. He'd won an apology: that what I'd said was false; that I'd been wrong in every respect. There were no conflicts of interest. He wasn't paid by a lawyer. Just like he said, all along. His twelve-child study was ethically approved, and the patients appropriately referred.

"We have been informed that defamation proceedings have been commenced," he read aloud from a 166-word statement of retraction he'd received, in which all of my findings were disavowed. "We apologize to Dr. Wakefield for any distress caused and, at his request, have paid an appropriate sum to selected charities."

This was Wednesday, July 20, 2005, on the grass of the National Mall. He leaned on a wooden lectern, which was festooned with microphones, wearing a pale blue shirt, sleeves rolled to his elbows, patterned tie, and khaki pants. He was ringed by a crowd—mostly the mothers—who clapped and whooped to hear he was cleared.

Dan Burton was there, plus three more from Congress: come to protest about the preservative thimerosal. By then it had been almost eliminated in the United States. Thoughtful House was planning research.

"Protect Our Children," shouted placards. "Autism = Mercury Poisoning."

But, as Lenny Schafer's newsletter would report to thousands, the joy for the campaigners, gathered in front of the Capitol, was:

British publication retracts slurs on Dr Andrew Wakefield

The achievement was masterful. Wakefield beamed—in front of those he now looked to for a living. Boosting his image as a man grievously wronged, he'd issued three libel claims over my investigation: against the *Sunday Times*, and me; against Channel 4, and me; and against briandeer.com, and me.

"Dr Wakefield's clinical report," his lawyers insisted in a nine-page demand for "substantial" compensation, "was sound and reliable in describing the history and clinical findings in a cohort of 12 children referred consecutively with regressive autism and bowel symptoms."

He stood more chance of that Nobel Prize. The apology wasn't from us. What he'd done was to threaten the *Cambridge Evening News*: a fragile local newspaper in eastern England, which had mentioned my stories in two sentences. Its circulation was five thousand (against the *Sunday Times*'s 1.2 million), and even the editorial time to process his complaint would have jeopardized its hand-to-mouth rhythms. So it groveled, retracting, within twenty-four hours, what it hadn't even printed in the first place.

"I was astounded when I was sent a copy of your publication," wrote Alastair Brett, legal manager of Times Newspapers, to the little evening paper on the same day as Wakefield's announcement in Washington, "which does nothing other than apparently apologise for material which has appeared in The Sunday Times."

The truth was that Wakefield *did* allege we'd defamed him. But, after that, he attempted a maneuver. My first reports had triggered a call from the British government's health secretary for an inquiry by the General Medical Council: the regulator for all British doctors. Shrewdly, Wakefield said he would "welcome" and "insist on" one. And after the GMC's officials took him at his word and launched an investigation into my first findings, he demanded that his lawsuits be frozen. He thought he could tell his supporters he was suing, but not actually carry it through.

So *we* took *him* to court—Channel 4 and me—to force him to put up, or shut up. If he was saying he was suing us, hell, he should *sue*. I wasn't going to have his allegations hang over me. So not only did we apologize for nothing whatsoever, but just seven days after his Washington triumph, we won our first ruling. He was *ordered* to file his suit.

Three months later, he was ordered again: to proceed, with due haste, to trial. "It thus appears," ruled Mr. Justice Eady, sitting in Court 13 of London's Royal Courts of Justice, "that the claimant wishes to use the existence of the libel proceedings for public relations purposes, and to deter other critics, while at the same time isolating himself from the downside of such litigation, in having to answer a substantial defense of justification."

His costs were being paid by the Medical Protection Society, essentially an insurance company. I, too, was covered, by a Channel 4 arrangement, but I was stuck with the upshot for nearly eighteen months, demanding almost full-time attention. There were countless briefings to draft for our legal team; hundreds of documents to be indexed and exchanged. There were meetings with counsel and hearings before the judge. And (although Wakefield later said that he'd never read my website) there were threatening letters to me from his lawyers—some delivered to my home by men in leather and crash helmets—warning me of ruinous costs.

My journalism shrank to two decent stories. One was a probe of Vioxx, Merck's killer of a painkiller, which took me about six or seven weeks. I remember five days in a public records office, running a ruler down columns of printed death listings, looking for a male in his seventies whose name was anonymized in an adverse event report with his initials, "KW."

And I found him.

Page 1 splash:

Vioxx death toll may hit 2,000 in UK

Inside, page 5, a "Special Investigation":

Victims of drug that took a hidden toll

My other success was a film for Channel 4: an investigation called "The Drug Trial That Went Wrong." It probed an experiment in which a monoclonal antibody, code-named TGN1412, caused near-death injuries to volunteers. The climax saw me chase the boss of the company responsible through the sumptuous hallways of the Four Seasons Hotel, Boston, much like my pursuit of Wakefield in Indianapolis.

I knew that his lawsuits would never be tested. Privately, that bugged me a lot. The last such crusader to appear in a London libel trial was a lying historian named David Irving, who sued New York author Deborah Lipstadt and Penguin Books for suggesting he was an apologist for Hitler. Not only did he lose, but her battle became a movie after the judge branded Irving a "Holocaust denier."

But one Tuesday afternoon in May 2006, I discovered I wasn't wasting my time. I was at Channel 4's lawyers, Wiggin LLP (all carpet, smoked glass, and "would you like coffee?") in the heart of London's West End. I was sipping a paper cup of redbush tea, when our formidable solicitor, Amali De Silva, dumped in front of me a stack of Xeroxed reports, disclosed to us by Wakefield's lawyers.

I counted nearly forty. Each documented a child who'd passed through Malcolm Ward. Each was about seventeen pages, crammed with diagnoses, histories, endoscopy findings, histopathology, and tables of blood tests. Frustratingly, their fronts were redacted in black ink, obliterating the patient's name and date of birth, which would make them effectively useless to me, since I couldn't match any against the twelve.

But as I flicked through the first, I nearly spat my tea when I spotted a name inside. After correlating court lists, news stories, and other sources, I'd learned the identity of all twelve *Lancet* kids, and in my hands was a report on a five-year-old boy who was anonymized in the paper as Child Six. Someone forgot to redact a pathology report. The rest in the stack were the same.

If an ATM machine had unloaded into my shopping bag, I couldn't have felt more grateful for a glitch. Although some were missing—including Child Two's and Child Four's—here were collections of the data behind the project that launched the vaccine alarm on the world. To the best of my knowledge (and I'm willing to be corrected), no journalist had ever obtained such a window of insight into anonymized biomedical research.

This was quite some payback for his Washington stunt, and just when he was getting a little comfortable. For himself and his family—Carmel and now four kids (aged seventeen, fifteen, eleven, and nine)—that month he'd purchased a house to suit his style, with views of the Texas hill country. There were no Roman gates or servants' quarters. But in five acres of woodland on Austin's west side, he'd gotten a Spanish-style foyer and marble floors, four living rooms, six bedrooms, and six full bathrooms. He'd a games room, gym, swimming pool, and hot tub.

Autism + vaccines = money.

Child Six wasn't the "sentinel" or "most compelling" case. But his mother was a person of interest. Like Ms. Two, she phoned Wakefield in the aftermath of *Newsnight*. She was a "founder" and "spokeswoman" of Jackie Fletcher's JABS group. And only four and a half months before the "apology" on the National Mall, she was a speaker with Ms. Two at a Thoughtful House event. The two mothers were in it together.

The report in front of me was an output from a database (maintained by a Royal Free research nurse) for Wakefield's pilot study. It was mostly Q&A requests for information to be inserted, with answers in labeled boxes. I thumbed to page 3 of Child Six's report, topped with the title "Summary."

Beneath the title was a single line, asking if the child's "initial development" was "normal." To claim vaccine damage, this feature was important. And I knew the *Lancet* paper was clear. In its "Methods" and "Interpretation" sections, it stressed that the twelve were "previously normal" children, with a "history of normal development."

But Child Six's report got off to a rocky start. "*Initial development—normal?*" it asked, and answered itself bluntly:

No

Promising, I thought. But this didn't detain me, because three inches below that, a six-inch-wide box went to the heart of Wakefield's behavior. It was labeled, in boldface, "Initial diagnosis" and was answered:

Aspergers Syndrome

Down the page was another box, "Current diagnosis":

Aspergers Syndrome (most likely)

I didn't need to check. That twelve-child paper reported *no* case of Asperger's syndrome. According to Table 2, column 2—"Behavioural diagnosis"—eight of the kids were diagnosed with "Autism," one with "Autism? Disintegrative Disorder?," one with "Autistic spectrum disorder," and two with "encephalitis?"

Asperger's had surfaced in the late twentieth century and would lose favor (at least officially, among pediatric professionals) in the early twenty-first. In the 1970s, the World Health Organization had pigeonholed autism among the "childhood psychoses." Then, in 1992, new thinking emerged, unveiling the "pervasive developmental disorders." Childhood autism was one, and Asperger's another: codes F84.0 and F84.5. "Disintegrative disorder" (in older kids) was F84.3, and when there was uncertainty (as often there was), the phrase "autistic spectrum disorder" became popular.

Notwithstanding lay talk, or the short words of news headlines, probably every pediatrician in the world would have known that Asperger's was a distinct diagnosis. "Pervasive developmental disorder," the Australian professor, John Walker-Smith, explained, for example, in his memoir *Enduring Memories*. "This includes children with autism and so-called autistic spectrum disorder as well as Asperger's syndrome. These latter children do not have the language delay and delay in cognitive development which is such a feature of autism."

Wakefield knew this. And, everywhere else, he routinely used the distinction. In his New Orleans conference abstract, reporting on thirty kids (which I drew on for data during my meeting at *The Lancet*); in a report to the Legal Aid Board on his clinical and scientific study; in a talk to a parent conference in Sacramento, California; at Burton's congressional hearing, speaking under oath; on the Thoughtful House website; and in documents in his lawsuit against Channel 4 and me. Every time, he distinguished them correctly.

"A fundamental aspect of Asperger's that distinguishes it from autism," he later explained in a book, "is the normal acquisition of speech, and a diagnosis of Asperger's requires cognitive function within the normal range for age."

This was nothing like the challenges of Child Two, or Child Four. As José Salomão Schwartzman (John Wilson's coauthor on the DTP paper) explains, when I meet him in São Paulo, Brazil, "It is our experience every day that you talk to the father, 'Your child has characteristics of Asperger's syndrome.' And the father says, 'No doctor, he's *exactly like me.*'"

The report in my hands at Wiggin LLP was so comprehensive it even revealed who had diagnosed Child Six. A box on page 3 named two pediatricians: one a consultant in a children's hospital's child development unit, fifty miles south of London. Another was a consultant developmental pediatrician in one of the capital's flagship centers. Then, at the Royal Free, the nonspecialist child psychiatrist, Mark Berelowitz, who'd spoken alongside Wakefield at the Atrium event, had concurred with the experts' opinions.

With my tea going cold, it appeared to me that Wakefield—a nonclinical, academic, adult gastroenterologist—had *changed* the pediatricians' diagnoses.

Why? *Why not?* He wrote up the data, and the change made his "syndrome" more convincing. The paper claimed to be a series of kids with "developmental regression": or, as his lawyers put it, "a cohort of 12 children referred consecutively with regressive autism and bowel symptoms." But Asperger's syndrome ("disorder" in the United States) was *critically different* in that—unlike autism— there was no recognized subgroup with *regression.*

Pediatricians reading *The Lancet* would have spotted that in seconds and realized something was adrift. "There is no such thing like regressive Asperger," Eric Fombonne, director of psychiatry at McGill University, Montreal, Canada, tells me later. "The presence of a regression of the type seen in autism would almost certainly rule out Asperger."

I carried on reading—past Child Six's "infection and vaccination history"—to page 5 and "Adverse reactions." Here the database report clashed again—and not only with the paper, published to such effect. It even clashed with the mother's account.

There wasn't much narrative in the report from Ms. Six. But she talked about her son many times elsewhere, with memorable color and consistency. "Within hours of being vaccinated with the MMR, he developed high-pitch screaming and a very high fever," she told, for example, a judge, after the collapse of Richard Barr's class action. "One thing that I noticed was that he was like a wild animal. That is the only way I could describe him. After his vaccine he screamed if anybody touched him, and he cried day and night."

She said the same to her member of Parliament: "high-pitched screaming" and "regressive autism." And, later, on an internet radio show, she gave more detail of her son's experience with MMR, which he received at *fourteen months*. "I took him the afternoon to have the vaccine done and, within a couple of hours, and I got him home, and he started having this awful high-pitched screaming," she said. "And it's like a cat scream. And I can still hear it. I wake up hearing it."

Strangely, however, such an experience with MMR wasn't listed in the box on page 5. A week after Child Six's shot, the report listed "fever," and "constant cold and blotchy rash." It said this lasted for two weeks, adding without timings, or specific detail, "Behavior became aggressive."

She wouldn't forget a scream that stalked her dreams. And it was a recognized vaccine reaction. It was noted in package inserts ("persistent screaming") and written-up as a rare phenomenon. A team from California and Maryland even crunched numbers: publishing in the prestigious journal *Pediatrics* with data on nearly sixteen thousand injections. They found 488 kids with persistent crying in the next forty-eight hours, and seventeen with a "high pitched, unusual cry . . . usually described by parents as a high-pitched scream."

This matched the mother's story. Picture perfect. The only snag with that picture was this: the package insert and the *Pediatrics* paper weren't reporting on MMR, but an entirely different vaccine. The scream was a known reaction to DTP, the diphtheria, tetanus, and pertussis shot. It was alleged in the Loveday trial and even described in media coverage, as the *Times* reported in October 1987:

> After the third inoculation, the baby screamed continually for two days. It was not a baby's normal cry, but a high-pitched scream.

"The high-pitched scream is pathognomonic of DTP," confirms David Salisbury, the by-now retired civil servant and pediatrician whom Wakefield phoned after the brand withdrawals. "Anyone who said that happened within forty-eight hours after MMR, in my mind, either made it up, or they read it somewhere. This is a classic DTP reaction."

I also remembered the "high-pitched scream," like I remembered "fourteen days." They were central, pivotal, unforgettable features of the case made against DTP. But, just as Wilson's fortnight seemed to migrate into Wakefield's, so the distinctive screaming appeared to move between vaccines in the account of Child Six's mother.

An easy mistake, if you didn't know the science. You might not know how different the vaccines were. The pertussis shot, at the time, was a quite dirty product: a big whole-cell bacterium, killed with formalin. It was known for reactions within hours. But the measles vaccine (like mumps and rubella) was a "live virus" shot, in which the components took *days* to grow in the recipient's tissue before being capable of doing much at all.

The *Lancet* paper included no screaming. Yet—getting weirder, as this story always will—a box in Child Six's report *did*. Deepening the mystery of his mother's recollections, it noted an incident—before she heard of Wakefield—that had allegedly occurred *ten months before* MMR, when the boy was only four months old.

> After 3rd DPT vaccination [Child Six] was described by
> [his mother] as crying too much and having a high pitched
> scream 5 minutes post vaccination. This persisted for
> 12 hours.

So, from the report, it appeared that it *was* DTP, and that not only had Wakefield changed the developmental diagnosis, but the mother had changed the vaccine.

There was plenty more in the stack that De Silva dumped on the table. So I fed her my impressions, and to Channel 4 executives, who planned to bring Wakefield to trial. We agreed that what we needed was an order for him to produce the twelve children's complete, unredacted records, and we made that application to the judge.

Ms. Six came to court to try to block us. But Justice Eady brushed her aside. "I'm not having the parents telling the parties who can have what documents," he said in November that year, from the bench of Court 13. "It seems to me clear that these medical records are central."

And so it transpired that on Tuesday, January 2, 2007, I was back at Wiggin's offices, reading the content of two hefty crates of clinical notes—while a lawyer supervised me at the table.

My conclusion that day was that Wakefield was finished. But I can't tell you what I saw to make me think so. Unlike the poorly redacted reports (which would be unsealed in the United States, when he unsuccessfully sued me again, in Texas, just to tell people he was suing), the full notes must remain unreported.

I didn't then know how it would all turn out. But heading home that evening, having studied the kids' notes, I felt the drudgery of the litigation lifting. Not only had I learned many secrets about that paper, but the past weekend I'd had a *Sunday Times* exclusive:

revealing the enormous, undisclosed sums of money in Wake-field's deal with Barr.

MMR doctor given legal aid thousands

It filled most of page 12, with pictures.

But I'd hardly got home for the six o'clock news when my land-line rang. It was De Silva. As I'd sat at Wiggin's offices with the medical records, Wakefield's lawyers had filed a Notice of Discon-tinuance, abandoning his claims that my journalism defamed him and agreeing to pay our costs.

- - - - - - - - - - - - - - - - - - - -

TWENTY-THREE

Sesame Street

A little girl waits on her favorite video. She can't take her eyes off the screen. She knows that, any moment, the music will start, and Big Bird, Cookie Monster, et al. will appear where so often they've appeared before. She's black-haired, Latina, dressed in pink and white, anxiously stretching from a sturdy high chair. Her name is Michelle Cedillo.

Her mother, Theresa, watches through a camera, recording on magnetic tape. And through that camera's lens, I'm watching her too: from a different place and time. Two and a half thousand miles east, and nearly twelve years later, I'm seated amid classical, dark cherry splendor, in room 201 of the Howard T. Markey National Courts Building, inside the green zone surrounding the White House.

Today is a session of "vaccine court"—a branch of the US Court of Federal Claims—now assembled to evaluate Wakefield's. Around me, in a chamber as cold as winter stone, sit lawyers, parents, experts, and public, facing a swing-gate bar and a raised, paneled bench, from which three adjudicators, or "special masters," gaze at monitors.

Like "fourteen days," and the "high-pitched scream," this court was a legacy of the DTP crisis, imported to the United States in April 1982 with NBC's *Vaccine Roulette*. In a more litigious culture than John Wilson ever knew of, the program had spurred an avalanche of lawsuits: from three filed in America in 1981, to more than two hundred per year four years later. Most manufacturers abandoned production, and in November 1986, Ronald Reagan signed a law reserving the disputes to the federal special masters and a no-blame compensation scheme.

Since the twelve-child paper—now nine years before—nearly five thousand families had been recruited across the country, from which lawyers had picked Michelle to lead. She was America's Child Two: their best-chance test case for an unchanged proposition that persistent measles virus from MMR was responsible for an epidemic of autism.

The music starts. Michelle reacts. And a gentle French accent offers calm guidance on what everyone in the room can see. "In the clip you see how she's fascinated by *Sesame Street*," says the Montreal autism specialist Eric Fombonne, giving evidence on day six of this twelve-day hearing in June 2007. "She gets very excited. We see all this sort of overflow movement—also hand movements, which are like flapping and stereotypic."

Six months have passed since Wakefield escaped his libel trial, but his claims have now made it to this courtroom. This is *Cedillo v. Secretary of Health and Human Services*: the latter being liable, on behalf of the government, for any appropriate compensation that may arise. If Michelle wins, Department of Justice staff calculate, the bill could be $15 billion.

Theresa, the mother, first heard of Wakefield in 1997. That followed his debut on the front of Bernard Rimland's journal, the *Autism Research Review International*. Then, in December 1998 (just two months after Richard Barr filed his lawsuit), she lodged a claim under the vaccine court scheme, charging that her daughter was a victim.

Primed to believe by the twelve-child paper, she finally met Wakefield in San Diego in October 2001. Much like the journey of Jane Johnson to Thoughtful House, Theresa attended a conference of Rimland's Defeat Autism Now!—at which the charismatic British doctor spoke. He told parents of his discovery, "autistic enterocolitis," and all but said that he'd found the cause. Theresa, standing, listening from the back, scurried after him as he exited the hall.

Under cross-examination on day two of the court hearing, she evidenced how that contact blossomed. "Have you ever exchanged emails with Dr. Wakefield?" she was asked by Lynn Ricciardella, counsel for the Justice Department.

"Yes, I have," Theresa replied from the witness stand: a chair between the bar and the bench. She was a well-presented lady, then forty-five, with spectacles, bouncing earrings, and a mop of black curls. Sophisticated. Cool. Like Ms. Two.

"Approximately how many?"

"Boy, I don't have a number," she said.

"More than ten?"

"Yes, more than ten."

"More than fifty?"

"Probably more than one hundred. But less than one hundred fifty."

The girl in the high chair—Theresa's only child—was born in the hospital near their home in Yuma, Arizona: twenty minutes from the Mexico border. She received a hepatitis B vaccine on the day of her delivery—August 30, 1994—followed, one month later, by a second.

At two months, she got three shots: the triple DTP plus *Haemophilus influenzae* (both by injection), and a polio immunization by mouth. She was given the same again the following December and March, and on the final occasion a third hep B. In September 1995, she was vaccinated against chicken pox. And on Wednesday, December 20, at the age of fifteen months, she received her MMR.

This was the typical United States schedule at the time. Her parents' case was that all of it injured. Theresa and her husband, Michael Cedillo, submitted through lawyers that thimerosal, the mercury-based vaccine preservative (in those days in the hepatitis and DTP shots) caused immune system problems that left Michelle vulnerable to the live measles virus in MMR.

The hearing was prepared around that proposition. But in the event, thimerosal was sidelined. Whether or not other vaccines seeded Michelle's problems, what her lawyers would call the "most critical issue" was a test for the virus in a gut biopsy sample at the Coombe Women's Hospital, Dublin.

"There is one key factual allegation," the presiding special master, George L. Hastings Jr., would explain. "All of the petitioners' causation theories depend upon the validity of certain testing that purported to find evidence of persisting measles virus in the biological materials of Michelle, and a number of other autistic children."

Wakefield was listed as the proceedings' star witness. And with John O'Leary's tests at the core of the case, you might expect both men to be here. They'd impugned vaccinations given to millions of children. But neither has come to explain.

In their place, the hard evidence was a sheet of white paper. Literally, *one sheet* of paper. It was dated March 15, 2002, and headed "Report for Measles Virus Detection." Signed by O'Leary for his company Unigenetics (from which Wakefield had resigned as a director the year before), it gave Michelle's name, date of birth, patient identification numbers, and stated:

Positive for measles virus

Nothing evidenced that this virus (if any) came from a vaccine. There was no strain given, or molecular sequence. Nor were there documents detailing the methodology—on an instrument that, as the manufacturer warned its customers, was "not for use in diagnostic procedures."

There were a few further details. The Dublin lab said it probed for strings of measles F gene (which coded little lumps that protruded from the bug). The sample, from Michelle's ileum, was reputedly "satisfactory." And the Apple computer attached to O'Leary's 7700 apparently reported the amount found thusly:

1.67 × 10^5 copies/ng total RNA

On learning this, Theresa had felt relief: validated, just like Ms. Two had felt after seeing the lymphoid hyperplasia on the endoscopy suite monitor when her son was scoped at Hampstead.

"I was overwhelmed," Theresa told the three special masters. "Because it was confirming—confirming to us—what we thought we had seen in her."

This certificate, however, confirmed nothing to scientists with long experience of measles virus. The quantity 1.67 × 10^5 copies meant 167,000 virions per thousand-millionth of a gram of RNA, and implied *overwhelming infection*.

"This number would predict that all of the cells in this section of the ileum were infected and actively producing RNA," wrote Diane Griffin, chief of molecular biology at the Johns Hopkins Bloomberg School of Public Health, in a report for the Justice Department. The Coombe figure, she said, was "suspiciously high," and "wasn't biologically plausible."

Meanwhile, Bertus Rima, head of biomedical sciences at the Queen's University, Northern Ireland, who'd earlier written a report for Barr's failed lawsuit, commented that, in the presence of such a quantity of virus, Michelle's cells would be so "stuffed" with measles RNA there wouldn't be room for vital cellular components.

The Cedillos' experts had nothing in reply to that. And they faced more on the molecular front. Although courts everywhere accepted lab results as evidence—in everything from product liability to driving while intoxicated—the Justice Department's lawyers had seen a news report by me on the controversy surrounding the Coombe.

Fresh doubts cast on MMR study data

Nine hundred words, on page 11.

I'd then supplied them with documents (my obvious public duty), and they enlisted the PCR geek, Stephen Bustin. "The dogged work of one journalist brought this to the fore," the government's lead attorney, Vincent Matanoski, a tall naval reserve officer, acknowledged my investigation to the bench.

By this time, Bustin had dug through more Coombe data and had come to Washington to say what he found. He alleged altered lab notebooks, and 7700 runs where its operators had failed to convert RNA to DNA, yet still reported amplifying the virus. He also compared results from batches of biopsies fixed in formalin (the standard preservative for hospital pathology) with others frozen in nitrogen by Nick Chadwick.

I felt extra fond of that last demonstration, as it wasn't too hard to explain. The frozen samples were taken because formalin degraded nucleic acids, making molecular amplification more challenging. So with formalin you would expect to run the machine for more cycles than with pristine frozen tissue to get any positive signal. But Bustin discovered that, for O'Leary's reported F gene, the average number of cycles was the same for both batches—unlike a "control gene," also checked.

That led him to submit that measles had infected the biopsies *after* the formalin fixing procedure by pathologists—therefore *after they left the children.*

"Whatever this is, is a contaminant," Bustin told Hastings. "This cannot be part of the original biopsy."

Seventeen witnesses, including Theresa, would give evidence. Hers proved to be the most impressive. As the court was aware, an essential element for claims of vaccine damage (dating back to the Stuart-Smith checklist, and beyond) was the claimed "temporal link" between shot and symptoms. And it would be over this—evidenced, as so often, by the mother's account—that the songs of *Sesame Street* rang out.

In a "narrative" Theresa wrote, years after the event, she said that her daughter had become ill with a fever *fourteen days* after receiving MMR. Later, she halved this to *seven days* after. And in an affidavit sworn before the trial began, she said that, from "seven or eight days" following the shot, her daughter would "cry inconsolably" unless a *Sesame Street* video was played.

"To the best of my knowledge, as an approximate, I would say one to two days into the fever, so that would be December 27, or December 28, 1995," she said under cross-examination.

"And could you describe how she would react to a *Sesame Street* video?" Ricciardella asked.

"It would calm her."

"Did she stop interacting with people during this time?"

"It began declining. Yes."

The mother said that, about two months later, Michelle began hand-flapping. And in the months that followed she became withdrawn, didn't respond to her name, pushed people away when they tried to hold her, and got "engrossed" in *Sesame Street*.

"What do you mean by 'engrossed' in it?"

"She would watch it and, I guess you could say, tune everything else around her out."

Her proof was of an order quite different to O'Leary's. I could see it in the courtroom for myself. The Frenchman, Fombonne, plays clip after clip of the family's home videos, in which the little girl's behavior, in the high chair and everywhere, correlates with the mother's impressions.

Here's Michelle, hands flapping to *Sesame Street*. Here she's not responding to a game of peekaboo. Here she's on a blue pony, with "no spontaneous action," and with colored balls she "doesn't explore." Then, at a birthday party, in a beautiful white dress, with her mother vainly calling, "Michelle . . . Michelle." We see unusual "finger mannerisms," hear a "guttural" sound, and we watch as she watches wheels spinning.

"This is a sample that I observed in multiple clips which are all consistent," Fombonne confirms. "In other words, it's not a highly selected series. All the videos show the same type of behavior."

The next day, another expert took the witness stand, and identified the same hallmarks of autism. Max Wiznitzer, a pediatric neurologist with a busy clinical practice and a teaching post at Case Western Reserve University, Cleveland, went through the videos again. "The parent is trying to engage her in making vocalizations, but we don't hear any response," he commentates. "There's no real response, or acknowledgment of the adults present, in terms of a social smile, or anything else."

There's no denying it. Even seated three rows back on the right-hand side, I can see what the doctors are getting at. The videos are powerful, with only one shortcoming: they were recorded *before* Michelle's MMR. Both Fombonne and Wiznitzer are witnesses for the government. And the tapes are date-stamped: from May 25, 1995, seven months prior to the girl's three-in-one, to December 17, 1995, three days in advance of the injection.

The recordings had been obtained through a government "motion for production." Videos were mentioned in a report by

Michelle's gastroenterologist—a New York pediatrician named Arthur Krigsman, who scoped for Thoughtful House. The family's lawyers opposed the federal application, but the special master, Hastings, overruled them. With down-brushed white hair and matching cowboy mustache, Hastings was a former tax lawyer and the father of three children. He said the tapes "could yield important evidence."

He was right. They did. And they weren't alone in raising doubt over the family's prospects. Medical records suggested that Michelle didn't smile for four to six months, or sit independently until eleven months of age. Her head circumference was assessed as larger than 95 percent of girls of her age, and—also before the shot—pediatricians' noted social delay, language delay, and intractable constipation.

There was nothing to establish that Theresa blamed vaccines before she heard of Wakefield. A better fit with the facts—as I found so often—was a feedback loop of confirmation. Parents, especially mothers, heard his claims and interpreted their children's histories in that light.

After the "opioid excess" fiasco in Barr's class action, Theresa's lawyers skipped the stoned rodent model of childhood autism, arguing instead that the virus directly attacked her brain. But the government side responded that this would typically cause death, and pointed out there was no epidemiology associating autism with outbreaks of measles.

The case was a bust. Just like Barr's. But like him—with Kirsten Limb and their class action professionals—the lawyers and experts would be paid from public funds (around $300 an hour for unsupervised preparation) even if, and when, the families reaped nothing but stress, suspicion, and bitterness.

For the three special masters, the evidence was overwhelming. Tragically, Michelle must get nothing. She was nearly thirteen now, and was wheeled into court, in baggy casual clothes and huge ear-protectors: a sobering sight for us all. On top of autism, epilepsy, and cognitive delay, she suffered with arthritis and optic nerve damage. She didn't speak, was fed through a tube, and hit herself on the eye socket and chin.

"I feel deep sympathy and admiration for the Cedillo family," said Hastings in his ruling. "And I have no doubt that the families of countless other autistic children—families that cope every day with the tremendous challenges of caring for autistic children—are similarly deserving of sympathy and admiration. However, I must decide this case not on sentiment, but by analyzing the evidence."

Two more test cases would follow this hearing: for Colten Snyder of Florida and William Hazlehurst of Tennessee. But the science, and the upshot, were the same. In 680 pages of rulings from the special masters, Wakefield was named (to my count) 360 times, as his reputation was torn to pieces by the US courts like a medieval hang, draw, and quartering.

"The result of this case would be the same even if I totally ignored the epidemiologic evidence, declined to consider the video evidence, and/or excluded the testimony of Dr. Bustin," Hastings said, in a 183-page ruling published later. "Unfortunately, the Cedillos have been misled by physicians who are guilty, in my view, of gross medical misjudgment."

Could there be a worse drubbing for a man of ideas?

Yes, there could. It was about to begin.

TWENTY-FOUR

Enterocolitis

From the time of my first stories, it took lawyers for Britain's General Medical Council (known to the nation as the GMC) nearly three and a half years to reinvestigate my early findings, conclude they were accurate, and bring Wakefield, John Walker-Smith, and Simon Murch to a hearing on charges of serious professional misconduct. And it would be another two and a half—on and off, with adjournments—before that saga finally resolved. In total, the proceedings ran for 217 days: longer than the trial of O. J. Simpson, then the most famous legal duel in history.

The original plan was for a snappy thirty-five days: centered on charges of dishonesty and fraud by Wakefield, and on a false claim, published in the twelve-child paper, that they'd had ethics committee approval. But his two gastro amigos threw the proceedings into turmoil by changing their stories about their roles in the affair. They now said the scopings, spinal taps, scans, and so forth were solely for the children's care.

That came as a surprise to parents, such as Ms. Four and Mr. Eleven. They'd gone to Hampstead for vaccine damage tests. And it surprised me, too, since those tests had been agreed on by a firm of lawyers before a single child was admitted. They were tests set out in the "clinical and scientific study," sliced into two papers, clinical and scientific, submitted to *The Lancet*, promoting the "new syndrome" at the core of Richard Barr's lawsuit.

But, for me, the clinicians' tactics were a gift. They literally opened the books. With Walker-Smith's lawyers, in particular, now arguing that every procedure was for the children's benefit, the hearing reviewed—in agonizing detail—every last diagnosis, vaccination, and symptom, including from the trove of confidential medical records that I read at my lawyer's office.

The dance began in July 2007. And what a dance it was. In an eight-story glass office building at 350 Euston Road, London, the ultimate data that launched the vaccine crisis would be spoken into the public record. Like Lord Justice Stuart-Smith, two decades before, I could review the children's cases, patient by patient. I could hear what was what. And what was not.

"I am going to turn to Child Ten, and the Royal Free records," counsel for the defense or the prosecution would say. And around a long third-floor room—with tubular steel furniture on a blue and ochre carpet—men and women would stretch toward stacks of cardboard crates, each crammed with three-inch-thick binders of documents. I counted fifteen stacks. Seven crates in each stack. And—*my word*—what secrets lay within.

This was some tool for an investigative reporter. On two sides of a hollow rectangle of seventeen tables, the three accused men and the council's five-member "fitness to practice" panel (three doctors, two lay members; three women, two men) faced each other across a lawn of empty carpet and surrounded by a phalanx of lawyers. I sat by the door, capturing what they said: the only reporter in the room.

"Child Seven . . ." They all stretched. "Child Nine . . ." Stretch again. Day after day. Month after month. "Now, I'd like to return to Child Ten . . ."

My first big break came on day thirty-two: Tuesday, September 14. Seated and sworn in the witness chair in front of me was a perky consultant named Susan Davies who'd led the pathologists in the project. She wasn't among the *Lancet* paper's original cast of authors but was added to the credits between its first submission and the version unveiled in the Atrium.

Right off, she explained the meticulous routines with which her department handled bowel biopsies. A slice from each snip of tissue, stained and mounted on glass, was examined by two doctors through a double-headed microscope, then described in reports that were printed and double-signed, discussed with clinicians at weekly meetings, and filed in the patients' records.

Those pathologists looked especially for any excess in populations of inflammatory cells—normally present, within reasonable parameters—and, most importantly, for damage, or distortion, involving the delicate epithelium and pit-like crypts, which surface the large and small intestines.

She was trucking along fine, with nothing too stimulating. But, at half past twelve, after the morning coffee break, binders for Child Two were yanked from the crates, and people turned to page 264. First came the report which had caused such excitement when Wakefield, Walker-Smith, and Murch had believed that—*yessss*—the eight-year-old had Crohn's. That was followed by another, when the buzz wore off, and a likely food intolerance was acknowledged.

I noted that change, which wasn't mentioned in *The Lancet*. Then, as more binders were pulled and flopped open on the tables, phrases began to drift between counsel and witness like tennis balls lobbed long and high. "No increase in inflammatory cells," I heard. "No abnormality detected."

As the paper's Table 1 had documented, years before, Wakefield's syndrome first rested on "chronic non-specific colitis"—

inflammatory disease of the large intestine—in children diagnosed with autism. Second was tabulated "lymphoid hyperplasia":
the ugly swollen glands, past the valve into the ileum, that so
shocked the children's mothers. Taken together, he proposed an
"enterocolitis"—inflammatory disease of the small bowel (enteritis) at the same time as the colitis in the large bowel.

"Enterocolitis," a source explains to me after the case, "is when
gastroenterologists get really excited."

In this, the paper claimed a "unique disease process" and sought
to link it with the three-in-one MMR. Chronic colitis was tabulated for eleven of the twelve, and the swollen glands were listed in
the ileum of ten, with the *Lancet* text summarizing the discoveries.

> We describe a pattern of colitis and ileal-lymphoid-nodular hyper-
> plasia in children with developmental disorders.

But through the rest of that Tuesday morning, and into the
afternoon, Davies was taken through her department's reports.
And most didn't square with *The Lancet*. Time and again, where
the journal reported disease—in the opaque phrase "non-specific
colitis"—her department's reports, of great medicolegal status,
noted humdrum, everyday findings.

> Large bowel type mucosa within normal histological limits . . .
>
> Minimal inflammatory changes. May be the result of operative
> artifact . . .
>
> No significant histological abnormality . . .
>
> No architectural abnormality. No increase in inflammatory
> cells . . .

So striking were the differences that an expert for the hearing—a professor of pediatric gastroenterology named Ian Booth—
filed a shocking assessment in a report. On the basis of what
he'd seen (and I would hear from my chair), he couldn't exclude
"scientific fraud."

"In six cases (3, 4, 8, 9, 10 and 12), the colonic histology is reported as normal, or virtually normal, but is presented as a colitis in the *Lancet* publication," he wrote, in a document I obtain through a Wakefield associate. "In two cases (2 and 5), there are minor histological abnormalities reported in the clinical pathology but presented in a more exaggerated, unqualified form."

Here, for example, is the report on Child Four: Wakefield's "most compelling" early case. The boy was listed in Table 1 with "chronic non-specific colitis" and "ileal and colonic lymphoid hyperplasia." But the hospital's findings, read aloud to the panel (and separately peer reviewed for my investigation) were *normal*.

The pathologists found no pathology.

I. Small bowel type mucosa with a lymphoid follicle.

II–VII. Large bowel mucosa, some with attached muscularis mucosae with no evidence of architectural distortion or increase in inflammatory cells in the lamina propria. Lymphoid follicles with germinal centres are present in many of the biopsies. No cryptitis or crypt abscesses are seen. The surface epithelium appears intact. No granulomas, ova or parasites are seen.

Comment: Large bowel series with terminal ileum, with no histopathological abnormality.

The leading lawyer for the GMC, a slender, blonde, and black-dressed Queen's Counsel, Sally Smith, asked Davies to explain her reaction when she saw the first write-up of the twelve-child study. "What was your overall view of the terminology used in relation to the histology findings in the *Lancet* paper? Just when you read the paper."

"I was somewhat concerned with the use of the word 'colitis.'"

"First of all, what did you understand that word to mean?"

Davies paused to gather her thoughts. "I personally use that terminology, 'colitis,' when I see active inflammation, or a pattern of changes which suggest a specific diagnosis. And it was not my impression that the children coming through in the spasmodic way that they had, I had formulated a sense of a distinct pattern warranting that terminology."

"Now, you say you were concerned. What was the nature of your concern?"

Another pause. "Well." She paused again. "As I've explained, the use of the word, predominantly, 'colitis.'"

I took advice on the diagnoses tumbling from the binders. And it seemed she was right to be concerned. "In the present reports and patients, overall," says Karel Geboes of the Catholic University of Leuven, Belgium, and one of Europe's most respected gastrointestinal pathologists (commenting on all but the American child's reports), "it is my impression that eight of the eleven were normal."

Wakefield, however, had been looking for his syndrome, and he had taken another stab at getting what he wanted by seeking a second opinion. During twenty-one days in the witness chair, he said the "ultimate conclusions," and "final determinant of the diagnoses" in Table 1, weren't from Davies's pathology department but from a longstanding associate in the medical school. His name was Amar Dhillon, who'd gained dozens of credits as a coauthor with Wakefield and had devised what he called a "grading sheet" to score these children's biopsies.

But after the doctor without patients finished giving evidence, I obtain copies of the sheets he said were Dhillon's. And I'm told by four specialists, in Europe and the United States, that these, too, were *overwhelmingly normal*. Essentially, Dhillon had captured the same picture as Davies, albeit expressed more in tickboxes than narratives.

"It is definitely not correct that the children had enterocolitis," Geboes comments.

"I'm astonished, really," says Paola Domizio, professor of pathology education at Queen Mary's College, University of London.

"These are the kind of things that we in our practice here would ignore completely," says Henry Appelman, professor of surgical pathology at the University of Michigan.

Then things got worse, as they so often did. Dhillon *denied* reporting colitis. "In none of my grading sheet observations have I stated 'colitis,'" he pointed out in a statement responding to an analysis of the sheets by me in *The BMJ*, which for some crazy reason had stopped calling itself the *British Medical Journal*. "The purpose of my grading sheet observations," he said, "was not, could not have been, nor was it intended to conclude, the final diagnostic assignment of colitis."

Wakefield stood his ground. He denied any error. But his reporting from the ileum was also strange. The lymphoid hyperplasia was considered off-topic for the disciplinary hearing and didn't figure much in the binders. So I headed east on Euston Road to the British Library's science section and reviewed a sample of ten papers and book chapters on this topic, which revealed a truth left hidden.

Ugly as they might look to parents on a monitor, the swollen glands were regarded by gastroenterologists as a "normal" or "benign" observation. They were like tonsil tissue, components of the immune system, in places clumping together in "coalescing masses" as so-called "Peyer's patches." Their total numbers varied, both by age and location, being most numerous in childhood and in the terminal ileum—right by that valve from the colon.

"They seem to be present in the majority of children," specialists from Buffalo, New York, published, for example, in the journal *Gastroenterology* in August 1980, with nothing to do with autism or vaccines, "and are now being appreciated clinically with greater frequency because both radiographic and colonoscopic techniques and equipment have improved."

Walker-Smith, of course, knew all about this. In 1983, he'd reported the swollen glands in the terminal ileum (of neurotypical kids) as having been termed "benign lymphoid hyperplasia" due to what he called "the frequency of its demonstration in asymptomatic children." And, nasty as they appeared to worried laypeople, in March 1994 he edited a textbook where two experts explained:

This is so common as to be a normal variant in children.

Wakefield, Walker-Smith, and Murch, however, revealed *nothing* of this background in *The Lancet*. Although space was cleared in the paper's final "Discussion" section for sixteen lines on the stoned rodent model, thirteen for Ms. Two's vitamin B_{12} notion, and about forty-five trying to pin autism on MMR, there were *none* that discussed the lymphoid hyperplasia. There wasn't even one reference in the "References."

These omissions were extraordinary. An oversight? *Unlikely.* This wasn't merely the first clause in the paper's title, but a sign that *defined* the syndrome. And, as ever, there was more to be noted from the records. Not only was the paper silent on the lymphoid hyperplasia, but the gastroenterologists didn't disclose that standard blood tests to check for inflammation were also found to be *normal*.

And there was more withholding of information. The paper included nothing—*not one word*—on the children's *principal gastroenterological symptom*.

What symptom was that? If it was the symptom of a syndrome, then that syndrome might literally be *shit*. As I sat by the door, watching the relentless flop of binders, I couldn't fail to miss it—month after month—in records for *ten* of the children. "Marked constipation," "Severe constipation," "Fecal impacted," "Significant constipation," "Chronic constipation," "Episodes of constipation," "His major problem is constipation." And on it went.

"We were realizing that constipation is a central aspect of these children," Walker-Smith acknowledged to the panel in July 2008, replying from the witness chair to one of his three lawyers, who'd wisely confronted this in advance of the prosecution. "Constipation," the Australian professor added to what by then was obvious to everyone, "is an integral and fundamental part of the clinical features."

But why leave out the "integral and fundamental" from a journal read mostly by doctors? For some, this knowledge might have aided patient care: raising the profile of an important issue for developmentally challenged children, including those without language to express it.

Yet, for specialists, it might also have raised questions, doubts, about the validity of the so-called "syndrome."

"Constipation is the exact opposite of what you would normally be looking for," Booth explained, "in a patient with inflammatory bowel disease."

Such a disease, of course, is what Wakefield claimed. It was integral and fundamental to Barr's lawsuit. And if mild inflammatory cell changes were reported in constipated children, it "raises the question," Booth told the panel, "of whether the constipation was responsible."

Constipation? *Not MMR?* Booth's analysis was far from speculation. Fecal stagnation behind intestinal obstructions, as well as abrasion of the intestines' surface epithelium (just *one cell deep*, in both the large and small bowels), had long been linked with inflammation. Indeed, nine years before the hearing, at the meeting at the Royal College of Surgeons, the Scottish gastroenterologist, Anne Ferguson, who'd asked about JABS, had also spoken of constipation and "little ulcers."

This would surely have been known to some of the paper's thirteen authors. But, to be fair, only one man wrote it. Strictly speaking, most of his colleagues weren't entitled to authorship, falling foul of stringent criteria. According to the *Uniform Requirements* for journal manuscripts, "substantial contributions" to multiple aspects were expected—which was true for hardly anyone but Wakefield.

None of the authors was eminent. Three were trainees. "In 1996–1998, you needed very little involvement to be named as an author," confirmed one of them, a junior pathologist, Andrew Anthony, in a statement. And the consultants were barely better placed. "I did not write the histology sections," Dhillon said in a reply to a story by me. Murch (who says he never saw the final version before printing) told me that "enterocolitis" was a "dreadful term" for what was found, while the swollen glands were "hugely oversold."

Indeed, when other authors sought amendments to the paper, before publication, it was left to Wakefield whether he took any notice. Mark Berelowitz, the child psychiatrist who'd spoken in the Atrium, not only said that he didn't know which of the children was which but that he didn't agree with Wakefield's descriptions of autism. It was "not a behavioural disorder," he told the panel, "and it was not clear that it was a regressive disorder."

Even Walker-Smith had accepted Wakefield's claims based on a secondhand data compilation. He said that Wakefield brought "all the clinical and laboratory details" to his office one day, prepared in a "sort of master chart."

"We all rely on trust," the Australian professor told the panel, on his twenty-fourth day in the witness chair, when asked about the descriptions in the paper. "I trusted Dr. Wakefield."

Whoaah. "I am sorry?" asked the black-dressed Sally Smith, from her position at the far end of the rectangle.

"We all rely on trust," the now-seventy-year-old pediatrician repeated, quietly. "Yes, and I trusted Dr. Wakefield."

"You trusted him in what context?"

"Just in general."

It was an emotional moment, on a bright August day. I think all of us knew what he meant. But there was more on the horizon regarding the pathology, from the next defendant in the chair. This was Murch, who would speak of an astonishing event—which Davies, Walker-Smith, and Wakefield all testified as having no recollection of happening.

Giving evidence on day 113, Murch spoke of a meeting between the paper's authors roughly three months before publication. Wakefield had circulated the latest version, he said, and several doctors, including Murch himself, Walker-Smith, and Davies, plus possibly two juniors and a few others in the department, gathered in a histopathology seminar room to look at the slides again.

Would the others forget this? Or did Murch imagine it? I can't gauge which would be the more incredible. This was around ten months after the last child left Malcolm Ward; about three months since a media storm over MMR had erupted, thanks to stories placed in the magazine *Pulse*; Wakefield and his mentor, Roy Pounder, had met with management; the Royal Free was gearing up for the Atrium event. And yet it seemed that, at least, someone influential still agonized over the accuracy of Table 1.

"I do have a very good recollection of the meeting," Murch told the panel, chaired by Surendra Kumar, a family doctor, flanked by Stephen Webster, a gerontologist, Parimala Moodley, a psychiatrist, Wendy Golding, an educationalist, and Sylvia Dean, a former local government chief executive. "I think the reason was initially that Dr. Davies had seen the draft of the paper and just wondered whether the description of the histology perhaps oversold it."

Think about that. Real or dreamt, this was remarkable testimony. If the descriptions were "oversold," what would be left to publish? Would the authors unnerve *The Lancet* by correcting Table 1? Would Wakefield tell the nation that he made a mistake? Everyone in the seminar room had résumés to think of. Would any junior raise a hand of objection?

Nobody present needed a PhD in psychology to know what Walker-Smith wanted. "Prof," as they called the top doctor in the room, who sat on committees with professors of medicine and surgery, wasn't only set for a tasty academic credit (which the university submitted to the Research Assessment Exercise), but he'd been putting all the children (apart from the American) on powerful Crohn's anti-inflammatory drugs that carried black box warnings to prescribers.

Wakefield, likewise. He was being paid at hourly rates to advance his "syndrome" in Barr's lawsuit. If he didn't find fault with the solicitor's target product, his lavish personal fees would stop. He'd filed for two patents claiming single measles shots. And, with Pounder, he'd already announced to the world, in *Pulse*, evidence that "confirm our suspicions."

Murch told the panel that the debate over the biopsies was led by the pathologists, Davies and Dhillon—who must have known their specialty's consensus. Mild elevations of inflammatory cells—as noted here and there in Davies's reports, and similarly scored on Dhillon's grading sheets—were frequent, *normal* findings in *healthy* guts, and shouldn't be reported as colitis.

"A common error is to diagnose 'mild chronic nonspecific colitis' in biopsies of normal colon because of the normal population of mononuclear cells," explains, for example, a landmark guide from the period, published in November 1989 in the *American Journal of Surgical Pathology*. (And I collect a small stack of papers saying the same.) "As a rule of thumb, the diagnosis should not be made unless there is evidence of injury to the colonic epithelium."

Davies, nevertheless, took an authorship credit, and Murch told the panel that the reporting was accurate. "All the pathologists present when the slides were reviewed," he said, "agreed that the wording was reasonable."

So, yes please, they'd have a paper with their names on it in *The Lancet*, the world's number two general medical journal.

TWENTY-FIVE

We Can Reveal

As what Wakefield would later call a "war" over vaccines spread from Britain to the United States, I began to get invitations to give talks. That meant PowerPoint, Microsoft's slide-maker, and weekends spent sizing and pasting.

From early days, I devised a less than lecture-like color scheme: orange and yellow on a solid black background, with a gambling theme in the artwork. The left bottom corner featured a card-fan motif: a hand with five aces, including two spades. And an opening run of photographs featured Wakefield with his base: an ever-increasing number of women.

One . . . four . . . five . . . nine . . . Then stock images of hundreds . . . and thousands.

At the start, my carbon footprint remained commendably small. Which was probably just as well. After revealing Wakefield's secret legal deal, the money he billed at hourly rates, his planned vaccines and products meant to make his fortune, how his own lab had failed to find measles virus genomes, and that he'd refused to perform a gold-standard study, what I had was too exhausting for a forty-minute presentation. It was more like a shopping list of conflicts and outrages than a hard news *"We can reveal."*

But all that changed on Sunday, February 8, 2009: five years after my first MMR splash. By now, the hearing on Euston Road was temporarily adjourned. And Wakefield was back on page 1.

I was at Heathrow Airport for a dawn flight to Detroit, Michigan, when I picked up the paper and spread it on the floor to read my latest installment. Around me, Terminal 5 was all but deserted as I gazed down at the front and scanned a couple of paragraphs, with my fists under my chin and my elbows on my knees.

MMR doctor fixed data on autism

It was about time, too. We'd probably waited too long. But we needed to be sure to get it right.

> The doctor who sparked the scare over the safety of the MMR vaccine for children changed and misreported results in his research, creating the appearance of a possible link with autism, a Sunday Times investigation has found.
>
> Confidential medical documents and interviews with witnesses have established that Andrew Wakefield manipulated patients' data, which triggered fears that the MMR triple vaccine to protect against measles, mumps and rubella was linked to the condition.

I wasn't sure about "the condition," but newspapers were team efforts. What followed, inside, was more so. I licked a middle finger, reached down, and turned pages, until I came to a spread at pages 6 and 7: three thousand words, across sixteen columns, plus two panels of further information. Reversed, in white lettering—upper case, boldface—on a gray background strip across the top of both pages, ran the headline:

HIDDEN RECORDS SHOW MMR TRUTH

Then a photograph of me, and an introductory standfirst:

> A Sunday Times investigation has found that altered data was behind the decade-long scare over vaccination

Neat.

Three color pictures ran from left to right: the inevitable baby crying after being stuck with a needle; the actors Jenny McCarthy and her then boyfriend Jim Carrey, waving their arms in "Green Our Vaccines" T-shirts; then Wakefield grinning, exposing a dental overbite, outside the hearing on Euston Road.

"Key Dates in the Crisis," one panel was headed. The other: "How the Scare Led to the Return of Measles."

I'd seen this coming. I'd gotten the interview with Ms. Two, which I'd not yet reported. I had the stack of poorly redacted reports from the pilot study database. I'd gotten expert submissions, filed in Richard Barr's lawsuit. I had transcripts of hearings before senior judges, countless documents obtained under the Freedom of Information Act. And, pursuant to court order, I'd read the kids' records at my lawyer's office on the day Wakefield dropped his claim for defamation.

Some of this stuff was legally sealed. And there were still gaps to fill in the evidence. Like a piano with missing keys, the recurring pattern was obvious. But I still couldn't play the tune.

The Australian professor came to my aid, however. His change-of-story strategy with the General Medical Council, to argue that the scopings were all pure patient care, meant his lawyers—and everyone around the rectangle of tables—rehearsed, over and over, sometimes a dozen times, every note and letter in those stacks of cardboard crates. Those three-inch-thick binders, stuffed with secret records, flopped and flopped far more than I needed.

Seated by the door, filling notebook after notebook, I not only had cases where normal pathology was reported in *The Lancet* as inflammatory bowel disease. I had kids, tabulated with diagnoses of regressive autism, who'd not been diagnosed with autism. I had boys who'd been listed with the first symptoms within *days*, whose records revealed nothing for *months*. And I had patients who'd been the subject of doctors' concerns *before* they received MMR.

I counted *not one case* where I could reconcile the records with what was published, to such effect, in the journal.

To me, it was pretty much what you might expect if you picked a bunch of patients from anti-vaccine groups' lists for a project supervised by provincial lawyers. And while our page 1 headline was shocking enough, when individual children's cases were drilled down through the records—histories, diagnoses, and claimed temporal links—the audacity of what had happened became staggering.

Each anomaly, in itself, seemed technical. Dry. A scratchy note here. A biopsy report there. But from this web of discrepancies had emerged a case series that had fooled *The Lancet*'s editors, peer reviewers, and readers, provoked a storm of publicity that ensured public funding for Barr's class action, and so created the engine for what would become a global crisis of confidence in vaccines.

One example was the case of the only girl among the dozen: a three-year-old, not only a JABS referral from the same town as Child Four, but a patient at the same general practitioners' office. "She was reported in the journal as having suffered a brain injury 'two weeks' after MMR," ran my story, on page 6.

> Her medical records did not support this. Before she was admitted, she had been seen by local specialists, and her GP told the Royal Free of "significant concerns about her development some months before she had her MMR."

A six-year-old boy's colon, reported in *The Lancet* as diseased, was revealed to be unremarkable in his records:

> He was reported in the journal to be suffering from regressive autism and bowel disease: specifically "acute and chronic

nonspecific colitis". The boy's hospital discharge summary, however, said there was nothing untoward in his biopsy.

Incredibly, two of the twelve (including Child Six, whose poorly redacted report I'd read at my lawyer's office) weren't merely similar cases, they were *brothers*. And, along with another boy, introduced to the research by the brothers' mother, they *hadn't been diagnosed with autism*. Indeed one, Child Seven, aged nearly three, was discharged from the hospital with a letter stating, "He is not thought to have features of autism."

There was so much stuff, we couldn't get it all in. Even the three thousand words were mangled. But pick-up was good, especially in the United States, where *USA Today*, *Newsweek*, the *Los Angeles Times*, the *Chicago Tribune*, and a string of other outlets ran reports.

And now I got more invitations to give talks on what I'd learned, where I could really dig into the detail.

My trip to Detroit let me do just that, starting on the day after we published. I'd been invited to give a week of lectures, seminars, and "grand rounds" presentations on the snowbound campus of the University of Michigan, Ann Arbor, where I unveiled my first-ever PowerPoint. I'd yet to get the colors right, and my formats were amateur: for the most part crude bullet points.

Wakefield's Assignment from the Lawyer

1. Establish a time link between MMR and disorders (historically 14 days)
2. Find a fingerprint of damage
3. Propose a mechanism for this damage

The Lancet Paper Delivers on the Assignment

1. 8/12 "MMR," with 14 days maximum to "behavioural symptoms"

2. A "new syndrome" of regressive autism and bowel disease

3. Proposal that the ultimate culprit may be measles virus

I also framed a Q&A quiz, which I would use in my talks ever after. Sharp observers might have noticed (although, if they did, they never said) an apparent contradiction in my narrative. If, as I reported, the children were recruited and brought to Hampstead to construct a case against MMR, why did *The Lancet* only report *eight* with the link? Surely the parents of *all twelve* would stake a claim?

"So why didn't all the kids' families name MMR?" I asked during my main event in Michigan: the Susan B. Meister Lecture in Child Health Policy.

I let that question hang, in the hope of raised hands. Then I answered myself, "*They did.*"

By now, the binders had been remorselessly scoured. The kids' records had been read into mine. And it was clear that when the parents gave their accounts at the Royal Free, *eleven* children's mothers or fathers blamed the shot. The one remaining family blamed a "viral infection" (first thought to be rubella, but then deemed to be measles), and even they later changed their story to finger MMR, after being visited at home by a lawyer.

Thus *three* allegations were *withheld* from *The Lancet*. Hence, *eleven*, not *eight* of *twelve*.

So now, when I asked the audience *why* the figures might be different, hands rose like spring-loaded umbrellas. The commonest opinion was that *eleven*, or *twelve*, would have given the game away. The cohort's parents would be exposed for who they really were: a group of marshaled, prescreened complainants against the vaccine, not a bowel clinic's typical work.

Much later, Wakefield raised a different explanation, however, citing a criterion not stated in the paper. "We reported on those eight who had made the link <u>at the time of their child's deterioration</u>

and excluded those who made the link later," he said, in a 148-page affidavit, with underlining.

> If a child's parents made the association later in time and not on their own because, for example, they had read about the issue in a newspaper article, their association was not included. To have included those who only came to this position more recently and "secondhand" would have clearly biased the *Lancet* paper's reporting.

He came up with that account when he was suing me again: this time, unsuccessfully, in Texas. At face value, it might seem to make some kind of sense, even if not revealed, as it should have been. However, while the maximum "interval from exposure to first behavioural symptom" for the reported eight was claimed to be *fourteen days*, it was between *one* and *three months* for those he omitted. So, including them would have blown his temporal link. But he was at least acknowledging that parents' stories might be *wrong*—an admission I never heard from him elsewhere.

But there was a whack-a-mole quality to Wakefield's explanation. The children's records revealed that, were his claimed criterion applied to all twelve, more parental claims would *disappear*. Ms. Four, for example, had gotten the idea about MMR and autism three and a half years after her son received his shot, inspired by a *newspaper clipping*.

So that was one case down. On Wakefield's professed formula, the paper was wrong already. "[He] did not have any initial reaction, and was not ill at the time," Ms. Four explained to lawyers in October 1998. She later sent me a Xerox of the clipping.

And hers wasn't the only child tabulated among the eight who didn't appear to meet the claimed criterion. Child One's local doctor wrote to Walker-Smith, describing MMR as the parents' "most recent concern" about their three-year-old son, who was vaccinated twenty-eight months before. And after interviewing Ms. Six in October 1996, the Australian professor wrote to Wakefield, saying that she'd only "relatively recently associated the change of behaviour" with a shot given to the boy three years before.

"In this child," Walker-Smith told the General Medical Council hearing, "although the mother did not associate the MMR with what went on, the mother became quite convinced latterly that MMR played an important role."

So was that *three* of the eight that, on Wakefield's claimed criterion, should have been omitted? *Yes.* Then there was Child Three. "Recently his mother has been told by Social Services that it is likely that the MMR might have caused the problem," the professor wrote to the local doctor who referred the boy, nearly five years after the shot was given, noting that Ms. Three "had been in touch with the organisation JABS."

And then there was Child Two, Wakefield's founding inspiration, whose mother seemed to surface everywhere. The first mention from the records of her raising any issue with professionals about MMR had flopped from the binders three weeks into the hearing, when her family doctor slumped into the witness chair in front of me and acknowledged a note he made in the boy's medical records, thirteen years before.

Nil obvious Re MMR story

He wrote that on Wednesday, November 2, 1994, when Ms. Two came to see him at his office. Her son had been vaccinated five years earlier. And on that day of her visit (five months ahead of the *Newsnight* broadcast), a half-page story had appeared in *The Guardian* newspaper, featuring JABS, Jackie Fletcher, and talk of compensation. It was headlined:

Painful choice of risks

Had Ms. Two read the story, from which there was nil obvious to the doctor? Did somebody tell her? Who can say? But it appeared that Wakefield's link between the shot and behavioral problems rested on shifting sands. His *eight* figure should have been *more*: declaring all parents who made the complaint at the hospital. Or it should have been *less*: based on thorough checks of the records. Either way, *Lancet* readers were misled.

That whack-a-mole phenomenon cropped up a lot. For example, over the three: the two brothers, plus one other (whose mother went to Wakefield on advice from the brothers' mother), who hadn't been diagnosed with "autism." Why were they listed in the paper's Table 2 as among nine of the twelve expressly stated to have been given a "behavioural diagnosis" of "autism"?

In his monster affidavit, Wakefield's answer to that argued that he didn't mean "autism" like he used it everywhere else: in his New Orleans conference abstract, which I raised at my meeting with *The Lancet*'s editors; addressing parents at a meeting in Sacramento; in his report to the Legal Aid Board; at Burton's congressional hearing; on the Thoughtful House website; in documents for the lawsuit against Channel 4 and me. Or even as he explained in his book.

Instead, he said, "autism" was used in *The Lancet* in a "generic sense," and as "a generic term," which, he said, was "appropriate" for a "disorder on a spectrum."

> In circumstances where the terms: "Asperger's," "autism syndrome," "autistic," "likely Asperger's," and "autistic spectrum disorder" are used, the label of the generic term "autism" is appropriate in the description.

But why would any medical professional think such a thing? It wasn't that Table 2 was too cramped to squeeze the words in. And the table contradicted his explanation. He'd used spectrum terms in it: "Disintegrative disorder?" as a possibility for Child Four, and "*Autistic spectrum disorder*" for Child Nine.

There was nothing "generic" about a diagnosis of "autism." Right, wrong, relevant, or irrelevant, the diagnosis was the diagnosis. Period. It was a considered form of words, which both parents and professionals often set great store by. And if his aim was really as he said, why would he want to change the *specific* to the *generic*, the *concrete* to the *vague*—deliberately disclosing *less information* (and less *accurate* information) to the journal's editors, peer reviewers, and readers? Why substitute the opinions of a lab worker and former trainee gut surgeon, who'd never examined the patients, and whose employment contract forbade clinical care, for the judgments of specialist pediatricians?

The clues, I thought, were in his paper and patents: where he claimed *all twelve kids* were "previously normal" and suffered a "regressive developmental disorder" (and "severe developmental regression"). Reporting the true diagnoses would contradict both. Pediatricians would spot that in seconds. If his motive wasn't to create the appearance of *regressive autism*—to go with *enterocolitis* to conjure his "syndrome"—why change the clinicians' words to his own?

He didn't explain that, but those changes also made a difference on Lord Justice Stuart-Smith's checklist. And after Ms. Two had told me, at the start of my investigation, that her son's head-banging began "about six months" after the shot (and, therefore, not within two weeks, as specified in the paper), I discovered more alterations impacting on the checklist in the critical temporal link.

Soon after my first story, I made a discovery that I never wrote up at the time. I obtained the early version of the *Lancet* paper, circulated in the medical school in August 1997: six months before the final publication. It made great PowerPoints: I created pretty pie charts to illustrate remarkable alterations. In these, the summer version of what would be unveiled in the Atrium, for instance, the number of kids whose parents fingered MMR wasn't *eight*. Nor was it *eleven*, as fished from the binders.

It was *nine*. Three out of four.

So, the figure started at *eleven*, when the parents spoke to doctors between September 1996 and February 1997, fell to *nine* by the following August, by which time Wakefield had allegedly invoked his exclusion criterion, and then to *eight* by January 1998, when the paper was ready to print.

And, yet—get this—with that ninth case counted, a striking phenomenon was evident. The additional boy's mother volunteered a *two-month* link and yet the combined figure in that early, summer, version *still involved fourteen days*.

Fourteen days: the figure picked by John Wilson for his 1974 paper that triggered the DTP alarm. Fourteen days: the time frame in Wakefield's paper, twenty-four years later (and three and a half miles north), doing the same with MMR. Fourteen days: the link cited by the Arizona mother, Theresa Cedillo, before she halved the time to onset to seven days. And now revealed from those binders, the "2 weeks" as volunteered by Ms. Two at Hampstead for when her son's head-banging began.

But the fourteen days in the summer version was different. It wasn't the claimed *maximum* time between shot and symptom. In the summer version, that was *fifty-six days*. The maximum wasn't two weeks, but two months.

Rather, with *nine* complaints included in the math, fourteen days was the *average* time to onset.

One child was then dropped—the outlier eliminated—and the *average* became the *upper range*. Eight of twelve. Fourteen days maximum.

Average = 6.3.

This was complex, tricky stuff. Tough to get your head around. But serious malfeasance may lurk in complexity. Ask anybody working on Wall Street.

Infectious agents, I assume, know little of fortnights. So, could that switch from *two months* to *two weeks* maximum, and the survival of two weeks as first the average, then the range, be just a coincidence, or what?

I sometimes wondered whether somebody whispered, "No, Andy, I meant fourteen days *max*."

But that was just me. And when I struggled with the detail, PowerPoint was my friend for presentation. The summer version also showed that, upon Wakefield's revision, bowel disease had skyrocketed among the children (who hadn't returned to the Royal Free to be scoped again) as the data were progressively changed. I could even use my pointer to make a pie chart movie, illustrating how the cases rose: from about three, to eight, to eleven.

Neat as it was, though, it was nothing compared with the power of human testimony.

A promising source was the Californian, Mr. Eleven, who'd dashed from Hampstead with a pot on his knees. I meet with him twice: the first time in London when he'd come to watch the annual tennis tournament at Wimbledon. He was staying at a hotel near Sloane Square, Chelsea, with Ms. Eleven, Child Eleven, and the boy's brother.

Seated in the lobby, I show the father Wakefield's paper, which he'd never seen or heard of before. I tell him that his son was eleventh in the tables, but give no further details (or mention that I'd read the boy's poorly redacted report) until I obtain his reaction *cold*.

According to Table 2, labeled "Neuropsychiatric diagnosis," "1 week" elapsed between Child Eleven's MMR and his first behavioral symptom. But looking at the table, the father objects. First, he says, he'd been told that his son was the *thirteenth* seen (I also spoke with a mother who says *her* son was the eleventh). Then when I assure him that my information is accurate on this question, he denies the one-week link. "That's not right," he says, pointing at the journal, open in front of us. "That's not true," he adds.

His son received the shot at fourteen months. And medical records, quoted in the poorly redacted report, gave two versions of when his development ceased to be what Royal Free pediatricians called "normal." One said *thirteen months*—which was *before* vaccination—and the other, itemizing the "initial behavioural abnormality," said:

18 months: slowed speech patterns; Repetitive hand movements

So that was *four months after* the shot.

The father had given Wakefield that time frame, *four months*, even before he brought his boy to London. "The onset of his autistic like behaviors," Mr. Eleven wrote from his home in January 1997, "began around 18 months."

Where the "1 week" came from, Wakefield couldn't explain. "It is not possible at this point to say exactly what the symptoms were," he said in his affidavit, filed in Texas. He continued:

I can say, however, that some behavioral symptom was reported to have occurred in a one week period or the statement would not have been made.

The father saw these things differently, however. After digesting the paper back home in California, he emails me a request that spoke his mind. "Please let me know if Andrew W has his doctor's license revoked." And later he's more specific in his opinion:

If my son really is Patient 11, then the *Lancet* article is simply an outright fabrication.

His was the only family not enrolled in Barr's lawsuit. The British parents—guided by Ms. Two and Ms. Six—weren't so easy to deal with. Although my investigation began after Barr's lawsuit collapsed, confused families were encouraged to blame me. But when Ms. Four broke ranks, made contact, and produced documents, another crack in the paper yawned.

She gave me everything, from diary notes reporting Wakefield leading ward rounds ("Dr Wakefield & team of 5 came in to explain things"), to an email from his wife, Carmel, asking Ms. Four to phone her as the GMC made inquiries ("I am sorry to trouble you but i am trying to help andy"). But what really made the difference to evidencing the truth was, again, a fatal disparity.

Child Four ("most compelling") was given special prominence, with text in a column, as well as an entry in Table 2. The summer version of the paper said that, following vaccination, his "mother described a dramatic deterioration in behaviour starting four weeks later." And this account was backed in the binders.

Yet in the *published version*, the link had tightened. Now the text said the first symptom was *"the day after"* the triple shot, and Table 2 reported (squaring the timing with fourteen days):

Dramatic deterioration in behaviour immediately after MMR

Nothing read from the binders supported that claim. And Ms. Four insists that it's untrue. Not only did she *not* make any link at the time of her son's immunization but, even before the hearing on Euston Road had begun, she'd written to Wakefield's lawyers (in an email she later gives me) *telling them* that his paper was wrong.

"I did not say [my son's] behaviour dramatically changed immediately after MMR," she informed them. "I said within weeks."

She had wanted to come to London to give evidence at the hearing: not least on the horrors of her son's time on Malcolm Ward.

But after Wakefield's lawyers took a written statement of what she would say, she learned that she wasn't required.

"My concern is the paper and what happened at the hospital," she emails me, adding:

I know that paper is not right and fraudulent. I can see that from what was written about [my son].

TWENTY-SIX

- - - - - - - - - - - - - - - - - - - -

Cry Smear

For all but three of the 217 days of the General Medical Council hearing, nothing outside 350 Euston Road betrayed the mammoth inquiry within. From Mondays to Fridays, the street scene was the same: a six-lane divided highway of blue-black asphalt, where westbound vehicles picked up speed—surging from the ramp of a cut-and-cover underpass—while those heading eastbound crawled toward traffic lights in a haze of hydrocarbon exhaust.

But on the other three days, there was a little extra interest. On the north side of this slice of London's official inner ring road, police erected steel barriers around revolving glass doors, and maybe fifty, or sixty, people—mostly middle-aged women—clustered with hand-painted placards.

We're With Wakefield

Dr Wakefield Cares

Stop Hiding Vaccine Damage

The first such gathering was on day one of the hearing: when, at the rectangle of tables on the building's third floor, ninety-three pages of charges were read aloud by a tag team of GMC staff. But it was another—the first day on which Wakefield gave evidence—that I'll always remember most vividly. For that was the occasion when I made a mistake, which taught me so much about anti-vaccine campaigners that, as they exported their hero's crusade to the world, forearmed me.

Never again.

My fail was epic—if, looking back, understandable. That world was changing so fast. Just two weeks before my first story about Wakefield, a couple of Harvard University students launched a website called Facebook. When he threatened the little newspaper, the *Cambridge Evening News*, the inaugural YouTube video had been up for two months. And when a court order allowed me to read the *Lancet* kids' records, the first Twitter post was sixty-three days old.

That velocity of change would take time to absorb. Although I started in journalism on mechanical typewriters, I thought I was an early adopter. I trailblazed on the internet in July 1990 and had published a website since June 2000. But the sum of the parts of the great transformation hadn't upgraded my biology. In particular, I hadn't guessed how it would all come together when every last shoulder bag and pair of long pants came packing a video camera.

My mistake went like this. As I passed through the protest, I paused to speak to a man holding a placard:

Witch Hunt

His name was David Thrower: brown beard, fifty-seven, a public transport planner from the north of England, who in Richard Barr's lawsuit had sued SmithKline Beecham on behalf of his autistic son, Oliver.

Thrower was the author of what he called "A Briefing Note," avidly circulated by vaccine campaigners, republished as a download by Lenny Schafer in Sacramento, and cited from Canada to

New Zealand. It was the most detailed document that I'd ever see that argued MMR caused autism.

I'd received a copy from Ms. Six, four years before, and was struck by its autistic quality. Thrower's "note," at that time, ran to 159 pages, with an "Executive Summary," an index, appendix, sections 1 to 130 (in Parts A to M), all crammed with excerpts, and interpretations of research.

But, more memorable to me than its systematization, was its title:

MMR and Acquired Autism (Autistic Enterocolitis)

It seemed to me that Thrower didn't know what that meant: that this man, who played guru to parents seeking answers, hadn't even the courtesy toward those who trusted him to at least get his first sentence right. By the time I saw him on Euston Road, more-over, his note had swollen to 427 pages, with a new, longer title—which told me that he still didn't get it.

MMR Vaccine, Thimerosal and Regressive or Late Onset Autism ("Autistic Enterocolitis")

So, with an entirely legitimate journalistic purpose, I ask him, "What's 'autistic enterocolitis'?"

Thrower is surrounded by placard-wielding protesters, and he repeats my question, half-shouting above the traffic. "What's 'autistic enterocolitis'? Well, we don't know, do we?"

Well, *yes we do.* "We know what Wakefield says it is," I reply. "What does Wakefield say it is?"

"We'd be here all day if I said what Wakefield says it is."

That wasn't true. But I settle for less. "What's *enterocolitis*?"

Thrower doesn't know. Above his beard, his face furrows. He burbles like a sinking ship.

I keep up the pressure. "You don't know, do you?"

"You tell me, you tell me," he flusters, gripping his placard. "I've never set myself up as a medical expert."

But he had. *Oh, he had.* He'd done just that. You could pick countless passages from his note. "Examination of children has identified a novel form of inflammatory bowel disease, ileal-lymphoid nodular hyperplasia," he'd lectured, incorrectly, in both versions of his document. "This condition is very rare in non-autistic children." *Wrong.*

Having confirmed my suspicion, I turn to go inside. But a circle of angry women close in. A few call out, "It's a bowel disease, a bowel disease." One waves a poster showing an x-ray of constipation. And then, foolishly, I double down on my error.

"They didn't have bowel disease," I reply to one of the shouters. "Have you been in the hearing?"

"No, I haven't."

"Those children," I repeat, "didn't have bowel disease."

All captured in video clips.

Abuse levels rose. One woman lifts a sign: "End the Witch Hunt, Time for a Deer Hunt." So I step inside the building where, at the rectangle of tables, Wakefield has twisted the witness chair slightly (forty-five degrees toward the panel), which I guess he felt made him look more honest. The events on the street soon fade from my thoughts as—sitting by the door—I take notes.

Then sometime later—I guess a year or two—that day came back to bite me. A man named Alan Golding, an amateur filmmaker, spliced the clips together with a bunch of parent interviews, in a confection of targeted untruth. He claimed, wrongly, that I wasn't being paid to attend the hearing (therefore, I was probably funded by drug companies). And his party piece of smear was my remarks about bowel disease: purported proof that I was a fool, or a liar.

He'd got two special interviews with which to harm me. And in those there's no doubt he succeeded. One was with a high-haired woman named Heather Edwards, who'd apparently been present on Euston Road. And she'd produced for him a picture of her fifteen-year-old son, Josh, whose large intestine had been surgically removed.

"Within ten days of being seen at the Royal Free they had him in and found that, yes, he had exactly what they were finding in other autistic children," she said. "It was so badly diseased that he would be better off without his colon."

In Golding's video (viewed 150,000 times when I last checked YouTube), he intercut this interview with my al fresco comments: "They didn't have bowel disease" and "Have you been in the hearing?" I should simply have kept my lips zipped.

The glory days of readers' letters to newspapers had waned. Haters lambasted me online. "One *Lancet* 12 child (now an adult) had to have his entire damaged bowel removed," one campaigner crowed—saying what anyone who saw the video would think.

Golding's other triumph was with the irrepressible Ms. Two, who read aloud a letter from *Lancet* parents, organized by herself and Ms. Six. With short-cut gray hair, circular glasses, and chunky bangles, the sentinel mother had gained a little weight since our interview. And she was nothing if not convincing.

"All our children were referred to Professor Walker-Smith in the proper way, in order that their severe, longstanding, and distressing gastrointestinal symptoms could be fully investigated," she read for the camera. "All of the investigations were carried out without distress to our children. . . . We are appalled that the doctors have been the subject of this protracted inquiry."

Game, set, and match to Golding's video. But his creation wasn't as it appeared. Unencumbered by editorial, or legal, supervision—which weigh heavily on journalists and program-makers like me—he'd exploited the trusted vocabulary of television to market a misleading account. Most notably, Josh Edwards wasn't among the *Lancet* twelve. He'd nothing to do with the hearing. And, according to a report in Britain's top-selling newspaper, *The Sun*, his colectomy was performed at a different London hospital, after a likely food intolerance was diagnosed.

Thanks to that video, I'd endure years of abuse. But some knew the truth when they saw it. One was Ms. Four, listed as a signatory to the letter, who was shocked that her name had been used. Not only was she adamant that her son *didn't* have bowel disease, and insisted that he'd suffered horribly on Malcolm Ward, but she resolved to come to my aid.

"A few times I had a strong urge to contact you," she explained, turning over to me more than one hundred pages of documents, diaries, letters, emails, and minutes of phone calls that evidenced the case against the doctor without patients, no matter what the hearing might decide.

She wasn't alone in changing sides, moreover. After studying my reporting, parents phoned our news desk, offering Wakefield's flight numbers for his trips from the United States. I got complaints about his lack of "family values" at conference hotels. And above all, one person, whom I call my "special source," turned double agent to betray him.

"I had a situation where there were two men," this source explains of a thinking process before he or she began a decade-long collaboration with me: leaking documents, reports, and plots meant to damage me, from the foxholes of Wakefield's network. "One was a doctor and one was a journalist. One of them was saying 'white' and the other 'black.' They can't both be right. One of them was an honorable man. And one of them was a shyster."

I'd long known that Wakefield's people were out to get me. Not least because one wrote to say so. At 3:54 on a Wednesday morning, just four months after my first report, my laptop chimed for an incoming email from a woman that I'd then never heard of. Her name was Carol Stott, then aged forty-seven, with a PhD in epidemiology. Barr had hired her for his lawsuit to counter the evidence of Europe's most eminent autism expert, Professor Sir Michael Rutter.

Her message, two lines, was headed "game on" and said:

Try me, shit head.
Beleive me, you will lose.

Five more followed, in the space of an hour. "So go fuck yourself" . . . "Got it yet shit head. Try me" . . . "Twathead" . . . "Stick that where it feels good. shit head." Then, at 9:34 a.m., when I'd still not responded:

well, ur a bit slow on the uptake . . . twat.

She didn't hide her malice. She wanted me to feel it. She was Wakefield's key lieutenant. "We referred to Stott as 'the colonel,'" my special source says. "She was behind everything. She was the pivotal member of his team."

Five months later, Stott launched an attack website, and a year after began preparing for the GMC hearing, spawning the gatherings where I'd questioned Thrower. In a "confidential" email to eight collaborators, including Ms. Six, she wrote that there was a mailing going out to their people "possibly funded by Thoughtful House."

I'm not sure if Wakefield came through with the dough on that. But Stott wasn't short of money. According to Legal Aid Board documents, the Barr lawsuit paid her £100,000 in fees. And Wakefield (who described her as his "dear friend") bizarrely appointed her "visiting professor" of his Texas dope 'n' scope shop—with accounts of his organization Visceral showing further payments to her totaling almost £200,000.

The "group," as Stott called it, was a secret society that she ran at Wakefield's pleasure. Named the New Autism Initiative, it was open only to those who were vouched for by a member, and it hid behind a public campaign that they called "Cry Shame," with a website, registered two months before the hearing, by the *Lancet* brothers' mother, Ms. Six.

At first, I assumed Ms. Six was the brains. For sure, I was top of her list. "I used to think the only organization she didn't approach to put you in the shit with was the cat protection league," my special source recalls of hundreds of hours that this mother spent complaining to editors, judges, politicians, hospital managers, and anyone who might keep me from the facts.

But, as documents poured in from my covert collaborator, I realized who pulled the strings. In control were individuals with no developmentally challenged children. The mothers were less players than played. Behind "Cry Shame," and the Initiative lurking behind that, were the night mailer Stott and Ms. Two's lawyer, Clifford Miller: as poisonous as a pair of cane toads.

Where Stott was brazen, Miller was sly and more adept in the new age of information. Secretly, he operated an anonymous website, which he called "Child Health Safety," pumping out falsehoods—I have to say *lies*—for others to pick up, and repeat. Claiming to provide parents with "reliable information on child health safety," among his tributes to the man he also advised, he planted every kind of smear against me.

He claimed I "made up" stories in the *Sunday Times*; that the editor, John Witherow's position was "looking untenable"; and that I'd *admitted* my reports were "speculation."

Among the tricks he played to amplify his impact was to post comments around the web in his own name, Clifford Miller, touting material that he anonymously published, as if offering independent endorsement. On websites ranging from *Eco Child's Play* to *Advances in the History of Psychology* he posted, "It turns out journalist Brian Deer made it up," followed with links to his own online creation. "The 'Child Health Safety' website has become widely recognised as a reliable source," he claimed.

Schafer, in Sacramento, lapped up this stuff, inflaming his readers across America. And Miller, fifty-three, went further with the group: not only spreading the lie that I was working with the drug industry, but that "it can be proved" it paid for my stories.

Documents from my source also identified others. In addition to Stott and Miller, and Ms. Two and Ms. Six, there was a man named Stone, a woman called Stephen, and Wakefield chipping in as he pleased. Then, within that circle was a yet tighter ring, including Stott, Miller, and Wakefield. And as the giant medical council hearing staggered toward its climax, they pressed their troops into action.

For years, Wakefield had retained PR specialists to maximize his campaign's impact. Now, with money from Americans, he hired a man named Max Clifford—a silver-haired millionaire and Britain's top celebrity publicist—to circulate ruinous smears. To whet Max's appetite, Stott brought him to the hearing and later briefed a freelance tabloid reporter (who tells me he met Wakefield at Max Clifford's offices) to prepare an exposé—of me.

"A media outcry will force action," Wakefield promised Stott and Miller, in an email green-lighting the offensive.

Among their weapons were three letters they created, making outrageous allegations against me. Headed "Confidential—Final Text" they were to be issued to parents (but only those deemed "sound") for them to mail to various bodies (including my employers and the Metropolitan Police) in a bid to end my career.

Each letter began, "I am the parent of a child," and accused me (in Miller's comedy legalese) of various "criminal" acts, including that I "aided and abetted counselled or procured or conspired" in "criminally illegal" and "clandestine" activities, such as the obtaining of medical records.

"I was told that there were vast sums of money from pharmaceutical companies involved," their celebrity publicist told me later when we talk on the phone—before Max Clifford was arrested for sex offenses and sentenced to eight years in prison.

But the plot backfired. No newspaper would touch it. Nor would the police, of course. And its betrayal to me revealed a nest of Russian dolls at the heart of the campaign against vaccines. Here was the manipulation of vulnerable parents, as complaints written by Miller, and approved by Wakefield, were filed (without a comma changed) by Josh Edwards's mother, Heather, and others on Euston Road.

- - - - - - - - - - - - - - - - - - - -

TWENTY-SEVEN

An Elaborate Fraud

On the day that his career as a doctor ended, he looked like he couldn't give a damn. Leaving his seat vacant at the hearing in London, he instead took a chair in New York City, at NBC's Midtown studios. With no prosecuting counsel, or investigative journalist rooting through the evidence, at 7:43 he settled for six minutes with "the face of the *Today* show," Matt Lauer.

"It may sound like a strange way to start the interview," Lauer began, like he was quizzing an old friend about a favorite breakfast cereal, "but do I still refer to you as 'doctor'?"

Wakefield grinned. Easy peasy. "Yes," he replied. "They can't take away the fact that I have a medical degree."

This was Monday, May 24, 2010. At the rectangle of tables, five hours ahead in London, the hearing panel's chair, Surendra Kumar, had just wrapped up day 217. He'd read aloud his panel's "determinations" and "sanctions": discharging as "misguided" the endoscopist, Simon Murch, while ruling that Wakefield and Walker-Smith's misconduct meant they should be "erased from the medical register."

The lists of offenses found proven—against a criminal standard of sureness—just went on and on. Among much else, Wakefield was found to have carried out research without ethical approval or safeguards; caused kids who'd had no reported history of bowel symptoms to undergo invasive procedures; and to have dishonestly misled the Legal Aid Board (including one charge his own counsel described as "fraud") by diverting money from the purpose for which he'd gotten it.

"The panel is profoundly concerned that Dr. Wakefield repeatedly breached fundamental principles of research medicine," Kumar read from the five members' determination. "It concluded that his actions in this area alone were sufficient to amount to serious professional misconduct."

But that wasn't the end of it. He'd failed to ensure that the *Lancet* paper was "true and accurate." He'd dishonestly published "a misleading description of the patient population," dishonestly claimed that children came through the "normal channels," dishonestly failed to disclose the conflict of interest in his funding through Richard Barr, and didn't reveal his measles shot patents.

The panel, Kumar said, had made "findings of dishonesty in regard to his writing of a scientific paper that had major implications for public health." And it agreed that his "continued lack of insight" meant that his medical registration must end.

Today show viewers were told none of this. Lauer pitched kindergarten softball. Facing his guest, in lightwood armchairs on a translucent blue set (with a few flowers and books arranged on a side table), he then introduced clips from a half-hour *Dateline* show on the early phase of my investigation. Here was Wakefield, lecturing at a conference. Here was me in the *Sunday Times* newsroom. Forensic inquiry was there none.

LAUER: "So you'll look me in the eye and say that, at the time you were doing your research, you were guilty of no conflict of interest whatsoever?"

WAKEFIELD: "No, not at all. And had I been, it would have been disclosed."

That answer was preposterous. But Lauer—at the time, every American's handsome uncle—moved on swiftly against the clock. I'd given the GMC a videotape I obtained in which Wakefield enthralled mothers at a lecture in California with how he bought blood from kids (some as young as four) at his eldest son's birthday party.

Dateline had screened a segment of this event, in which, to Wakefield's audience's laughter, he'd joked about kids crying, fainting, and vomiting. *Hilarious. Ha ha. Go, Andy.*

"Were they paid for the samples?" Lauer asked in the *Dateline* excerpts.

"They were rewarded; they weren't paid," came the response.

"How were they rewarded?"

"At the end of the party they were given five pounds."

"Why isn't that paying them?"

"Well, it's not saying up-front, by coercing them, 'You do this and we're going to give you money,'" Wakefield replied. "It's saying, at the end of it, 'Here's a reward for helping.' It's a different thing, in ethical terms."

There had never been a market for blood in Britain. But *Today* made it look as if the campaigner had lost his license merely for this bizarre lack of ethics. Notwithstanding Lauer voicing that his guest had been found to have acted "dishonestly and irresponsibly," he moved on to argue about this and that, leaving Wakefield safe in his chair.

"Your study involved twelve children," Lauer said. "I've seen studies that involved hundreds of thousands of children that do not replicate your findings. And so, today, will you sit across from me and tell me that you believe there is a possible link between that particular vaccine—the MMR vaccine—and autism in children?"

A duel of studies? Wakefield's specialty. All he'd ever needed was to split the difference—*they* say *this*; *I* say *that*—and he'd win more adherents to his war. "Not only do I think it, but the American government has conceded that it exists," he said, in flat contradiction to that government's statements. "The point is, despite denying it in the public relations campaigns that they waged against me, and against the parents, they are conceding these cases in vaccine court."

The court, again, would expressly deny this. No case had ever been conceded over autism. And, with regard to his own views, he couldn't keep the story straight, even for twenty-four hours. While telling America one thing, he told Britain something else, as reported that day in the press. "I never made the claim at the time," he was quoted by both *The Guardian* and *The Telegraph* newspapers, "nor do I still make the claim that MMR is a cause of autism."

Later, he would tell a BBC radio network, "I have *never* said that vaccines cause autism."

His performance was as confident as a cat swatting flies. He knew he could handle any TV presenter, bypassing both media and medicine. He spoke to his base—confused, wounded mothers—to whom he'd looked for his living and meaning in life since refusing to replicate his research.

But journalism hadn't slept through the hearing on Euston Road. I'd got the changed pathology; the altered diagnoses; the kids with symptoms starting before, or *months* after; the secret contract with the Legal Aid Board; plus a mass of material from my investigations: the deal, the business schemes, and all of that. And one Wednesday in April—his eighteenth day in the witness chair—I'd observed an admission, wrung from his mouth like a molar without anesthetic.

"What I now want to ask you is where you make it clear that the children had come to the Royal Free in the first place, at least in the majority of cases," he was asked about his paper by counsel for the prosecution, the black-dressed Sally Smith QC, "because their parents, or in some cases their doctor through their parents, thought that MMR might have caused the damage?"

By this time, we'd heard the evidence, over and over. There was nowhere left to hide. "That is implicit to anyone reading this paper," he responded. "The group is self-referred because of the symptoms manifest by the children, including the history of a possible exposure to a vaccine, or an infection that has led to the problem."

Smith's question was dry. But it was, nonetheless, a killer. She wasn't a breakfast show anchor. If the parents had gone to the hospital to finger the vaccine, then the paper's first *finding* was invalid. The connection between the shot and autism wasn't *found* by vigilant doctors, as *Lancet* readers thought. It was an artifact of selection. *It was rigged.*

She put it to him twice. He'd once sued me for saying it. But, at last, he said it himself. "The patients, children, are self-referred based on their symptoms and their history," he told the GMC panel, itemizing his study's true inclusion criteria, and with me now emphasizing the news. "That contains the *three key elements* of an *environmental exposure*, gastrointestinal problems, and developmental regression."

One version for the hearing, painfully extracted. Another for America, and the world.

The medical council's findings vindicated my own. And now I received an unexpected request to set out details for a professional audience. My PowerPoint slides would now be augmented by a commission from *The BMJ*—*The Lancet*'s main competitor in the United Kingdom.

I'd already written a four-pager on the pathology: "Wakefield's 'Autistic Enterocolitis' Under the Microscope." Then, following the council's verdicts, and his appearance with Lauer, *The BMJ*'s chief editor, Fiona Godlee, a doctor, suggested a three-part series. Born in San Francisco and educated at one of England's more eccentric private schools, she was a mischievous intellectual mother figure of medical evidence, who'd fearlessly taken on drug companies and other interests with take-no-prisoner investigations.

So I did it—a series titled "Secrets of the MMR Scare"—which, including references and summary tables, totaled twenty-four thousand words, across nineteen pages, including an elegant front cover. They took six months to write, check, and check again. Six or seven editors went over the copy. Godlee's deputy examined the medical hearing record. A pediatrician and a pathologist carried out peer review. A lawyer billed for sixty hours of work.

I met with Godlee many times over those months. And one afternoon, she uttered an F-word I suspect was rarely heard at the journal. We'd been going through my copy with the lawyer, Godwin Busuttil, when the editor-in-chief made an observation.

"It's fraud," she said. "You need to say that clearly."

This wasn't wholly news, since the GMC found the same in the dishonesty rulings on the paper. I stated it on my website, and in the *Sunday Times*. There could be no doubt of the facts.

"Well," I responded to Godlee's judgment, "if you think that, it's you who should say it."

So, emerging on the first Thursday of January 2011, a press notice went out from *The BMJ*'s London offices to provoke more than breakfast-time banter. Announcing publication of my first installment (which kicked off with the Californian Mr. Eleven's reaction to the *Lancet* paper), it quoted from an accompanying *BMJ* editorial: denouncing Wakefield's study as what the journal's editors judged to be "an elaborate fraud."

> Who perpetrated this fraud? There is no doubt that it was Wakefield. Is it possible that he was wrong, but not dishonest: that he was

so incompetent that he was unable to fairly describe the project, or to report even one of the 12 children's cases accurately? No. A great deal of thought and effort must have gone into drafting the paper to achieve the results he wanted: the discrepancies all led in one direction; misreporting was gross.

First to pick up was CNN. The reporter: Anderson Cooper. This was no schmooze job. This was America's news bloodhound, on the scent of drama. And he got it. "Just hours ago," this media prizefighter, youthful beyond his age, spoke into the camera, face stern, eyes narrowed, "the *British Medical Journal, BMJ,* did something extremely rare for a scientific journal. It accused a researcher, Andrew Wakefield, of *outright fraud.*"

Cooper explained how this wasn't just "any" researcher; that the 1998 study had "literally changed the way many parents think about vaccines"; and how it was based on just twelve children. "Many parents, desperate for answers around the world, embraced Wakefield's claims," he said.

Clips showed the actors Jenny McCarthy and her then boyfriend, the zany Jim Carrey. Another followed: of the congressional committee chair, Dan Burton. And then—Cooper's coup—came a live interview with his subject, from an anti-vaccine conference in Jamaica.

Blinking out of darkness via Skype, split-screen, this time Wakefield wasn't in control. "Well, you know, I've had to put up with this man's false allegations for many, many years," he said of me, speaking uncommonly fast, for him. "I've written a book . . ."

"But this is not just one man," Cooper interrupted. "This is published in the *British Medical Journal.*"

"And I have not as yet had a chance to read that. But I have read his multiple allegations, on many occasions. He is a hit man. He has been brought in to take me down because they are very

concerned about the adverse reactions to vaccines that are occurring in children."

"Sir, let me stop you right there. You say he's a 'hit man,' and
he'd been 'brought in' by 'they.' Who is 'they'? Who is he a hit man
for? This is an independent journalist who's won many awards."

Wakefield snorted. "And he's, you know, who's brought this
man in? Who's paying this man? I don't know. But I do know for
sure that he's not a journalist like you are."

"Well, he's actually signed a document guaranteeing he has no
financial interest in any of this, or no financial connections to anyone who has an interest in this."

Now for the smear. Where else could Wakefield go? The
"pharma shill gambit," as some call it. "Well, that's interesting he
should say that because he was supported in his investigation by
the Association of the British Pharmaceutical Industry, which is
funded directly and exclusively by the pharmaceutical industry."

I'd last dealt with this trade group in 1993—about sending me
its compendium of product data sheets—and I'd *interviewed one
doctor* who did consultancy work for a related company, regarding the European Clinical Trials Directive. But either Wakefield
repeated this absurd fabrication, cooked up on the network that
my special source betrayed, or he'd no explanation for his predicament. By this stage of his unmasking, one thing was clear: that
one of us was fooling the world.

But could it be me? Could I—a man who has never bought a
car—have tricked the editors and lawyers of a world-ranking
newspaper for which I'd worked on staff, contract, shifts, and freelance for almost thirty years? Could I have bamboozled the executives, producers, and lawyers of the UK's Channel 4 network,
a five-member panel of the General Medical Council, Mr. Justice
Eady, sitting in the High Court, and the editors, lawyers, and peer
reviewers of one of the world's top five medical journals? Could
documents published on my website be faked? Could I have per-

jured myself in a Texas legal deposition? Could my investigations of Big Pharma be a charade?

Cooper's report struck the spot like a crossbow arrow, shuddering as it thumped into the bulls-eye. And, for the next three days, Godlee and I taxied around the London bureaus of the North American networks, and Al Jazeera, while the press roared the story around the planet.

Backing the coverage came a slew of punchy editorials: from the *Wall Street Journal* to the *New Zealand Herald*; from the *Toronto Star* to *The Australian*.

The *New York Times* was among many who honored me with a namecheck from the editorial board:

> Now the *British Medical Journal* has taken the extraordinary step of publishing a lengthy report by Brian Deer, the British investigative journalist who first brought the paper's flaws to light, and has put its own reputation on the line by endorsing his findings.

That was some pick-up, with its impact calibrated in a survey two weeks later. According to the Harris polling organization, 47 percent of Americans—almost 145 million people—were aware of the *BMJ* verdict. "Forty-seven percent is a huge number," commented the pollster's chair, "and this is a relatively new thing, so it's remarkable that they have heard of it."

A result, I'd say, for old-fashioned journalism. And, in the months that followed, I went on the road, after a flurry of speaking invitations.

The first was with the Canadian Journalism Foundation, which, in February of that year, asked me to spend a week in Toronto: the city of Wakefield's founding epiphany. On top of my talks, there was a college dinner, a chat show, a meeting with the board of the *Globe & Mail*, and another with the national broadcaster.

"I shook hands with Brian Deer," tweeted a perceptive young man at Ryerson University, from a vast, crowded lecture on investigative reporting. "This is to me what meeting Madonna is to idiots."

And yet, in the glow of a job well done, I felt more melancholy than satisfied. It was right that my investigation had spoken truth to power. But, as my career-defining story, I would have been happier to have proved that vaccines cause autism. That would have been something: a much bigger splash. And, for all of the benefit that would have accrued to children in unraveling some part of the mysteries of autism, to my kind of reporter, the story was the name of the game.

Is it new? Is it true? Do we have it to ourselves? Read all about it. *Exclusive.*

And there and then, in Canada's metropolitan heart, with the February sidewalks piled with snow, I skipped a dinner, planning to nurse my jet lag with a movie at the Holiday Inn. Then for maybe twenty minutes, I blew steam along Bloor Street, contemplating Wakefield's thoughts, a quarter century before, as he pondered the cause of Crohn's disease. If I bought a pint of Guinness, I amused myself, and gazed hard enough for where my life would go next, maybe in the froth of Ireland's famous black beverage, I too might find a big idea.

As a teenaged student at the University of Warwick, I used to drink Guinness, in a bar called Frank's Bar. It cost fifteen and a half pence a pint. But as I'd grown older, I found it gave me indigestion, and my alcohol of choice switched to bourbon. Nothing seems impossible if you drink enough of that. And should any inspiration settle upon your aspirations, you have to hope you only hurt yourself.

Alone with a pint of Guinness on a freezing Toronto night? *Nah.* I went to bed.

AVENGED

TWENTY-EIGHT

- - - - - - - - - - - - - - - - - - - -

Rock Bottom

The British are a famously apologetic people. "Sorry" seems to be the easiest word. A polling organization found, for instance, that if you bump into a Brit, and it's not their fault, they are 50 percent more likely to voice self-blame than would a similarly innocent American. The exclamation in Her Majesty's United Kingdom, moreover, is rarely "Excuse me." It's: "Sorry."

At the hearing that canceled his medical license, Wakefield was sorry as hell. "Sorry, could you take me to the page?" he'd ask. Or, "I am sorry, I cannot remember." On the April Wednesday when he, finally, admitted that MMR concern was an inclusion criterion—and therefore not a *finding*, as he claimed in *The Lancet*—he used the word fourteen times.

But he still wouldn't regret any matter of substance. He didn't do guilt, or shame. Even when confronted with a letter *he* wrote, for instance, stating that his research for the twelve-child study was commissioned from him by the Legal Aid Board, he said it wasn't true, and the reason he gave was that he was "only communicating to an accountant." He called no witnesses. No parent, coauthor, colleague, or admirer. And after a parent, Ms. Twelve, gave evidence for the prosecution (as with the vaccine chief, David

Salisbury), his leading counsel, Kieran Coonan, rose to say, "No questions."

He did make a concession when the paper was published. Readers spotted that "abnormal laboratory tests" he'd listed in Table 1 were actually normal ("These errors do not affect the conclusions," he replied). But the only thing—*the only thing*—he conceded to my findings was that the man in the video, laughing about buying blood at a children's birthday party, was, indeed, himself.

"Mr. Deer's implications of fraud against me are claims that a trained physician and researcher of good standing had suddenly decided he was going to fake data for his own enrichment," he said in a fifty-eight page complaint about my *Sunday Times* reporting, which he abandoned after I pressed for adjudication. "The notion that any researcher can cook such data in any fashion that can be slipped past the medical community for his personal benefit is patent nonsense."

In response to my "Secrets of the MMR Scare" series, he mirrored the allegation, much as he'd done with his conflict of interest charges against government doctors and scientists. "There was fraud," he'd say. "And the fraud was not on the part of me, or my colleagues, but on the part of Brian Deer, and the *British Medical Journal*, who concocted a story of fraud, in order to discredit me."

The traditional British way might have served him better. There was nothing at the hearing about whether vaccines caused autism. Nor was that the focus of my investigation. He could have appeared on Euston Road, or the Brooklyn Bridge, and acknowledged "misunderstandings," "confusions," or "slipups." He could have taken a course on ethics, or professed new insight. And then the GMC, after a doctor-friendly interval, might well have restored his license.

But he just couldn't do it. It wasn't in his nature. So, instead, he told supporters, with no evidence I know of, that he was "framed by the pharmaceutical industry." He blamed the media, especially the mogul Rupert Murdoch, whose family controlled the group whose UK subsidiary published the *Sunday Times* (and also Fox News, who platformed Wakefield a lot). He besmirched judges, including "someone very high up" in Texas. He even insulted the GMC panel (including two senior professionals from outside medicine), claiming it aimed to "discredit" doctors investigating vaccine safety.

In short, he sought comfort in the status of *victim*. A victim of the sinister *they*. "There was this very incestuous cabal involving government, media, and the industry, that all wanted this outcome," he announced online. "Against them there was *me*. Now, accuse a researcher of fraud in thirty seconds, and it takes a lifetime to turn that around. And *they* know that."

They would be the government that, through its legal aid scheme, paid him to manufacture a case against MMR; the media (including Murdoch's) that championed him for years; and the drug industry that funded him, and flew him, for a decade. And *thirty seconds*? More like *seven years*. But, instead of saying "sorry," came this pity-me narrative: repackaging his unmasking as proof of conspiracy, and his ruin as evidence of integrity.

It worked, too. After he toured the conferences, where for years he'd drawn the confused and vulnerable under his influence, abuse poured into my inbox.

> I believe one day soon the truth will come out regarding dr Wakefield and his research. You know what you have done and it's possibly on par with hitler. Evil beyond belief!

And:

> You are one of the most evil, lying awful men that has ever lived. So many children are sick or have died because of you. You will answer to God one day.

And:

> You are pure scum. You ruined a persons life. You are complicit
> in furthering the harm done to millions of children around the
> world.

The establishment, in which he'd once longed for prominence, wasn't as easily impressed. The Royal College of Pathologists, where he gained a fellowship by the submission of papers,
stripped him of its letters after his name. The Royal College of
Surgeons would have done the same, if he hadn't already resigned, years before, by not paying his fees. In the United States,
he was asked to quit Thoughtful House. And the *American Journal of Gastroenterology* retracted the data he presented on Capitol Hill.

Even gastroenterologists working with autism piled in at the
time he was weakest. In the same month that the medical council announced its findings, twenty-seven specialists from across
the United States published an eighteen-page "consensus statement" on bowel disorders in autism, in which they shredded his
purported syndrome. Pointing out, among other things, that lymphoid hyperplasia was found in "children with typical development," they ruled:

> The existence of a gastrointestinal disturbance specific to persons
> with ASDs (eg, "autistic enterocolitis") has not been established.

Here was disgrace—and with a big red stamp applied to the research at its heart. From bottom left to top right, on each online
page, a single word, in uppercase:

RETRACTED

"It was utterly clear, without any ambiguity at all, that the statements in the paper were utterly false," Richard Horton, *The Lancet*'s chief editor, told *The Guardian*. "I feel I was deceived."

In the absence of remorse, there could be no insight. Therefore, no comeback was possible. But, despite a now sometimes bedraggled appearance, with bloodshot eyes and hobo haircuts, the ex-doctor wasn't quite down and out. There was severance income from his various jobs, probably some residue of the deal with Richard Barr, and the benefit of a land deal—including the building of a five-bedroom house in west London—which he'd pursued as a sideline to medicine.

Plus, of course, he retained that famous "charisma," enhanced as an Englishman in America.

First up in the wilderness came a big idea that took him to the state of Minnesota. For some reason, it boasted the United States' biggest community with origins in Somalia, and anti-vaccine groups hoped to gain a toehold. At several appearances in a Minneapolis restaurant—with attendances estimated at around one hundred—he was reported as explaining that, while the incidence of autism was rocketing in the US Somali community, their old country had *no known cases.*

"It is solvable, it has a cause, it had a beginning and it must have an end," he told his new audience, in December 2010, as captured by Minnesota Public Radio. "We cannot accept the damage that is being done to all of these children. It is completely unacceptable."

The hint he brought was of an *environmental exposure.* But he punched beyond his reach. What he didn't know—or didn't think mattered—was that the Somali language had no word for "autism," and so it couldn't be reported in Somalia. Even in developed countries, it was only a construct (rescued from "brain damage," "mental handicap," and "retardation" by pick 'n' mix menus of late twentieth-century psychiatry). No surprise, the Horn of Africa lacked the lingo.

"We have 'schizophrenia,' 'crazy,' or 'not crazy,'" explains Marian Ahmed, cofounder of Somali Parents Autism Network, in a

YouTube video. "That's it. Every Somali will tell you that. We don't have 'autism.' There's no name, no word, for us. We need to create one."

He couldn't help with that. And, crazy or not crazy, he was a herald of misfortune in Minnesota. Just six weeks after his first event, a US-born boy of Somali descent returned from Kenya, incubating measles, and triggered a small outbreak in Minneapolis. He was thirty months old, and hadn't received MMR. Twenty-one cases were identified in the community, and linked through PCR sequencing.

Historically, immunization had been trusted by Somali families. In 2004, 91 percent of children of that descent in Minnesota received MMR as recommended. But, as Wakefield's claims had crossed the Atlantic, with Dan Burton's hearings, Lenny Schafer's newsletters, and lawyers' recruiting for the vaccine court fiasco, the proportion had slumped to just 54 percent by the time he appeared in person.

Nobody died. But here was a warning of what was coming—and his next expedition wasn't so lucky. Following his trajectory, on which everything gets weirder, he'd started a relationship during the medical council hearing with an autism entrepreneur. Her name was Polly Tommey, who followed him to Texas, bringing her family (including her husband), where with Wakefield she launched a media enterprise—the Autism Media Channel—which became ensnared in a horrifying incident.

Tommey—blonde and lithe—was ten years his junior. She'd worked as a body double in movies. The parent of a boy, Billy, with developmental issues, she mixed for-profit businesses with charitable ventures, allowing her to make a living from campaigning. Departing England, she left a memory of her upper body on roadside billboards, gazing full-face from above low-cut, black lingerie, with the slogan: *Hello Boys . . .*"

Husband, Jonathan, was a fitness instructor, who set up as a "clinical nutritionist." And, together, they'd hit it big on British TV, promoting the pig hormone "secretin" (later reported in manufacturers' trials to be useless). They scored two appearances in a tabloid current affairs show, called *Trevor McDonald Tonight*, where their first slot was sixteen minutes, and the second twenty-five, with the presenter reading aloud full-screen captions advertising the couple's website. From this they spun a glossy magazine and were on their way to making a living off of autism.

Before long, Polly Tommey was shifting forty thousand copies of the monthly *Autism File*. And, stateside, this became the base for ambitions with Wakefield for a reality TV show. For the pilot, they filmed children sent for scoping in New York City by the former Thoughtful House endoscopist, Arthur Krigsman. He was the doctor who'd mentioned the family videos in the Cedillo affair (and who fled Lenox Hill Hospital, in Midtown Manhattan, after management inquiries into his practice).

The show wasn't picked up. But, as destiny beckoned, they got footage to shape their future. They filmed a fourteen-year-old Chicago boy, Alex Spourdalakis, who was profoundly developmentally challenged. On camera, he was rushed to Krigsman for ileocolonoscopy, and later filmed in a hospital, restrained naked to the waist, with Wakefield speaking from his bedside.

Twelve days later, the boy was dead, at the hands of his mother and godmother. Stressed beyond coping (and I've seen that filming), they'd first tried to poison him with sleeping pills. Then they stabbed him four times in the chest with a kitchen knife, almost severed his hand while trying to slit his wrist, killed the cat, and tried to take their own lives.

More bad luck. But now the ex-doctor had found a new vocation. It was to serve him well in his next career move: to extend his reach from the United States to everywhere that people had screens. "If you want to beat the media, you become the media," he'd declare. "*I am now a filmmaker.*"

But he'd hit rock bottom. His speaking schedule became strange— appearing with climate change denialists; "truthers" who said the World Trade Center attack was an inside job; and a man who claimed that aircraft trailed toxins to control the masses. Then he turned up on a "Conspira-Sea Cruise." It set sail for a week from San Pedro, California, with one hundred eccentrics paying three thousand bucks, and a fellow speaker who was arrested upon landing.

"Brian Deer—and please, you can write this—is a *psychopath*," Wakefield told journalists, who joined the cruise for cheap laughs. "I say that not in a pejorative way, I say that is what Brian Deer is. He's a psychopath. He manifests all the characteristics of a psychopath."

Could it get any worse? Well, yes, it could. Crazy or not crazy, a yet greater humiliation had been steaming quietly forward in London.

As the work of a tribunal set up by Parliament, the medical council's findings of professional misconduct were subject to re- view by the courts. Wakefield's lawyers didn't support any appeal on his behalf, but the Australian professor's were rightly optimis- tic of overturning their client's conviction. In John Walker-Smith's case, the panel had committed a procedural error in the way it set out its findings.

Because he changed his story—from arguing that the scopings were ethically approved research to claiming that they were solely for patient care—he wrong-footed the panel, which didn't appre- ciate how profoundly this impacted their task. The flopping of binders was great for me. But it meant that each child's case would need to be evaluated separately—essentially a dozen hearings, just on them, back to back—with the reasoning for each conclusion set out.

That wasn't the burden of the charges facing Wakefield. His research was unarguably research. "My case was related to entirely different issues to those that concerned Dr. Wakefield," the Australian pointed out in a statement. "Every investigative procedure I ordered was to find out what was wrong with the children."

If that wasn't true, and he was really doing research, then he wouldn't just be wrong. He'd be *lying*. "The panel had no alternative," explained Mr. Justice Mitting, the judge who heard the appeal at the Royal Courts of Justice, "but to decide whether Professor Walker-Smith had told the truth."

And yet it didn't. Overwhelmed by the scale of the three doctors' indictments, the panel skipped this foundational decision. Like in the trial of *Best v. Wellcome*—in which the drug company submitted that the mother was "confused"—the panel hadn't grasped the nettle.

Wakefield, of course, pounced on his accomplice's acquittal: telling his supporters that, by implication—if only his own—*he* was acquitted too. But that wasn't the judge's view. Nor the professor's, who as a result of the hearing, and no doubt my journalism, had gotten a new view of the man who persuaded him to leave Barts Hospital for Hampstead. And, now aged seventy-five, he would have his say in the most devastating, silent critique.

In his autobiography, *Enduring Memories*—published a few weeks before I interviewed Ms. Two—he'd simpered like a teenager with a crush on his teacher. "Shades of Princess Diana," he'd gushed.

He is tall, handsome, fluent, charismatic and above all a man of conviction. He is a man of utter sincerity and honesty. In reality the out of fashion term "crusader after truth" would best describe him.

Now, retired from medicine, at home in north London, John Walker-Smith reread those words: a hymn to the blight of his career. He then calmly deleted them, closed up the surrounding paragraphs, and dispatched his memories for reprinting.

TWENTY-NINE

Payback Time

In what I've called the golden age of ink on paper, Wakefield's disgrace would have been the end of the matter. The crisis over vaccines would have been shut down—just like it was in the 1980s with DTP—once nothing new to excite readers remained.

Neurologist John Wilson had accepted his fate. "There was a very wise doctor who made the introductory observations to a new batch of medical students," he tells me, when I catch up with him in the 1990s, "that, in twenty years' time half of what you now learn will be proved to be wrong. But the problem is: we don't know which half."

For sure, the "MMR doctor" was finished in the press. Britain's editors had got the message that for years they'd been duped. And even those who'd given him the most favorable coverage signaled that they'd had enough. As the *Daily Mail* reported in April 2013, during a measles outbreak in which one man died:

> The MMR vaccine controversy was a case of scientific misconduct which triggered an unwarranted health scare.

But Wakefield wasn't done. They couldn't shut him down. With the emergence of epoch-changing, peer-to-peer social media, anybody could narrowcast, exploiting algorithms that lured the unwary into markets of misinformation. Thus it was that, on Monday, August 18, 2014, when (just as we thought he was all washed up) a post appeared on his Facebook page that would herald an incredible new chapter. Over the next two years, he was to achieve the biggest impact on public attitudes to vaccination that had been seen in the United States since the 1930s, when President Franklin Roosevelt's legendary "March of Dimes" launched a nationwide crusade against polio.

GET THIS OUT!!!!!

With five exclamation marks! Andrew Wakefield's fight back had begun.

Those who clicked on a link reached a video-sharing site and were hit with a dramatic countdown. To the *whirring* sound of a twentieth-century projector, feeding celluloid film from spool to spool, a rotating clock arm swished in one-second circles, window-wiping images in black and white, like the start of an ancient newsreel.

They went: **7**—*swish*—a group of African American boys with President Obama; **6**—*swish*—a *New York Times* report about Minneapolis Somalis with autism; **5**—*swish*—the nameplate of the US Centers for Disease Control and Prevention, in Atlanta, Georgia; **4**—*swish*—a silhouette face; and **3**—*swish*—a needle.

"Oh, my god, I cannot believe we did what we did," comes a disembodied male voice, in telephone quality. "But we did. It's all there. It's all there."

That was for the ears. This was for the eyes, a simultaneous sensory input:

CDC Whistleblower Confesses to Vaccine-Autism Fraud

Then:

an Autism Media Channel exclusive

"This is a real story of a real fraud," Wakefield says, now appearing full face in a pressed white shirt, with spectacles hung from a button. "Deliberate, high-level deception of the American people, with disastrous consequences for its children's health."

For nine and a half minutes, his "exclusive" continues with—at face value—remarkable disclosures. A scientist at the CDC's headquarters in Atlanta had turned "whistleblower," Wakefield says, to reveal "fraud" in the execution of a ten-year-old government study of whether the MMR vaccine caused autism.

"So troubling was the fraud," Wakefield, now aged fifty-seven, explains, "that one of the CDC researchers broke ranks."

Now another man appears, in three-quarter-face close-up, to confirm the ex-doctor's account. This is one Brian Hooker—not the "whistleblower" himself—but a science teacher at a Northern Californian Christian arts college, with a PhD in biochemical engineering. Wakefield announces him as the "father of a vaccine-injured child" and a "vaccine safety researcher."

Hooker, fifty, is overweight, receding, with a craggy, mustached face and a chin sinking to his neck. The shot cuts to reveal him in a brown plaid jacket and a yellow high-collared shirt. He says that one day he'd received an unsolicited phone call and, "lo and behold," it was "Bill Thompson," the scientist.

"Dr. Thompson had appointed me his priest," Hooker says. "And when he appointed me his priest, then he started confessing. And we have had many, many phone exchanges. We've exchanged dozens of emails. And he has released quite compelling information regarding fraud and malfeasance in the CDC."

Thompson, also fifty, and a psychologist by training, had coauthored the study in question. It was published, with little fanfare, in February 2004 in the high-rank journal *Pediatrics*. Using painfully convoluted methods, it had sought to investigate Wakefield's proposed link by comparing the age of vaccination among Atlanta children with autism against those who were developmentally typical. More than six hundred records from the first group were studied, plus three times that number from the second.

"The assumption," the eight-page paper explained, "is that if the MMR vaccine increases the risk of autism, which usually develops before 24 months of age, then children who are vaccinated at younger ages would have a higher risk."

Wakefield's nine and a half minutes don't address such detail. They focus on snippets from Thompson. On the ex-doctor's advice, Hooker had surreptitiously recorded four conversations, in which the scientist had talked about his government research and life at the public health agency.

"It's the lowest point in my career that I went along with that paper," he's heard telling Hooker, in one of ten brief clips sprinkled through the video. "I'm completely ashamed of what I did," he says in another. And, "I'm not going to lie. I basically have stopped lying."

For an internet video of the mid-2010s, Wakefield's was uncommonly slick. With his business partner and special friend, Polly Tommey, he'd hired a Canadian editor who'd worked on commercials and who knew a thing or two about pace. And with somber tone and sinister music, those nine and a half minutes would evolve into a project that would erupt across America and around the world.

Documents are screened, including one marked "restricted access." But the meat is a string of abrupt clipped-and-spliced phrases, sometimes repeated for impact. "It's the lowest point in my career that I went along with that paper [00:25] . . . It's the lowest point in my career that I went along with that paper [03:41] . . . It's the lowest point in my career that I went along with that paper [08:36]."

On analysis, it's really that obvious.

The gist of Thompson's concerns—barely mentioned in the video—was that the paper had left out statistically significant data that he felt should have been included. In raw figures on the kids, an excess of autism had shown up in a subgroup: African American boys vaccinated with MMR within certain specified age bands.

His fellow authors, however, thought the finding was implausible, and that a smaller sample, predefined in the protocol, gave a more valid comparison. These were children on whom additional information was available (from birth certificates) but among whom any "race effect" was weaker.

I read Thompson's documents, and study *Pediatrics*. To me, what he'd gotten was terrific. In the paper's Table 3, the CDC researchers had left out two lines of data that, had they been favorable to the vaccine's safety profile, I'm pretty sure they would have included. I'm also pretty sure that, if the scientist had taken his worries to the *Washington Post*, the *New York Times*, or even to me, any of us would have written up the story.

It touched so perfectly on a longstanding debate about the nature of the Atlanta agency. Many observers had argued that the CDC's immunization role was strategically conflicted: tasked not only with researching vaccine safety, but also for promoting the shots. Here was an opportunity to reopen that debate with an example of how this might work.

"The question would have to be, is the reason why that data is not given in that table," I ask a former senior CDC manager, who supervised Thompson's project, "because the team working on it had an eye to public opinion, and public concern? Because journalists might pounce on that and say, 'Look, there's a "race effect"?'"

"I think that's a good question," my source agrees.

To any half-decent journalist with a front-of-the-paper beat, even that concession was explosive. At the time, the agency was weathering controversy, after a researcher, Poul Thorsen, who worked on MMR studies, was indicted for allegedly stealing CDC grants worth a million dollars, and spending them on everything from a Harley Davidson to a house.

The way I saw it was that, if Thompson was right and CDC staff had sanitized Table 3, what else might they sanitize in *any other* table that didn't suit institutional goals? But Thompson told Hooker, Hooker told Wakefield, and Wakefield seemed to see the matter as less about the challenges of conflicts of interest, and more about his own situation.

GET THIS OUT!!!!!

SENIOR GOVERNMENT SCIENTIST BREAKS 13 YEARS OF SILENCE ON CDC'S VACCINE-AUTISM FRAUD

AFRICAN AMERICAN BOYS WILLFULLY EXPOSED TO HIGH RISK OF AUTISM FROM MMR VACCINE

Now I'm thrown back onto my earlier investigation into "the world's first AIDS vaccine," AidsVax. After that surefire flop, in February 2003, the ex-CDC staffers behind the company VaxGen had likewise rooted among subgroups. "There were 78% fewer HIV infections among black volunteers," they breathlessly reported to financial markets on the day their trial was unblinded. "The results are statistically significant."

Most likely the complaint against the *Pediatrics* paper was another such dredging from subgroup analyses, and the data the result of a mistake. The CDC study had long been recognized as defectively designed and, three years before, had been excluded from a review of vaccine safety carried out by the prestigious US Institute of Medicine on grounds of "very serious methodological limitations."

But, within hours of Wakefield's post, it was rippling online as an *"OMG! Must Watch."*

Whistleblower admits CDC fraud, lies and deceit. They knew MMR was causing autism.

Even the future president, Donald Trump, leapt in. "The doctors lied," he posted on Twitter.

The video would later be revamped as a feature-length movie, where the impact of its claims would be explosive. But even for the environment of social media—among the sayings of Einstein, and dogs playing piano—Wakefield went so heavy on the crazy in his script that he nearly strangled his creation at birth. Two minutes were devoted to the Tuskegee syphilis experiment of the mid-twentieth century, in which African American men were left untreated for the disease. And he likened Thompson's coauthors, most of them women, to that century's most brutal mass killers.

"You see," Wakefield snarls, over images including children in Auschwitz camp stripes, "vile as the crimes of Stalin, Pol Pot, and Hitler were, these men were not hypocrites, their motives ambiguous, or their rhetoric glazed with apparent care and compassion."

The only snag was: his story wasn't true. The allegations of fraud were his own. Thompson himself—who'd not known that his musings were being secretly recorded—issued clarification soon after. His concerns, he said, in a four-hundred-word statement, were that, apart from omitting significant data, he felt the original study plan wasn't stuck to.

"Reasonable scientists can and do differ in their interpretation of information," he said, in words that any competent and honest journalist, but not Wakefield, would be obliged to quote in any reporting. And, "I want to be absolutely clear that I believe vaccines have saved and continue to save countless lives. I would never suggest that any parent avoid vaccinating children of any race."

Remarkably, given the mischief that was to follow the video, apart from Thompson hand-wringing, ripped out of context, all Wakefield and Hooker had of substance from the scientist was a five-word phrase, used at 03:46 and 05:37, upon which they'd hung their own meanings.

We didn't report significant findings.

Obviously, that wasn't a claim of fraud. Things may be *wrong* for all kinds of reasons. Indeed, the recordings of the psychologist (which I obtain soon after) show not only that Hooker had sought to *provoke* such a claim, but that he failed, three times in a row.

Hooker's billing as a "vaccine safety researcher" didn't do justice to his status. For twelve years, he'd been suing through the vaccine court system on behalf of his autistic son, Stephen. Hooker worked with a campaign called Generation Rescue, fronted by the actor Jenny McCarthy, which (at the time) blamed autism on thimerosal. And the day before the phone call, from which all but one of the clips was harvested, he'd been presented by Wakefield, at a conference of mostly mothers, with the Andrew J. Wakefield Award for Courage in Medicine.

Thompson—with cropped gray hair and wire-framed glasses— *hadn't* made Hooker his "priest." Like me, he was garrulous and made the same mistake that tripped me on Euston Road. Just like I'd interacted with a litigant father (he of the massive "note," which he didn't understand), the scientist had engaged with another such parent whose behavior should have raised a red flag.

Using the US's powerful, but slow, freedom of information laws, Hooker had filed more than one hundred applications with the CDC, many of which were passed to Thompson for processing. Since joining the agency in 1998, his most acclaimed work had been on vaccine safety, including not only the 2004 *Pediatrics* paper, but also a twelve-pager in September 2007 on thimerosal, in the *New England Journal of Medicine*. But, as study after study dismissed any autism link, Thompson's managers had lost interest in his area of achievement, and he longed to regain their attention.

"I want to be a resource," he told Hooker, hoping to renew public pressure. "I want to be valuable to you. I want you to have someone in the system that can give you feedback."

If he'd been half as cautious as he proposed for his studies, he would likely have been better off. He was captured in the recordings laughing inappropriately, bad-mouthing colleagues (a veteran epidemiologist was "like a used car salesman," a female researcher "a twenty-five-year-old bimbo"), and discussing his personal health. Self-describing as "mentally ill," and "blowing up and stuff like that," he spoke of human resources issues and a "delusional episode," using "delusional" in its clinical meaning.

"But I am settling down," he tells Hooker. "The good news is I am settling down."

His new bestie replies, "I need you sane."

Under pressure within himself, Thompson was vulnerable. And, behind Hooker, was no stranger to treachery. Fifteen years before, a British government doctor hiding behind a pseudonym— "George" he called himself—had secretly met Wakefield and Richard Barr (at the same railway station where I met Ms. Four) to allege foot-dragging over the two brands of MMR whose recall first launched this saga. But out of concern for his family, George wouldn't go public.

So Wakefield first threatened then betrayed him. "As this broadcast is going out on the internet, I hope 'George' gets to see this," the then doctor without patients told a delighted conference crowd, before revealing the man's identity on YouTube. "Because I was very tempted to disclose his name and address, and contact details to this audience [laughter]. And I will do that, if he feels he can't come forward spontaneously [applause]."

That was the voice of the doctor who fooled the world. He reveled in his power to terrorize. And he saw in Thompson the opportunity that it was: to mirror the complaints found proven against himself, by accusing the government of fraud. "*They say this, I say that.*" Here was a chance to reclaim familiar territory— and in the months that followed, he did.

"So I said to Brian, 'Brian, are you recording these conversations?'" he boasted later of his advice to Hooker. "'Whistleblowers can disappear as easily as they came. They are like a fish on a hook. And your job is to get them into the boat.'"

And how they tried. After the call in the video, Hooker phoned Thompson again. All they'd got so far was loose talk. No fraud. So, three weeks later, the teacher had another go—sounding to me like he was working from notes.

Within barely one minute of Thompson picking up, Hooker got down to business. "I want to talk to you about the MMR study," he said.

The psychologist's response was, "Yep."

Then a little back-and-forth. A bit of "right . . . yep . . . yep." Then Hooker tossed a barbed, leading, question. "And then you basically deviated from that particular plan in order to reduce the statistical significance that you saw in the African American cohort?"

In order to reduce. An admission of *intent*. All Thompson had to say was, "Yep."

But Thompson didn't. The interpretation was Hooker's. He hadn't got his fish on the hook. "Well, we, we um, we *didn't report* findings that, um, all I will tell you is we didn't report those findings," the CDC man replied. "And I can tell you what other—I can tell you what the other—coauthors will say."

The next question for a journalist would be, "What will they say?" But Hooker merely responded, "Uh-huh."

"They will say that they didn't think the race variable was reliable," Thompson continued, "is what they're gonna say."

Hooker moved on. Briefly argumentative, he spoke of spread-sheets, and stuff like that, before closing in on the topic of thimer-osal. "I mean I've got all the records," he said. "I see that on the *New England Journal of Medicine* paper you were pressured to downplay the relationship between thimerosal and tics."

Pressured to downplay. Again, *intent.* But, again, the fish didn't bite. "Well, er, let me just say this," Thompson replied, referring to a minor paper he'd published with a student. "I did a follow-up study, 'cause I wanted my opinion on the record."

How Wakefield's heart must have sunk with these responses. Then his associate tried for a third time. "So, did you feel in the 2007 paper that you were pressured to downplay significant results?"

"No," replied Thompson.

Damn.

In fact, during that same follow-up call, on June 12, 2014, they even stumbled toward a possible reason why the autism rates among some vaccinated black kids had appeared to be significantly different. African American children tended to get worse health care, and when they eventually turned up with developmental issues, they were offered the shots they'd missed.

It likely wasn't vaccination causing their autism, but their au-tism causing vaccination.

In short, the study was badly designed (using data collected for quite different reasons). Its results could never have been solid. "So, in fact, you could argue the [*Pediatrics*] paper is like a bunch of crap because the better educated moms get their kids vacci-nated earlier," Thompson said, laughing. "We had a crap study because we weren't even adjusting for the appropriate variable."

"Right, right," Hooker replied.

"I never even thought of that."

Yep.

Wakefield and Hooker must have known they were struggling. But cold as revenge is reputedly best served, for the ex-doctor even the smell was delicious. For not only had the *Pediatrics* report targeted his *Lancet* paper, but another man in this stew, if that's what it was, had been on Wakefield's menu for years.

Thompson was first author of the *New England Journal* paper. But not of the *Pediatrics* report. In pride of place on that was an epidemiologist: Frank DeStefano, whom I interview within days of the video. And he was one of the two senior CDC experts who in 1998 had been invited by *The Lancet* to contribute a response to the twelve-child paper, in which they dumped on the Royal Free research.

DeStefano et al.—the *Pediatrics* paper—was "the worst fraud in the history of medicine," Wakefield claimed later, and "the greatest medical fraud in the history of the world."

Now, that was some projection. Investigations found nothing. But the entrapment of Thompson was a triumph. Forget controversies over any individual shot: DTP, HPV, even MMR. Those clipped and spliced snippets of the "CDC whistleblower" would now be leveraged for an unprecedented crusade: to persuade the world that *all* vaccines were suspect.

- - - - - - - - - - - - - - - - - - - -

THIRTY

Vaxxed

The voice is female. And relatively young. Maybe thirty, or thirty-five. It rises from a crowd gathered in Santa Monica, California. As soft as a mother's kiss. "We love you."

Up four stone steps outside the entrance to City Hall, Wakefield calls back, "I love you too."

A second woman shouts, "We're sticking up for our children."

I hear another yell simply, "Yes."

It's a Friday in July, 2015, at shortly after five p.m. Maybe two hundred people—overwhelmingly women—have gathered in this wealthy, west of Los Angeles beach community to vent fury over a change in the law. After an outbreak of measles at the Disneyland amusement park—forty minutes southeast on Interstate 5—the government of California has resorted to coercion against a tiny awkward squad of young parents. If their children aren't vaccinated according to schedule, they may in future be barred from school.

The crowd began assembling, hours earlier, on Ocean Avenue, beside a twelve-foot Civil War cannon. Then they'd marched two blocks to the municipal headquarters—built in the 1930s, with the clean lines of a steamship—chanting, "The parents call the shots, the parents call the shots," and waving Magic Marker placards at passing cars.

Health freedom

Stop forced vaccinations

Repeal SB-277

Five speakers are listed, but it's Wakefield they love. Without him, the day would be lacking. He greets his audience with an *aw shucks* grin, like a naughty (fifty-eight-year-old) boy. He wears a baggy white shirt, with two buttons undone, and firm creases in the fabric that suggest, at least to me, that he might have just bought it this morning. It's what Men's Wearhouse would market as "regular fit," with plenty to tuck where the mound of his belly meets his too-tight, beltless pants.

"We stand at the moment, I believe, in a defining moment in the history of this country," he begins, glancing left and right through hooded gray eyes, as a breeze catches his hair like the fronds of nearby palm trees. He fingers a microphone stand.

A cheer goes up, with applause, cries of "*Yes,*" and high-pitched whoops. "*Wooo-ooo.*"

"And I think future generations will remember that this was the beginning of the end of the first republic of the United States of America."

A state senate bill as the end of the republic? Now there's an idea. But he drops it. His topic today isn't the latest law (which bars exemptions from vaccination on any but medical grounds), but a more immediate concern to himself. Now stripped of any medical or scientific status, he's thrown back on these women as the source of the power that he has wielded for the past twenty years.

"You have had something taken away from you as a people," he says, looking out and down at the latest contingent, who grin at him in T-shirts and sunglasses. "And I'm not talking about your rights in SB-277. I believe your innate instinct for the well-being of your children has been usurped by pediatricians and doctors who think they know better, when they do not."

More cheers and whoops. "*Woo-oo-oo. Woo-oo-oo.*"

"There is *no one* who knows a child better than her mother."

So far, so good. He spoke to the mood. Many of the faces that he probes from the steps are of "health freedom" activists, "alternative practitioners," and parents riled up over "choice." But, while making sense to these, his targets are others: mothers of children with developmental issues.

"And I read the other day an anecdotal story of a patient who had died from exposure to measles," he continues, stabbing the air with a ringless left hand. "An *anecdote*. And that anecdote made the news. But your anecdotes are irrelevant, apparently. Your hundreds, your thousands, your tens of thousands, your millions of anecdotes about what happened to your children."

Parents' anecdotes. Vaccine damage stories. They had long been his faithful standby. Study after study, after study, after study, had reported no link between vaccination and the numbers of children diagnosed with autism. Massive class actions had come and gone. And yet there remained these reports of injuries— recollections, assumptions, even some deceptions—much as there were when *Newsnight*'s woman in scarlet had sent him his sentinel case.

Back then was Child Two, and the mother, Ms. Two. But now, in the years that he'd lived in the United States, his parent followers had swelled to many thousands. And if they didn't blink, and stuck with their stories, what doctor, scientist, judge, or journalist was equipped to prove them—or him—wrong?

"Because *everything* I have learned about vaccine safety, and about autism in particular, comes from you," he says from the steps. "It does not come from my profession. All they have taught me is what we don't know. What I've learnt from you is what we *do* know, and what we *should* know, and what we should continue to pursue."

Here was his creed since the start of his crusade: that (notwithstanding those who'd accused him of fraud and fabrication) the parents were *always right*. Even in September 1997, he'd told an anti-vaccine conference in Alexandria, Virginia, that the "first lesson" in medicine was to "listen to the patient, or the patient's parents," because "they will tell you the answer."

I thought that was likely something his father had once said—a neurologist trained before the age of scanning—as a joke to a medical student son. If you don't know what's wrong, ask the patient to tell you (and then bill them for the diagnosis, if you can). Certainly, when I try it at a lecture to a roomful of pediatricians, those who don't laugh look at the ceiling.

But as the years had passed, and science had let him down, he'd turned to the infallible mother. "Keep faith with your instincts," he'd urged at a rally in Washington, DC. "Trust your instincts," he told the group to whom he'd praised Italian opera. It was "the most powerful force in the world." And in a blog, he went further: sourcing this knowledge to a land of impossible proof.

> Such instinct operates in a realm, and according to a set of rules, that are not accessible to the physical laws of the universe.

Parents vs. science. Faith vs. facts. A religion: with him as the priest. "So my message to you, please people," he calls from the steps, "is you must go back and you must trust your instincts. You must believe in yourselves as you have never done before, and do not let that be taken away from you."

He must have used that argument many hundreds of times, as he trekked round autism conferences. But that Friday afternoon there was fire in his speech that drew air from something unsaid. Still unknown to most present, his script would soon change, as anecdotes would be joined by the whistleblower story, in a bid to revisit old triumphs.

By now, William Thompson had issued a second statement, challenging Wakefield's account. It was true that the psychologist believed his CDC colleagues had "intentionally withheld controversial findings," but he didn't agree about the upshot. "The fact that we found a strong statistically significant finding among black males does not mean that there was a true association between the MMR vaccine and autism-like features," he said, striking at the heart of Wakefield's latest argument. "This result would have probably have led to designing additional better studies."

He'd got that right. DeStefano et al. had designed a defective study. In comparing cohorts of kids with and without autism to see which was vaccinated *earliest*, they failed to account for the way the onset of symptoms might impact on the first group's behavior. Simply put, some children (especially those, like African Americans, with lower vaccination rates) might have received their first shots *after* their parents joined the desperate quest, loading misleading associations into the stats.

As the 2004 *Pediatrics* paper explained in its "Methods" section, instead of trying to match symptoms against the dates shots were given, the project had compared *age bands* for the children—as if this wasn't a fatal mistake.

> Other studies have tried to address the possible relationship to MMR vaccination by examining the temporal relationship between vaccination and onset of initial parental concern, date of first diagnosis of autism, or onset of regression (if present). We had incomplete information on these events, so we compared the distribution of ages at first MMR vaccination between case and control children.

Asking the wrong question, they got wrong answers, generating what Thompson described in a phone call with the father,

Brian Hooker, as "something they couldn't understand." The misconceived study (which one senior pediatrician tells me he thought was a "job creation scheme for epidemiologists") had been hugely expensive, and might have provoked public disquiet if abandoned. But two decades on—thanks to the psychologist's office politics and Wakefield's dishonesty—it had resurfaced to ignite the most damaging immunization controversy since NBC's "Vaccine Roulette."

You say "fraud," I say "fraud." Wakefield mirrored his critics. And standing among the mothers, at the foot of the steps at Santa Monica, was just the man to polish his glass. His name was Del Bigtree, aged forty-five: dressed in a purple T-shirt, with a mane of wavy gray hair, holding a 35mm camera at nose height.

He was gathering material to repackage the crusade and finish what Wakefield started with his video.

At the time of the Facebook "*Get this out!!!!!*," Bigtree had worked as a TV producer for a daytime magazine show, *The Doctors*. His credits included "Late Night Snacking Mistakes" and "Chest Wrinkle Cream Put to the Test." Brash, fast-talking, and prone to flights of fantasy, he presented himself as an "Emmy Award–winning producer," in which guise he'd gone to work for Wakefield. In fact, the network ranked him at position twenty-eight in a thirty-six-strong team that won the prize for CBS. And his mother chips in that he acquired people skills from "a lot of years he did waiting on tables."

Bigtree's instinct was to make the most of what he'd got. And in the whistleblower story he'd got plenty. In the months that followed the Santa Monica event, he took the ex-doctor's nine-and-a-half-minute video, scrubbed it of Stalin, Pol Pot, and Hitler, made Wakefield the star, inserted human interest, gave it a name, *Vaxxed*, stretched it to a running time of ninety-one minutes, and launched it as the centerpiece of an assault on vaccination of a like never seen before.

As ever, it drew on parents' grim anecdotes. "She lost all acquired speech," "Within days he stopped talking," "She had seizures every day for the rest of her life until she died in my arms."

But such pain was now threaded into a whistleblower narrative—in which its creators interviewed each other. Omitting Thompson's statements that contradicted their claims (information any ethical filmmaker would be obliged to include), front and center was its "director"—Wakefield—playing himself as a vindicated victim of injustice.

In twenty-four appearances—from seven seconds in length to nearly three minutes—he was presented as merely an ex-bowel researcher, approached out of the blue by a random mother, and then selflessly dedicating his life. Years later, he's approached by Brian Hooker, as if a stranger, with the news of Thompson proving him right.

"*Wow, really?*" Wakefield recalls, onscreen, as his reaction to the psychologist's information about the *Pediatrics* study. "After everything that had happened. Everything we'd all been through. Everything that the families had suffered for the last fifteen years. And the CDC had known all along there was this MMR-autism risk."

Also onscreen were Bigtree and Polly Tommey, the English autism entrepreneur. The former—*Vaxxed*'s producer—appeared sixteen times, sometimes speaking as if a medical expert. And the latter—co-owner of the film's production company—supplied the boutique anecdote. In seven appearances, totaling eight minutes, she and her husband, Jonathan, said their son didn't "wake up" to the child he'd been after a seizure on the day of his shot.

Here was home video meets *Triumph of the Will*. "We have a piece of the movie that was cut," Wakefield would tell an overwhelmingly black audience, for instance, in the Compton district of Los Angeles. "And it's a picture of Red Square, at the height of Soviet power. And there are thousands of people marching in precise step. There are missiles and tanks. And the power of the structure is massive, and could never be overturned. Yet it disappeared in the blink of an eye, led by one man."

Bigtree's advice was, wisely, adopted. But Wakefield was no passenger on the project. Much like he won drug companies to fund him at Hampstead, he turned his charms to raising enormous sums of cash, which would only be revealed, in June 2019, by reporters Lena Sun and Amy Brittain, in a *Washington Post* investigation. A New York hedge fund millionaire, Bernard Selz, seventy-nine, and his wife, Lisa Selz, sixty-eight, were reported to have given $3 million to Wakefield, Tommey, and Bigtree—including two hundred thousand for Wakefield to sue the *British Medical Journal* and me.

And then . . . and then . . . *Vaxxed* hit the big time. That dependable *charisma* paid off. He got himself introduced to an actor, Grace Hightower (it was said that he slipped onto a movie set where she worked), who wasn't only the mother to a teenage son with autism, but was married at the time to the boy's seventy-two-year-old father: the A-lister Robert De Niro.

Here was a name to add a footnote to history: De Niro threw his weight behind *Vaxxed*. First booking it for a festival that he produced in Manhattan, and then withdrawing it after a deluge of condemnation, he brought publicity the Selzes' money couldn't buy. He even appeared at breakfast on the NBC network, recommending that viewers "must see" it.

"There are many people who will come out and say 'No, I saw my kid change, like overnight,'" the double Oscar-winner told *Today* host Willie Geist, three days after *Vaxxed* was released in New York City, on April 1, 2016.

"Is that the experience you had, Robert?" Geist responded. "Something changed overnight?"

"My wife says that. I don't remember."

Now Wakefield was *made*. One way or another. With the Selzes and De Niros, he was laughing. Hardly had *Today* taken its next commercial break than the ex-doctor had a deal with a Los Angeles distributor to take his crusade from city hall steps into movie houses, coast to coast.

No question, something remarkable was happening: a transformation in anti-vaccine campaigning. In the next six months, *Vaxxed* reportedly grossed more than $1.1 million, playing some weeks at nearly one hundred locations. And employing an app, Gathr—a theater-on-demand service (which booked multiplex screens if enough customers reserved tickets)—some audiences were six hundred strong.

It was an extraordinary feat, thanks to the De Niros and Selzes, igniting parents' fear of children's vaccines not seen since the 1980s. With celebrity and money they overrode science, achieving in the United States what was accomplished in London with that twelve-child paper in the Atrium.

To get Wakefield's team from location to location, a long-wheelbase Coachmen motorhome was bought, sprayed black, and driven from city to city. It was emblazoned with the film's title and slogans in red and white:

Where there's risk, there must be choice

We are not government property

Trundling freeways and throwing open its doors at parking lots and gas stations, here was a road trip like a band on tour: a nationwide mobilization. And with advance publicity through social media, at key pit stops, the vehicle became a studio: spreading in real time through Facebook and Periscope visitors' stories about "what happened" to children.

"When suddenly law and order breaks down, and I can get away with some shit that I can't now," says a man named Curt Linderman, who climbs into the bus with talk of the "fascistic Deep State" and produces a loaded pistol, "I'm gonna come looking for you. It's as simple as that. I want retribution, and I want revenge for my son."

Until I learned of their funding from the New York investor, I thought the trio's demeanor remained eerily upbeat for the dark stories being collected on the tour. Tommey, in particular, laughed, giggled, and chirped, plainly having a wonderful time. "You guys are amazing," she tells the gunman and his wife. "I think we've never been so high on YouTube."

More money poured in, and a new message poured out: now Wakefield ruled that *all* shots were suspect. As the "documentary" credits rolled at the end of each screening, he, Bigtree, and Tommey often pulled out chairs, to sit and field questions. And there they led audiences beyond the *Vaxxed* script into a frenzy of escalating allegation.

For a while, the ex-doctor remained relatively cool. Returning to Santa Monica, two weeks after the film's release, he lectured audiences in near-professional tones. The hepatitis B vaccine was "noted to be associated with multiple sclerosis," he claimed. Thimerosal was "a major player in neurodevelopmental disorders." Aluminum as an additive "had the potential for great harm," and injecting it into children was "insanity."

But, as the tour went forward, he grew ever bolder, until half the population were victims. "We are dumbing down the nation," he declared, four months later, in Austin, Texas, flailing his arms in a black *Vaxxed* T-shirt. "And people are saying it's the schools. It's not the school system, but it's a biological phenomenon. You don't see it in girls. Girls aren't failing. Boys are failing. Why are boys failing? *Why?* Because boys are susceptible to these toxic insults early in life."

Those insults, he argued, weren't just injuries. They were injuries intentionally inflicted. "They decided to lie and to cheat and to deprive you of informed consent for your children," he railed at his audience, "and to damage the brains of millions."

Tommey followed his lead, like she followed him to America. "No more killing of our babies," she'd say. "They give our kids the injection, and we go back and tell them what's happened to our child. And they can see it. It's not just your child, or my child. It's millions of children. So they know exactly what they're doing."

Here was the journey that led to Donald Trump, then crisscrossing America like themselves. In that year of rebellion—2016—when the United States was stunned by Trump's defeat of Hillary Clinton, and Britain narrowly voted to leave the European Union, here were campaigners who grasped the paradox of the age: that the more incredible and outlandish their claims, the more these might spread and be believed.

Screenings were packed—sometimes in big theaters. And, at the end, they delivered more spectacle. As closing credits rolled, and house lights rose, Bigtree stepped forward and offered an invitation: part daytime host, part revivalist minister, and part purveyor of some miraculous remedy.

"Will every parent, or family member, with a vaccine-injured family member, please stand up at this time."

Or, "Would everyone who has a vaccine-injured family member just please stand up, right now."

His words varied slightly from screening to screening—from Nashville to Boise, San Francisco to Pittsburgh—but the request and the response didn't change. Dozens among the audience—overwhelmingly women—rose from their seats, alone, or in clusters, to declare a vaccine victim. There was one over here, two over there, and a family at the back, in the gloom. Soon it would seem that maybe a quarter of those present were silently affirming their instincts.

"Look how many people just stood up," Bigtree continued, here in small-town Utah. "The official statement by our medical community is that one in a million children is injured by a vaccine. Do you realize what the population of Provo would have to be if that is true?"

To any parent unsure about the cause of a child's issues, here was surely a moment of decision. If so many present gave such visible testimony—primed by ninety-one minutes of Andrew Wakefield—wasn't this a time to stand? *Why not?*

"I had a woman grabbed me last night," Bigtree told one local TV station. "I was walking out of the Q&A and she just grabbed me, and was *sobbing*."

Nobody could doubt the showmanship. But, at best, those mothers were guessing. Right or wrong, they assembled two-and-two together, just like those before them in England. And here was the product of the same optical illusion as I exposed behind the twelve-child paper. Even before the black bus had set off across country, nearly six thousand families had filed with the vaccine court to sue for compensation over a child's autistic issues: easily enough to salt these screenings, with parents, grandparents, siblings, and friends.

Who would ever guess at how it was done? *He* said *they* said; *they* said *he* said. Together, they agreed: *it was true*. Behold, a cauldron of self-verification. And so it went on.

Woo-oo-oo.

Anecdotes were scooped, standings were recorded for a sequel, *Vaxxed II*, and Q&As delivered to bounce online, narrowcasting the spectacle around the world. And as the mothers—some weeping—filed out into the dark, vox pops were captured and contact names taken to package and export their pain.

THIRTY-ONE

Wakefield's World

As the *Vaxxed* bus trucked across the United States, back in Washington, DC, a different note was sounded over the merits of vaccinating children. On the last Tuesday of September 2016, speeches rang out from beneath forests of furled flags. A certificate was signed and cradled in display. Group photographs were posed for participants to take home. Even a cake was cut.

Adiós Sarampión y Rubéola
Bye-bye Measles and Rubella

Those present had flown in to represent two continents at a meeting of the Pan American Health Organization (PAHO). That day, its tail was up. With the last cases mopped from an outbreak in Brazil, measles was officially declared "eliminated" from their region, meaning that transmission of the virus had been halted for more than a year from the Canadian Arctic to the Chilean Cape Horn.

"To the ministers of health assembled here today," proclaimed Merceline Dahl-Regis, chief medical officer of the Bahamas government, from the ceremonial room platform of PAHO's curving, modernist headquarters building next to the US Department of

State, "your colleagues, your children, your grandchildren, and generations to come will be able to see you in that photograph, on this day, when we have declared the Americas free of endemic measles."

This moment had been targeted for twenty-two years: since PAHO—one of six regions of the World Health Organization—vowed to send measles the way of smallpox: into extinction. That triumph might be the next step—from *elimination* in the Americas to *eradication* from Earth—when the virus would be entombed in high security labs and, after more certificates, speeches, and photographs, vaccination against it might end.

Everybody hoped that one day this might happen. PAHO had blazed the trail. The biology was hopeful for the RNA microbe. Its closest relative had already been caged. In June 2011—five years before that Tuesday—flags had been out at the United Nations Food and Agriculture Organization at the funeral of rinderpest: only the second infectious disease to be eradicated. A member of the same *Morbillivirus* genus of paramyxovirus bugs, it raised the dream that measles (along with the enterovirus polio) might eventually be immunized into oblivion.

"Measles can be stopped," the WHO's director-general, Margaret Chan, told applauding PAHO dignitaries from thirty-five countries and four associate members, following Dahl-Regis's speech from the platform. "It is my hope that other regions of the world are encouraged by the success of the Americas."

They had reason to clap. The stats told the story. PAHO ran one arm of a worldwide campaign that, in fifteen years, had seen measles deaths fall from half a million children, annually, to a little over ninety thousand. The projects they'd rolled out across North and South America had proved a showcase of what vaccines could achieve.

But even as Chan spoke—of "strong national immunization programs," "dedicated financing," and "political commitment"—

beyond the sumptuous wood-lined ceremonial chamber, with its semicircle of seating, and four official languages, measles was making a comeback.

The first sign was bureaucratic. Just three weeks after the *adiós* to *sarampión*, a report was discussed at the WHO in Geneva, warning that progress to eradication was "slowing." Then six months later, in April 2017, came a full-on outbreak, with nearly eighty cases, in the heartland of PAHO's biggest member. In Minneapolis, Minnesota—where Wakefield had shared his wisdom in the winter of 2010–11—the Somali community was blighted for a second time with a disease that seemed to follow him like a smell.

By now he was an openly anti-vaccine campaigner, publicly declaring, "If I had a baby, I would not vaccinate them." And with many taking such advice, and skipping protection, the Somalis were easy prey. WHO models showed that, to irrevocably break the bug's transmission, 95 percent of a community need to be immune. Yet, among these African American citizens, the reported vaccination rate had fallen to 42 percent in the aftermath of his intervention.

"Anti-Vaccine Activists," headlined the *Washington Post*, "Spark a State's Worst Measles Outbreak in Decades."

Wakefield told the newspaper, "I don't feel responsible." But, just weeks after the publicity for his earlier visits, his supporters had launched a group targeting the Somalis: the so-called "Vaccine Safety Council of Minnesota." This had talked up vaccine risks and belittled clinical measles, with many of the same arguments that were fashioned in England for Richard Barr's newsletters and fact sheets.

"It's funny how they try to make this 'outbreak' look like a big deal," was how one supporter shrugged off a disease that could sometimes cause pneumonia, blindness, deafness, brain damage, or, very rarely, a lingering death. "With proper nutrition and rest, the measles is a nasty cold with a rash. It's not fun but it's also not a crisis."

Wakefield didn't reappear. He was busy with *Vaxxed*. But his associates couldn't resist. After reports of children getting sick, a friend of his, Mark Blaxill—who'd started a national group, Safe-Minds, and who accompanied the ex-doctor to Donald Trump's inauguration ball—flew to Minneapolis, like a tornado chaser, drawn to the thrill of the danger. "Parents have rights," he was reported telling a meeting of mostly Somali Americans, in the same city restaurant where Wakefield had spoken. "Families have rights. And that's what's important to protect."

But this wasn't how those working for eradication saw it. Minnesota was but a volley in a bounce back of disease to defy the WHO. In Europe, major outbreaks had been spattering from the East, like cluster bombs popping in a jungle. Romania, then Italy, Greece, Serbia, France, and Britain were hit. In South Asia, too: the Philippines, Vietnam, India, Thailand, and Myanmar.

Wakefield appeared to be pleased with himself. "I have been in this battle, this war, for twenty-two years now," he said, in a mood of calm ecstasy, at a public meeting in Paris, France, in February 2017. "And this is the first time, in all that time, that we are truly winning."

Through 2017 and 2018, measles cases soared around the globe. Poland, Kazakhstan, Georgia, Albania . . . Europe reported the worst figures in two decades, linked to faltering levels of immunization. Italy experienced a six-fold jump. In France, four hundred reported cases became twenty-five hundred. And Ukrainian government data showed that, in a single year, five thousand leapt to fifty-three thousand.

"We risk losing decades of progress," warned WHO deputy director-general Soumya Swaminathan, in a statement from Geneva in November 2018. "The resurgence of measles is of serious concern, with extended outbreaks occurring across regions, and particularly in countries that had achieved, or were close to achieving, measles elimination."

It wasn't all Wakefield. In addition to the virus's mysterious ebbs and flows, Italy was bewitched by a comedian, Beppe Grillo, who, before storming into politics, had made a film attacking vaccines, released weeks after the twelve-child paper. In Thailand and Indonesia, Islamic clerics condemned the use of pork gelatin in some shots. In Uttar Pradesh, India, a rumor went around that immunization caused impotence. And in a slew of countries, from Poland to Venezuela, political upheavals took a toll.

Yet, seemingly everywhere, his name was invoked: as I learn most forcefully in Brazil. There, monthly measles reports jumped from none in December 2017 to six thousand the following November. And, as I climb into a taxi to cross São Paulo, a magnificently named epidemiologist, Cristiano Corrêa de Azevedo Marques, turns to me in the back seat, introduces himself, and states the problem, as he sees it.

"It's amazing, that paper of 1998," he says, "is still having an effect here in the popular mind."

Brazil had been lauded as Latin America's high achiever. Since the year 2000, its measles immunizations had tracked PAHO's targets. But in 2017, the picture abruptly changed, and uptake graphs, previously flatlining success, slumped to little more than 70 percent, as parents became scared, or indifferent.

"It was a shock to me," says Helena Sato, a pediatrician and head of São Paulo state's immunization programs, when we meet in September 2018 amid a cluster of hospitals and academic and research units at the state's Centro de Vigilância Epidemiológica. "People just didn't show up at the clinics."

"And that's new?" I ask.

"That was something that happened first last year," she replies. "It was completely unexpected."

PAHO's crowing may have encouraged complacency. If measles was eliminated, as media reported, then maybe parents saw no reason to vaccinate. But that was a decision that, in those changing times, was weighed with Wakefield's fingers on the scale.

Pediatric neurologist José Salomão Schwartzman didn't doubt it. He blamed the ex-doctor and *The Lancet*. "Every day in my practice I hear this question, 'Is there a relationship between vaccinations and autism?'" he tells me, six thousand miles from London, in his office at Mackenzie University, São Paulo. "Once you create an urban myth, it is very difficult for people to forget it."

Yet it wasn't only echoes from far away, and years ago, that had spooked Brazil's young families. Wakefield's influence was here and now. He'd *become the media*, as he'd said he would. As he achieved resurrection in the United States, he spawned clickbait globally for countless online presences: now mixing English with a cacophony of languages (Mandarin . . . Spanish . . . Arabic . . . French) promoting him and his masterwork, *Vaxxed*.

In Brazil, Facebook pages were easy to find: with names like "O Lado Obscuro Das Vacinas" (The dark side of vaccines) and "Vacinas—Por Uma Escolha Consciênte" (Vaccines—a matter of personal choice). The platform hosted his messages in a mix of Portuguese and English, consumed by tens, or hundreds, of thousands. And now, like in many countries, his reach was greater still: entering the lives of those who hadn't even searched— through autism, baby care, or family groups—via messaging networks such as WhatsApp.

Here were reports of *Vaxxed*'s New York premier; links to downloads subtitled in Portuguese; false claims that a "CDC whistleblower" admitted to "fraude"; Robert De Niro's appearance on NBC's *Today*; pictures of the black bus on its United States tour; and video bloggers hailing the "documentary."

Such material, moreover, wasn't here and there, now and then. It was recycled, over and over, sometimes day after day, from bedrooms and kitchens, laptops and phones, by obsessed, anonymous individuals.

Robert De Niro é Ameaçado Pela Máfia Farmacéutica

Autismo após vacina da MMR

Here too were videos of Wakefield lecturing ("I believe that vaccines cause autism," he says) and his associate, Del Bigtree (now earning $146,000 a year, plus expenses, funded by the New York millionaire Bernard Selz), claiming conspiracy as the reason why so few doctors and scientists agreed with him.

"The really sad thing is the amount of doctors that I've spoken to that say to me, 'Del, I know that vaccines are causing autism. But I won't say it on camera because the pharmaceutical industry will destroy my career, just like they did to Andy Wakefield.'"

And it wasn't just dissemblers who touted the agenda. Tech behemoths such as Amazon and Apple pushed the product, as the *Times* of London reported in a splash:

Web giants profit from anti-vaccine fraud's video

But what did Wakefield care now about the *Times*?

Favored jurisdictions were blessed with personal appearances. Polly Tommey drew the long straw and was dispatched to Australia. And just as Blaxill had chased the tornado to Minneapolis, Wakefield turned up in Poland.

He was having a great time. He'd found no cure for Crohn's, or remedy for autism, no vaccine, no nothing in medicine. But now he was a man delivering fear, guilt, and disease to everywhere with an internet connection. "It was only yesterday that the president went on television to sing the praises of vaccines," he laughed into Periscope, from a restaurant in Bologna, Italy. "So the film has got them terribly, terribly worried."

He was right about that. He'd gotten governments worried. By the turn of the year into 2019, the WHO was listing what it called "vaccine hesitancy" as among the top ten "threats to global health," and the United States faced its worst tally of measles in more than thirty years.

In the wake of my investigation, Britain had seen confidence rebound. But now planners watched graphs plunge once more. The National Health Service warned of a "time bomb" of disease, and the government's health secretary said he would "require" social media to take down what he called "lies."

Internationally, talk of compulsion was now commonplace—although some governments had long invoked it. Poland, for instance, had levied fines on nonvaccinators under rules from the Soviet era. And most US states barred children from attending school if they weren't immunized to a CDC schedule or been granted specific exemptions.

France had taken the plunge in January 2018, when an existing list of three compulsory shots was expanded by eight more, including measles. Months later in Australia, a prevailing "no jab, no pay" law was toughened to cut tax benefits for the noncompliant. And, soon after, a populist coalition ruling Italy (home of websites such as "Movimento Contro Autismo") upended the ideas of the joker Grillo and launched an "emergency" campaign to vaccinate eight hundred thousand children and young people.

Initiatives varied. Fines, school bans, loss of benefits. Some systems, such as Britain's, remained voluntary. But then came a game changer in the United States, when local public health chiefs went nuclear.

The trigger was an outbreak in Rockland County, New York, a suburb of New York City. Some accounts tracked its origins to an epidemic in Ukraine, which in 2017 had seen the beginning of a toll of measles infections unmatched anywhere else. Gene sequencing traced the virus to likely pilgrims to Jerusalem, where, in the fall of 2018, the disease had spiked. Then, from the holy city of the Abrahamic religions, it was flown to America's East Coast.

Rockland's response was, to say the least, brutal: akin to measures that I'd read of from an outbreak of bubonic plague in seventeenth-century London. County bosses issued an "emergency order" forbidding anyone under eighteen "to enter any place of public assembly," if he or she couldn't be validated as vaccinated against measles, unless holding an exemption from a doctor.

Within days, the law was amended to any *indoor* place. But hard-line thinking hadn't passed. In New York, the city decreed that parents living or working in any of four zip codes must take any child, aged six months or over, who hadn't had MMR, for the shot within forty-eight hours.

Such panic measures captured a global mood. But they harbored risks of which history had spoken. It was British enforcement of smallpox vaccination (with hefty fines, or even imprisonment, for noncompliance) that, in the 1860s, had spawned the first anti-vaccine movement. Individuals stood defiant. Tens of thousands joined rallies. And when the English crusader William Tebb spoke in New York City, to launch the Anti-Vaccination League of America, he was reported telling his audience, in October 1879, that if the US authorities "could only be persuaded to pass an anti-vaccination law," it would *strengthen* the movement he championed.

Brazil had a similar rite of passage. An "obligatory" smallpox vaccination law, passed by the national assembly in October 1904, erupted onto the streets of Rio de Janeiro in a week-long mass insurrection. Sticks, stones, and guns were ranged against troops in what would be remembered as the "Revolta Contra Vacina."

"The revolt did not result merely from a fear of medical treatment, but rather an ideological opposition," writes American historian Thomas Skidmore in a textbook, *Brazil: Five Centuries of Change*. "The *Revolta Contra Vacina* was for many of its combatants a fight of the poor against state interference in their private lives."

Wakefield was some way from that big idea. But street demonstrations were spreading in Europe. Italy witnessed protests in June 2017, involving thousands in Rome, Milan, Bologna, and other cities. Hundreds protested in Paris months later. And, in the summer of 2018, a great column of protestors snaked through Warsaw, insisting on their right to say no.

Here was no small legacy for an ex-doctor without patients. On videos, he grinned and chuckled. The resurgence of disease wasn't entirely down to him. But, just like you can't make gunpowder without sulfur, charcoal, and potassium nitrate, he knew he was essential to the explosion.

To reprise the line from the *New Indian Express*: "Can one person change the world? Ask Andrew Wakefield."

- - - - - - - - - - - - - - - - - - - -

THIRTY-TWO

Cause and Affect

The United Kingdom of Great Britain and Northern Ireland once preened as the ruler of the biggest empire in history. With ingenuities fueled by coal and a cool climate, it was the anvil of the worldwide Industrial Revolution. It was the cauldron of a language that all humanity would come to share in. It was the first home of football, or "soccer" as some called it. And it was the birthplace and nursery of scares over vaccines. Not once. Not twice. *Three times.*

In the nineteenth century came fear of immunization against the often fatal or blinding smallpox. A century later it was the shot against pertussis, or whooping cough, in DTP. Then, from the late 1990s, it was Wakefield's targets: first MMR, then pretty much any vaccine that might earn him applause and income. And because these began in England, it's in England that I end: concluding the investigation of that twelve-child paper that will doubtless be remembered on my death.

I caught a train to Merseyside, in the English northwest, to visit with the mother of another among the twelve. For the usual reason, I'll call her Ms. Three. But her son, Child Three, in Table 1 and Table 2, had, in fact, been the first to be brought to Hampstead for recruitment to the vaccine research.

He'd been referred to the Royal Free—like nearly all the others—through *Newsnight*'s woman in scarlet. Child Three's sole GI problem was profound constipation. His blood tests for inflammation came back normal, and pathologists didn't report colitis. Upon her son's ileocolonoscopy, however, Ms. Three saw the swollen glands ("blotches," she called them). Then, three months later, the boy's records were altered, he was experimentally prescribed drugs carrying black box warnings, and tabulated in the journal with the "syndrome."

My journey was the third I made to Ms. Three's home over the space of a little more than ten years. London to Liverpool—two hundred miles—then a twenty-minute bus ride through working class suburbs to a rented, two-story, mid-terrace house, with a gold-colored letterbox, number, and knocker, like every other door on the street. At the back was a yard like I'd never seen elsewhere: a rectangle of clipped grass that met fencing on three sides. No bushes. No flower beds. *Nothing.*

Ms. Three was a quiet-spoken, slightly built lady, by this time fifty-eight years of age. Child Three was her second son (with two brothers and a sister), who by now was anything but a child. He was twenty-nine years old, on the cusp of middle age, and had long ceased living at home.

He was a great-looking guy. Black hair. Blue eyes. Were his face to smile up at you from a dating app profile, you'd think he'd be snagged within minutes. He'd got what I call "the Liverpool look," which I imagined I saw in the late Beatle John Lennon. In my mind, it seemed to speak to some mysterious, wry wisdom to be found on the streets of that city.

But he'd no app profile. No *right now* encounters. No walking, hand-in-hand, beside the Mersey. "He could be kissing your face off one minute, and within the space of half an hour he'll just change," says his mother, as we sit in her living room. "Sometimes I'm scared. I lock myself in the garden, because I know how hard he can hit."

His conversation, too, would be less than romantic. He'd lost any speech in his second year of life: which was also the time he began to eat carpets, and obsessively flick his fingers in front of his eyes. Now his core vocabulary was to tap his lips to mean "yes," or "give me." And he recognized, but didn't use, a gesture for "no," or "can't": when his mother would cross and uncross her hands, like a referee disallowing a goal.

"If he wants somebody to leave, he will open the front door," Ms. Three had explained, during the second of my visits. "If he wants a cup of tea, he will give me the cup, or he will put four tea bags in his cup and try to make his own . . . But the thing with [him] is he doesn't know when to stop. When he gets to the top, he just keeps pouring, so it's all over the place, it's too dangerous."

Dangerous, he was: both to himself, and to others. Which meant that, by my last visit, he no longer came home. Rather, he lived among strangers in one of a string of seedy care homes, where he head-butted window glass, slit his own wrist, and broke the nose of a member of staff. Even on a cocktail of three antipsychotics, he was as unpredictable as any lifer jailed without blame: one minute listening to his music in sunshine, the next sending someone to the hospital.

"What makes him happy is having a bath," his mother tells me. "He's had about twelve baths in six hours."

This wasn't Asperger's, or "neurodiversity." The gulf of his aloneness was too vast. His wasn't a difference to be celebrated by advocates (worn like a badge, as in "I'm a bit autistic"), or likened to being gay, or part Native American. It was what some parents called—to personal grief, and a little criticism—full-spectrum, "train wreck," autism.

But could it be a vaccine that explained his predicament? His mother didn't doubt that it was. For the past quarter century she'd made the same case: that at the age of fourteen months, he received MMR, experienced a nosebleed immediately after the shot, then suffered a high fever within forty-eight hours, and a measles-type rash within a week. After that, he began rocking back and forth in his cot, lost speech, and became aggressive.

A neurologist, writing when Child Three was aged five, and who diagnosed him with a combination of "severe learning difficulties and autistic behaviour," said *no*, the mother was wrong.

> She is very sad and is looking both for somebody or something to blame and also for specific treatments for [her son], and I'm afraid I have not been able to help her on either count.

That opinion aligned with the prevailing wisdom. Developmental pediatrics 101 said that the first symptoms of autism usually surfaced, or were recognized, sometime in that second year of life. Scientists argued, meanwhile, that the viruses in the shot took days to multiply under the skin, so it was biologically implausible for measles, mumps, or rubella to have the sudden impact the mother described.

Epidemiologists, likewise, weighed in to cast doubt on parental "anecdotes" like hers. Study after study, from country after country, reported nothing to support Wakefield's signature claim—illustrated in his report with the falsified graph—that MMR was a major cause of autism. Papers from Finland and Denmark had each looked at records of more than half a million children and rejected any association. A project from Yokohama, Japan, found that, during a spell when MMR was suspended, autism diagnoses kept climbing.

As Wakefield campaigned, the disparity grew. "Parents versus science," was how the media framed it. From Montreal, Canada, a team found that pervasive developmental disorder diagnoses "significantly increased" when MMR uptake "significantly decreased." And doctors in Krakow, Poland, tracking development and intelligence, reported no differences in outcomes.

But big-data studies gave results for *populations*. Not *individual cases*, like Child Three's. Maybe they were so rare they slipped under the radar, undetectable to epidemiology. Could that boy— now a man—have a biological trait or a passing vulnerability to a vaccine-induced event? Every medicine that works hurts somebody. And reports, like his mother's, of a fever shortly after, was the commonest recollection in anecdotes from parents who blamed the three-in-one.

> That night he was so cranky and had such a high fever that he was given Tylenol . . . The next day when he woke up he couldn't move and couldn't crawl. He just kept punching himself in the face and ears.

> Two days later he spiked a fever of 105. He was a typically developing child to that point, laughing, making lots of noise, trying to roll over. After the shot we watched him melt before our eyes.

Observations like those weren't parents versus science. They were evidenced in solid research. A study of twins in Finland had documented symptoms, including a striking incidence of fevers after the shot. Publishing in *The Lancet*, back in April 1986, Helsinki pediatrician Heikki Peltola and epidemiologist Olli Heinonen devised a brilliant, placebo-controlled, double-blind study of the immediate aftermath of MMR.

Each child was randomly allocated to one of two groups, splitting the twins between each. One got the vaccine, then the placebo three weeks later; the other got the placebo, then the vaccine three weeks later. And data were analyzed from 581 pairs of twins, tabulated in columns for "days after injection"—revealing an awful lot of fevers.

In the column for *days 1 to 6* (which would cover Child Three), the Finns tabulated a rate for children experiencing "mild" fevers to be *163* per thousand MMRs. They rated a "moderate" fever at *eight* per thousand and a "high" fever at *one* in a thousand. No wonder such events set so many bells jangling among parents of children with autism.

But here came the beauty of the Finnish research: the twins' temperatures after the *placebo*. For mild fever, the rate was 162 per thousand: just *one less* than after MMR. For moderate fever, it was again *one less*. And for high fever there wasn't any difference. So the likelihood of an immediate fever caused by the vaccine was negligible.

There were causal fevers later—peaking at ten days—but, overall, true side effects were rare. "The results of the present study show that adverse reactions to the widely used MMR vaccine are much less common than was previously thought," Peltola and Heinonen commented.

But even this doesn't *prove* Ms. Three was wrong: only that anecdotes aren't sufficient. And it was in anecdotes that Wakefield, Tommey, Bigtree, and other campaigners now took refuge against doctors and scientists: graphically presenting horror stories, and claiming parents' rights to self-certify victims on the principle that mothers *just knew*.

"If ten thousand people say the same thing—ten thousand mothers—anecdotes ultimately *become* science," was how the lawyer Robert Kennedy presented this argument at an anti-vaccine rally in Atlanta. "These women know what happened to their children. They *know* what happened to their children."

Which was, I suppose, where I entered the controversy: by now so many years before. Did Ms. Two *know* in September 1996, when she told Royal Free pediatricians that her son's head-banging began two weeks after MMR? Or did she *know* in November 2003, when she told me that the time elapsed was "about six months"? Or did she *really know* in November 2001, when she filed a statement of her case in court.

She sued a drug company. Her lawyers hoped to win a settlement. But Big Pharma rarely came quietly. In legal papers, given me by another parent in the action, Ms. Two, whose phone call alerted Wakefield to autism, accepted a submission from the defendants, SmithKline Beecham. There were *no symptoms* in the boy's medical records associated with autism, or any purported sign of any "new syndrome," for *nine months* after the shot.

Facing that fact, any "temporal link" went out the window. She was left with John O'Leary's measles tests. And, through her lawyers, she made another concession in the lawsuit that would make any sound mind wonder. "The Claimant's case," she submitted at England's Royal Courts of Justice, "is that symptoms of autistic spectrum disorder and bowel disorder do not necessarily present themselves within days or weeks of the vaccination."

> It is the Claimant's case that the significant feature is that the symptoms occur after and not before the vaccination.

That was about the strength of the sentinel case: "clearly vaccine-damaged," Wakefield said. And Ms. Two wasn't alone in her mirages of memory as the anecdotes of Ms. Six unraveled. This was the mother (she of the "high-pitched scream") who enrolled two of her children in the Royal Free research and also recruited another. Thus (unknown publicly until my investigation), she was responsible for *one-quarter* of the dozen in *The Lancet*, and *one-third* of those tabulated with "autism."

Behind the awesome veil of medical confidentiality, Ms. Six had caused concern from the start. Professionals were so worried over the veracity of her assertions that the pediatrician Simon Murch traveled sixty miles from London to meet with local clinicians. Social workers considered putting the two boys on an "at risk" register. And an independent panel of lawyers, reviewing the termination of Barr's class action, opined that neither child appeared to have any established medical condition to give grounds for their mother to sue anyone.

"She was a very confusing person," her family doctor told the General Medical Council panel, "and the story would vary between consultations."

Both Ms. Two and Ms. Six were close Wakefield retainers: working with him, campaigning for him, and doing their best to thwart my investigation of his research. And Ms. Six was also a confidante of another in his network: Ms. X, a flamboyant liar. Although she wasn't among the parents of the original twelve, she'd taken her son for scoping at the Royal Free bowel clinic, joined Barr's lawsuit as a frequent court-attender, and turned up on Euston Road.

"He saved our children," she yelled above the traffic. "Dr. Wakefield saved our children. Dr. Wakefield, and his colleagues, saved our children. Dr. Wakefield saved our children."

The only snag was those pesky medical records, as many mothers would learn, to their dismay. Ms. X's anecdote began with her eighteen-month-old son spiking a fever after MMR, then losing speech and eye contact "immediately." The shot was followed by six hours of seizures and vomiting, she said, then six months in a "persistent vegetative state."

But after scrutiny of records, a judge wouldn't have it, and used an F-word disliked by lawyers. "The critical facts established in this case can be summarized," he ruled. "[Child X] has autistic spectrum disorder. There is no evidence that his autism was caused by the MMR vaccination. His parents' account of an adverse reaction to that vaccination is fabricated."

And why not, indeed? Ask yourself the question: if you could swindle yourself to millionaire status by stealing from the government, or a pharmaceutical company—and be sure that, if you fail, you won't even face criticism, let alone go to jail—would you maybe give it a go? *Well, would you?* And now, if you don't have a developmentally challenged child—with all that turmoil, worry, and expense on your mind—if *you did*, would that impact your moral calculation, if it meant misrecalling a few facts?

Here was grim accountancy on the human condition. Didn't people stamp on the brakes to get their cars rear-ended, fake gastric disease after ocean cruise meals, and pretend to have been present during terrorist attacks—to get their hands on compensation? And would it even be a crime in the balance of injustice if Wakefield had convinced them that on the other side was a conspiracy: by drug companies, corrupt doctors, lying scientists, and "shill" journalists?

Surely, here was a morality wild card.

But such sad reckoning was light years from Ms. Three's. I never thought for a second that she lied. Wouldn't any parent believe in the link after what they'd seen, and couldn't explain about their child, and heard from the charming Dr. Wakefield? Decent as she was—as with countless, countless others—it didn't mean she was right, or wrong.

Over the years, I noticed how, with the passage of time, parents' stories so often morphed. Memories faded, events became telescoped, and recollections scrambled, like lab DNA when amplified with too many cycles. Then, there were cases where information surfaced that provoked more questions than answers.

Take the account of Wakefield's special friend, Polly Tommey, who said that her son, Billy, was damaged by MMR, and who toured the United States in 2016 with talk about doctors killing babies. In *Vaxxed*, she and her husband, Jonathan, explained that on the day of the boy's shot, at *thirteen months*, he'd begun "uncontrollable shaking," had a feverish seizure, and "didn't really ever wake up" to himself.

Maybe so. But seventeen years earlier, when they pitched a pig hormone for autism on British television, the account broadcast was appreciably different. Everything was "fantastic" up to the age of *nine months*, when Billy's development appeared to falter. "We thought his speech delay was purely because he couldn't hear," his father told the program (which made no mention of vaccines or seizures). "And everybody kept saying, 'Oh, he's not talking because he's had glue ear, and how can you talk if you can't hear?'"

Can't hear? A classic first confusion in the early recognition of autism. And there's more between the dates of the Tommey's two accounts that cause me to press the pause button. In February 2010, I received a phone call from a close friend of the Tommey family, who approached me through the *Sunday Times* news desk.

"Has she ever really sat down," I ask this source, in a recorded conversation, "and looked at her son's medical records?"

"Oh yeah, oh yeah, oh yeah," the friend replies.

"And she remains convinced it was the MMR?"

"*No, no, no.* Never actually was."

I was past surprise over such responses. So often I found that time impacted narratives: as another Wakefield admirer—the actor Jenny McCarthy—may have experienced with regard to her son. She'd long held him out—in books and on TV—as an MMR-injured child. But the boy's paternal grandmother came forward later and told a Milwaukee-based writer, Ken Reibel, that she noted classic early autistic behaviors *before*.

She said *before*. So what about *without*? I may have stumbled on a case of that, too. It was of the JABS campaigner, Jackie Fletcher. She, who first put Wakefield and Ms. Two together, who was among the first to sign up to Barr's nascent class action, and who referred most of the *Lancet* twelve. For years, her son had been the UK's poster child for MMR vaccine damage.

Again it was records: this time court papers plus an entry with the US government's Vaccine Adverse Event Reporting System, which another mother drew to my attention. Fletcher had linked a febrile seizure to MMR, and even evidenced her anecdote with a vaccine batch number, G0839, which she submitted had done the damage. But doctors attributed the boy's seizure as secondary to a chest infection; the manufacturer disclosed the batch as a *tetanus* vaccine; and tests noted that her son's immune system had produced no antibodies to measles, mumps, or rubella virus, but *had*, weakly, to tetanus toxin.

Memories, understandably, fray with time. But often I found it was parents who made the most noise whose stories, when probed, underwhelmed. And I think lawyers, too, must have felt something similar when they found their test cases as tragically threadbare as Child Two's and Michelle Cedillo's.

Ms. Three didn't campaign over causality issues. I don't think I ever saw her in the media. But while she didn't rage on Facebook, or shout in the street, she was an unstoppable crusader for her son. She would fight to have his medication adjusted and reassessed, protest when his clothes were stolen from his room, and battle to close the shittiest care homes. Without her, who knows where he'd be?

By the time of my third visit, we focused on that: the life of Child Three as a man. But at an earlier meeting, we'd talked more of MMR, as we sat in her living room with her partner, Mr. Three, who once worked as forklift driver.

"Do you really believe," I asked them, with my mind on Wakefield's most toxic allegation, "that there are doctors, and people working in the government, who *know* that MMR is causing problems like your son's, and are *covering it up?*"

"Yes," she said.

"I don't," he said. "I don't."

"I do," she repeated. And she did.

The moment passed. But the father said something else that hinted at a difference of opinion. "Actually, I think, we were just vulnerable," he said. "We were looking for answers."

And who wouldn't?

Ms. Three, however, never lost faith, as she makes clear when we meet for the last time. She "didn't trust the MMR." She "still wouldn't trust it." And she also believed what Wakefield had said, decades before, when he spoke at the press conference in the Royal Free's Atrium to set loose his epidemics on the world.

"I honestly believe," she says, echoing his advice about the triple vaccination, "that giving it separately would have been the better answer."

But even she doesn't swallow the whole Wakefield hog. She doubts his biggest idea. The way she sees it, the ultimate culprit for her son's situation *wasn't* the measles virus in the three-in-one.

"I always thought it was the rubella," she says.

- - - - - - - - - - - - - - - - - - - -

A Wonderful Doctor

The last I heard of him, he was shacked up in Miami, Florida, with a supermodel, divorced wife of a billionaire. Which only goes to show that, once you've fooled all of the people some of the time, and some of the people all of the time, your next big idea had better be good.

The lady was Elle Macpherson (a.k.a. "the Body"), a fifty-five-year-old mother of two from Sydney, Australia, and patron of numerous good causes. Best known for a record-breaking five appearances on the cover of *Sports Illustrated* swimsuit issues, she reportedly bagged $53 million in cash and a $26 million home after a four-year marriage to her last husband.

Wakefield, sixty-two, was first sighted in her company in November 2017. The occasion was an anti-vaccine event in Orlando, Florida, where they met in what appeared to be a calculated introduction, having been seated together for dinner. Just two months later, they were spotted for a second time, at a similar kind of gathering in Red Bank, New Jersey. Then, once more, in May 2019, at another in Chicago, Illinois.

Few who weren't rock stars were showcased in circumstances as were lavished on Wakefield at such events. Thronged by women,

mostly the mothers, who clapped and hooted and jostled for self-
ies, he was their Nelson Mandela (to whom he'd taken to comparing himself) returning from the grave to pass among them. In
New Jersey, they gorged on a ninety-minute video, lauding their
champion as a family man (chopping wood, cracking eggs, and
browsing the internet) at the Texas home he soon abandoned for
Macpherson.

I didn't care. To be frank, I never did. I'd never asked for the
assignment. It had given me little pleasure. What I'd long most
hoped for was an exit. If the things that we dwell on become the
shape of our minds, who'd want to spend years on this? But, once
he'd begun suing and sliming to cover his tracks, I'd no choice but
to stay on his trail.

Is it new? Is it true? Do we have it to ourselves?

The rest of it: not my problem.

Medicine was for doctors; science for scientists. My responsibility was to question. And if that meant digging till his house fell
down, then, corny as it sounds, better journalists than me have
lost their lives for untold truths. All I'd risked was forfeiting my
home to legal bills (since I republished my stories at briandeer
.com) if the facts didn't check out. Which they did.

And then, when I figured, at last, *that* was *that,* he bubbled up
again, after months out of sight, like an alligator from Macpherson's swimming pool. This was a Monday evening in May 2019,
when he graced the digital stream with an appearance, via Skype,
during an outbreak of his favorite disease.

The location was a ballroom: the Atrium Grand Ballroom, in
the hamlet of Monsey, in Rockland County, thirty miles north of
Manhattan. Better known for weddings with single-sex dancing,
readings from the Torah, and stamped-on wine glasses, this shopping mall venue was the hub of a community of ultra-Orthodox

Jews. It was among these that the virus once slated for eradication had erupted that spring and provoked the extreme measure of a public ban on unvaccinated kids.

By now Wakefield realized that Donald Trump had betrayed him. Before the Rockland outbreak, and its New York City cousin, the president had said nothing publicly about immunization at any time since entering the White House. Then, at the height of the reporting of that year's alarm, Trump commented on what families should do. "They have to get the shots," he called out to journalists, on the way to his chopper. "The vaccinations are so important. This is really going around now. They have to get their shots."

Wakefield knew better, and his mission that Monday was much the same as it was, years before, with the Somalis: he was targeting a troubled community. In his sights were neighborhoods where immunization rates were low, and he wanted to keep them that way. Vaccines, he now preached, were "neither safe, nor effective," and the historic decline in deaths and sickness from measles, was "nothing to do with vaccination."

His appearance looked strange: like the face of a sweating ghost, materializing from out of the ether. On a screen, erected in the fifteen-hundred-seater ballroom, his shiny forehead and cheeks glowed lobster-red raw, like he'd been making full use of the nearly two acres around Macpherson's waterfront mansion. But two zones of his complexion remained spectral pale: one striping horizontally, narrow at the nose, wider around the eyes; the other like a bib, around his mouth.

"I want to reassure you that I have never been involved in scientific fraud," he announced to the ranks of Haradi Jews, who'd been summoned to the Atrium by robocall phone messages. "What happened to me is what happens to doctors who threaten the bottom line of the pharmaceutical companies, and who threaten government policy, in the interests of their patients."

The ever patientless doctor must have forgotten the Australians, Warren and Marshall of *H. pylori* fame. They shared the Nobel Prize after slaughtering drug markets, dining out on dissing Big Pharma. And it must have slipped his mind that he'd only criticized MMR after British researchers found fault with two brands. John Wilson was elected a fellow of the Royal Society. The CDC whistleblower still worked for the government (with a pay raise). None had been charged with fraud, or dishonesty. Only him. And he knew why.

"I want to let you know that you have been misled," he told his audience, following an address by the "Emmy-winning" *Vaxxed* producer, Del Bigtree, funded by a Manhattan financier. "I'm going to talk specifically about measles."

Only forty-five seconds made it onto Twitter. But I found his latest angles on YouTube. During the months that I'd thought he was sunning in Miami, he'd not merely been counting the ways he loved Macpherson. He'd also repackaged himself as a tutor, making a series of video lectures.

I counted twenty-one, bought a tub of strawberry ice cream, and spent an afternoon making notes. Measles was now *good*, apparently. Vaccines made it *worse*. "Herd immunity" was a dangerous delusion.

His YouTube audiences were impressed by the performances, spoken to camera, hands clasped near his chest. "What a great series," "You are a blessing to humanity," "Great to hear from you again."

To me, his epistles didn't make a lot of sense. On one hand, he said the worldwide fall in deaths and illness wasn't as a result of immunization but because the disease was evolving to be milder. But then he also claimed that measles was doing *more harm*, as a result of immunization.

Please, I thought. *Who's got a wet towel?* I honestly couldn't take much more. So the illness was getting milder, and shots made it more dangerous? Was this the lesson of the outbreaks then exploding around the globe? Ninety-five percent of confirmed cases among the Somalis were unvaccinated. Figures reported from Rockland County were likewise.

Even I knew that, for an RNA genome, measles was a comparatively stable virus. "I am not aware of any changes that would affect the pathogenicity," says, for instance, a virologist and professor of molecular biology, who, unlike Wakefield, had published countless research papers on paramyxoviruses. *If* there was any progression toward a milder infection, he tells me, the most likely reason was the advance of vaccination.

But, he was an expert. So what would he know? The question for me wasn't *who to believe*, but what should have been asked, two decades before, over Wakefield's performance in an Atrium. Like, *who was* this guy to call the shots on children's safety? *Who was he? What did he want?*

He didn't like doctoring, that's for sure. Nor was he a scientist: as researcher after researcher lined up to point out after I nailed him. "It was junk," says one of his former team members, who'd worked alongside Nick Chadwick in the tenth-floor lab. "I think he just read about measles in a textbook. That's not how science is done."

Others pointed out that they'd tried to help him, only to find their efforts rebuffed. An internationally renowned authority on measles virus, a pathologist with deep experience assessing children's biopsies, and a world-class clinician in inflammatory bowel diseases, all said they explored collaborations with Wakefield that fell apart after advice he didn't like.

"I did some fecal calprotectin levels for him," a professor of gastroenterology emails me. "He then drafted his hypothesis with my name on it, where the central mechanism of damage was vaccine induced increased intestinal permeability, leading to absorption of neurotoxins affecting the brain. It was all gobbledygook, and I put it right but, because it interrupted his belief, he took no notice and published the paper and took my name off it. He is now rich, famous and lives with a sex goddess."

A senior virologist told me he was commissioned to peer review the *J Med Virol* paper, which launched the whole measles thing. "It's burned on my memory," he says, twenty-three years later, explaining that he asked his lab's electron microscopy specialist whether what Wakefield had photographed was measles. "So my man said, 'No it's not, it's microfilaments,' which is a normal component of cells. [Wakefield's] got: 'This is a T-cell eating something else.' And my man says, 'No it isn't. He's got the picture upside down, and it's the other way around.'"

Countless sources told me how important it seemed to Wakefield that he shouldn't be questioned or contradicted. And no fewer than three (possibly four) recounted a spectacular incident when he was orally examined in a "viva" session over a master's degree dissertation. Notwithstanding his customary grand demeanor, they said he was so rattled by the quizzing he got that he "walked out," or "stormed out" (the verb varies between accounts), and so failed to obtain the qualification.

"He reckoned the examiners were ignorant, and didn't understand what he was doing," one professor tells me over lunch. "Now, I have never, ever, heard in forty, fifty, years of clinical science, of *anyone* who's walked out of a viva."

That reported incident showed character revealed under stress: where character is usually revealed. And it wasn't only Wakefield where its marks were left, but in a trail of dented reputations and damaged careers among those who fell for that charisma.

Roy Pounder, his mentor, and Arie Zuckerman, the dean, (who both refused to speak to me) had lost their chance of being honored with knighthoods (and thus donning the glorious prenominal "Professor Sir") in the aftermath of the Royal Free scandal. The first stood for the presidency of the Royal College of Physicians—and lost the election after my first findings. The second presided over the launch of a health crisis that his peers could never forgive.

"This has been dragging on now for eighteen years," Zuckerman had practically wept, after rising from the witness chair at the end of his evidence to the General Medical Council panel.

Among the rest, of course, was *The Lancet*'s editor, who would forever be taunted over his decision to publish. And the Australian professor, John Walker-Smith, who, despite escaping conviction due to procedural error, would regret ever entering the concrete castle with its views across Hampstead Heath. Barts, *Barts*. He should have stayed at Barts. "The mother hospital of the Empire." What a dope.

But these men's humiliation was nothing to the collateral of Wakefield's gift to families. That, in my opinion, should be carved in yellow limestone and erected by the entrance to that villa on Beacon Hill, ninety minutes by train west of London.

> *Here lived Andrew Wakefield*
> *A doctor without patients*
> *He brought us fear, guilt, and disease*

For medicine and the media, it was fear and disease that were the be-all and end-all of the saga. Parents got scared, kids went unvaccinated, illness bounced back among those left unprotected, occasionally with brain damage and deaths.

For me, however, it was the overlooked suffering: the gnawing horror of guilt. Sure, I wrote about failing confidence and outbreaks of disease. I even reported the first British death (a thirteen-year-old boy) from measles in fourteen years. But thanks to a conversation with *Newsnight*'s woman in scarlet, I'd seen the crisis a little differently from the start.

I phoned her first—the day before Ms. Two—and invited her to walk me through her story. "It was dreadful," she told me, of what happened with her son, which I noted on page 19 of my notebook 1, in September 2003. "I had taken him while he was vaccinated, and so there was a major guilt side that I should have done all this research before the vaccine was given."

Richard Barr and Kirsten Limb had long spread this anxiety, as if they thought their clients needed reminding. "We know that many parents find it difficult to come to terms with the fact that their child might have been damaged by a vaccine," they'd announced in a "fact sheet" before the twelve-child paper was published. "If the damage is caused by some natural illness then it is something over which they have no control; but if it was caused by a vaccine then inevitably many parents will feel guilty for agreeing to have their child vaccinated."

Shrewd advice. Parents blaming themselves was an agony that I found everywhere.

"No matter who I interview," said Wakefield's business partner Polly Tommey, for instance, summarizing what she'd heard on the black bus tour. "They can't sleep at night. They are racked with guilt." And, "along with the guilt," she added, they were "rocking in grief," grabbing "anything they can to numb the pain."

She'd found her analgesic. Her painkiller was Wakefield, whom she wanted to share with the world. What would it take, she asked, during a video in which he featured, for the "powers that be" to own up and admit that vaccines had "injured and killed so many people"?

Tommey had a point. If maybe not the one she thought. And I pasted both her comments into a pair of matched slides, which I could click back and forth in PowerPoint. Both featured a block of identical *Vaxxed* artwork, including her face and an alliterative slogan:

Listen to the Parents, Not the Pediatricians

In other words, listen to *her*.

On one of my slides, I typed her quote on guilt; on the other, her "powers that be." Back and forth, I'd click. Back and forth. Back and forth. Her face looking out, unmoving.

And that was her choice, like for so many of his followers: beat yourself up, or accuse someone else. It was the trap, I believe, that made him. Within that awful space between guilt and accusation, he'd risen to be all that he was. *If you'd listened to me, your child wouldn't have autism.* It's *them.* It's *them.* It's *they.*

Professionals with long memories had seen it before. It was the face of the "refrigerator mother." It was blame the parent: lay the charge on *their choice*, and make a living out of selling them redemption.

"Trust your instincts," he'd say when science had failed him. But what I thought he really meant was *trust mine.*

And they loved him for it. He was a "wonderful" physician: so caring, professional, and *wronged.* But victims also said that of the serial killer Harold Shipman. His admirers were one and the same as his prey. "He was so popular," noted a patient who didn't die at Shipman's hands. "Everyone thought he was a marvelous doctor."

Wakefield's mothers felt guilt so that he didn't have to. They bore remorse and shame on his behalf. And why that's important isn't just because they suffered—shouldering a pain they surely didn't deserve—but because it let him mobilize their misery.

The weaselly insinuations behind Barr's failed lawsuit—that doctors and scientists weren't playing it straight—had eaten at parents' hearts since the 1990s. And like a pyramid sale in bitterness and hatred, Wakefield had conscripted a global militia, armed with modern weapons—Facebook, Twitter, WhatsApp, YouTube—undreamt of in the golden age.

Planners and professionals couldn't see how it was done—like they couldn't with that twelve-child paper. Indignant at the impertinence of a doctor doubting vaccines, they missed even asking the right questions. And now faced with a phenomenon they still didn't understand, they ran opinion surveys on "vaccine hesitancy," backed legal bans, and beat the drums of disease. But they talked past his army of the tormented and heartbroken, who wouldn't quit anytime soon.

The man, meanwhile, untroubled by conscience, addressed hundreds of Jews in the Atrium Grand Ballroom, sure to take from them more than he gave. He craved the attention. Yes. He loved his voice. Yes. One of the professors who taught him at medical school described him as "one of the most attention-seeking individuals" he'd ever met.

Wakefield even had the chutzpah to cast himself as the victim, the most classically malignant projection. "I lost my career," he'd bleat, as if it wasn't his fault. "I lost my job, I lost my income, I lost my country, and I lost my reputation."

Poor, poor Andy. Too bad.

But I thought there was more. He was *owning* that outbreak. In his dark confusion of subject and object, he wanted us to know that *he* controlled events. He reveled in the dance to his tune. And, like one of those fantasists you used to hear of, back in the day, who snuck into hospitals, stole a white coat, and stepped out onto the wards to diagnose and treat, I believe that, inside, he was laughing.

His own mother revealed something that I'd mulled over for years. We were talking one evening, my tape recorder running. I think Bridget may have sipped a dry sherry. And she made reference to Edward Matthews, he of *Sex, Love and Society*, when explaining her second son's character. "He's very like my father," she said. "If he believed in something, he would have gone to the ends of the earth to go on believing."

To go on believing. Not to search for solutions. He'd always been making a case. And the case he made—which was rarely not for profit—was that *his* big ideas must prevail. No matter his betters, no matter the truth, no matter the outbreaks of fear, guilt, and disease, *nothing* would obstruct his path.

The way I saw it, it was never about the science, the children, or the mothers. It had always been about himself.

November 1988: One month after the three-in-one measles, mumps, and rubella vaccine, MMR, is launched in Britain, Andrew Wakefield returns to London to work at the Royal Free medical school, Hampstead, after a training job in Toronto, Canada.

September 15, 1992: The media reports the British government's discontinuation of two MMR brands due to the mumps viral component causing sporadic cases of meningitis.

September 23, 1992: Wakefield asks the government for money to research MMR measles component and Crohn's disease, warning of possible media involvement.

April 1993: A science journal publishes a paper in which Wakefield claims to photograph measles virus in bowel tissues from Crohn's patients.

January 1994: A British mother, Jackie Fletcher, launches a campaign group claiming that MMR damaged her infant son's brain. She plans to sue the manufacturers and seeks similar cases to her own.

September 1994: A small-town lawyer, Richard Barr, is awarded a contract by the British government's Legal Aid Board to represent litigants in a potential class action lawsuit over MMR.

February 19, 1996: Wakefield accepts a deal to work for Barr at lavish hourly rates to construct a case against MMR. This deal remains secret until exposed in Deer's investigation.

February 19, 1996: On the same day, two hundred miles from London, a doctor refers the first child to Wakefield's research project after the six-year-old's mother is advised by Fletcher.

June 1996: Before any children are admitted for his research, Wakefield applies to the legal board for a grant to test for vaccine damage, predicting that he will find a new "syndrome" of bowel and brain disorders caused by MMR.

June 1997: Wakefield registers for a patent on his own single measles vaccine, plus treatments for both autism and inflammatory bowel disease.

September 1997: After flying to the United States, Wakefield speaks at an anti-vaccine meeting near Washington, DC.

February 26, 1998: At a press conference to announce a paper in *The Lancet*, Wakefield attacks MMR, urging parents to avoid it in favor of single measles vaccinations. His legal deal stays secret.

February 28, 1998: *The Lancet* publishes Wakefield's paper claiming discovery of the bowel-brain "syndrome," putatively caused by MMR, that he said he would find before he performed the research.

March 3, 1998: Wakefield meets to discuss a private company of his own to develop putative products, including a measles vaccine, which only have any prospects of success if public confidence in MMR is damaged.

October 1998: The first court claims are filed in the UK class action lawsuit against MMR vaccine manufacturers. Wakefield is the principal expert, creating the underlying hypothesis and pivotal evidence for the case as if he is an independent scientist.

July 1999: The US Public Health Service and the American Academy of Pediatrics urge the withdrawal of a mercury-based preservative, thimerosal, from vaccines. Lawsuits and anti-vaccine campaigning follow.

December 1999: Wakefield's university and medical school ask him to replicate his research claims with a gold-standard scientific study. After months of delay, he refuses.

April 2000: Irish pathologist John O'Leary appears on Capitol Hill to give "independent testimony" to a congressional committee that Wakefield, seated beside him, is "correct." Neither man reveals they are business partners, and that O'Leary, too, works for the lawyer Barr.

November 2000: Appearing on CBS's *60 Minutes*, Wakefield claims, wrongly, that autism "took off dramatically" in the United States and later in Britain when MMR was introduced.

January 2001: British newspapers launch campaigns backing Wakefield after he publishes a purported review of vaccine safety studies, and repeats his calls for single vaccines.

January 2002: As Wakefield's campaign moves to the United States, media outlets announce his appointment as head of a "multi-million dollar" research program, which turns out to be a Florida family doctor's office.

October 2003: Barr's class action lawsuit against MMR makers collapses in London for lack of evidence. The total cost of the action, which drove the crisis, converted to rough 2019 figures, was one hundred million US dollars.

February 2004: The *Sunday Times* of London runs Deer's page 1 story disclosing Wakefield's contract with Barr and the litigant status of children in the *Lancet* study.

January 2005: Wakefield, funded by a UK medical insurer, announces and then stalls a libel lawsuit over Deer's revelations. But, after a London judge finds the suit driven by "public relations purposes" and orders Wakefield to trial, he drops the action and pays costs.

April 2006: As measles outbreaks follow Wakefield's campaign, Deer reports the first death in Britain from the disease in fourteen years.

September 2006: Complaints begin to surface about a Wakefield business in Austin, Texas. Parents say they feel pressure to have children without bowel symptoms undergo colonoscopies.

February 2009: The *Sunday Times* of London runs another of Deer's page 1 stories revealing wholesale discrepancies between the *Lancet* paper and medical records.

May 2010: The UK doctors' regulator, the General Medical Council, orders Wakefield to be banned from medical practice. Charges found proven include dishonesty, fraud, and a "callous disregard" for children's suffering.

January 2011: A US media firestorm erupts after CNN's Anderson Cooper reports an editorial in the *British Medical Journal* denouncing Wakefield's research as "an elaborate fraud."

March 2011: Wakefield appears in Minneapolis, addressing Somali Americans. Outbreaks of measles follow.

January 2012: Wakefield, funded by investment millionaire Bernard Selz, sues Deer and the *British Medical Journal* in Texas. The defendants reject the suit as frivolous, and counter-sue for their costs. But the case is thrown out for lack of jurisdiction.

May 2013: Wakefield appears in a video from the bedside of a developmentally challenged Chicago fourteen-year-old, Alex

Spourdalakis, ferried to New York for a colonoscopy. Days later, the boy is killed by his mother.

June 2014: Anti-vaccine campaigner Brian Hooker, acting with Wakefield, tries and fails to entrap a CDC scientist, William Thompson, into alleging fraud in US government vaccine research.

April 13, 2016: Actor Robert De Niro appears on NBC's *Today* urging viewers to see *Vaxxed*, a ninety-one-minute video by Wakefield claiming that Thompson had alleged fraud at the CDC.

November 3, 2017: Wakefield meets and begins a relationship with wealthy Australian supermodel Elle Macpherson.

November 2018: The World Health Organization warns of a global resurgence of measles. Two months later, "vaccine hesitancy" is named as one of the top ten threats to human health.

May 2019: At the center of major measles outbreaks in New York, Wakefield appears via Skype dismissing risks from the disease. He says, "I have never been involved in scientific fraud."

December 2019: Ending a year marked by measles outbreaks around the world, the tiny Pacific islands of Samoa report more than eighty measles-related deaths in less than two months, after many years of none. Almost all are among children under five. Authorities in the Democratic Republic of Congo notify nearly five thousand measles-related deaths for the year.

NOTE TO READERS

In an essay on the craft of journalism, the celebrated writer Tom Wolfe decried the output of what he called "the literary gentleman with a seat in the grandstand." Plenty of such books have been written about vaccines, autism, and the integrity of science. *The Doctor Who Fooled the World* isn't among them.

This is a work of reportage, fact, analysis, and some opinion based on what I believe to be the most extensive investigation by a reporter into an aspect of medicine ever undertaken. From my first, routine, assignment, in September 2003, to my writing of this note in October 2019, my life was dominated (albeit with breaks) by the *who*, *what*, *when*, *where*, and *why* through which epidemics of fear, guilt, and infectious disease were manufactured and exported to the world.

Before laying out that story for the first time in this book, my inquiries into the research and claims of Andrew Wakefield and his associates generated more than two dozen reports for the *Sunday Times* of London, Britain's market-leading quality weekend newspaper. Prompted by those, I was invited by *BMJ*, the *British Medical Journal*—one of the "big five" general medical journals internationally—to deepen the evidence with peer review and fresh editorial checking for a specialist readership. This effort produced seven reports running to tens of thousands of words in text and footnotes.

I also benefited from a commission to make a one-hour, prime-time *Dispatches* investigation for the United Kingdom's Channel

4 TV network—as well as from the broadcaster's determined efforts to meet Wakefield at trial in the English courts—to avoid which he paid our costs and walked away.

Underpinning my reporting lies a trove of more than twelve thousand indexed documents that I gathered over the years. Some five hundred video and audio recordings are also archived. And I ordered more than 200 items from storage at the British Library. At my suggestion, for editorial validation, more than two thousand of these materials (including letters, emails, interview transcripts and recordings, legal papers, business reports, patents, etc.) were submitted for cross-checking against the pre-publication manuscript of this book, allowing my evidence to be examined by the publishers, at arm's length from me.

Were it not for the exhaustive indexing of documents (obtained by painful extractions under freedom of information legislation, and gathered from diverse sources, including the parents of children involved in Wakefield's research, court papers, and what I'm told is a six-million-word transcript [I've never counted] from the longest-ever medical misconduct hearing), I could have finished this text, at twice the length, in half the time. But at its heart are real people and specific facts potentially impacting on the safety of children.

I've filed more than two hundred pages of statements in district court, verified under penalty of perjury, and have been deposed under oath for six-and-a-half hours by Wakefield's lawyers. This story is, and would have to be, true.

ACKNOWLEDGMENTS

- - - - - - - - - - - - - - - - - - - -

On my personal website, briandeer.com, I've hosted, for some years, a video featuring an environmental microbiologist named Dr. David Lewis, who claimed to exonerate Andrew Wakefield. In the video, he explains the logic by which he purported to expose my journalism as a sham: on grounds that it was *too good to be true*. "Brian Deer, a reporter with no training in medicine or science, *supposedly* wrote these articles," he told an anti-vaccine conference in Chicago. "It doesn't make sense. These are well-written articles by someone who has considerable expertise in medical practice."

I wrote those articles. And I wrote this book. Nevertheless, journalism is always a team effort, and many people have contributed to the enormous undertaking that lies behind it. Unlike those who so often seek to mislead the public, my work has been subject to phenomenal scrutiny, perhaps exceeding any comparable project in the annals of journalism or medicine.

First, the team at the *Sunday Times*, led by its editor, John Witherow, and after he departed for the top job at the paper's sister, the *Times*, his successor, Martin Ivens. Then hands-on, the executive editor, Bob Tyrer, whose continuing support over more than a decade ensured that this investigation was never lost amid fierce competition for space. It was also he who rescued me from *The Lancet*'s spoiler, when the journal did its best to frustrate my findings and substitute what would be proven to be untrue. Paul Nuki, the paper's "Focus" editor, was there at the beginning and reappeared at the end to read my manuscript, for which I'm indebted. Richard Caseby, then managing editor, most notably tackled attempts by Wakefield's inner circle to spread false information. And among others, Alan Hunter, Jack Grimston, Charles Hymas, Mark Skipworth, Sian Griffiths, Angela Connell, Peter Conradi, Richard Woods, Rosemary Collins, Robin Morgan, and Graham Paterson all played important roles over the years. Sorry to anyone I've missed.

Channel 4 Television, one of the UK's five terrestrial networks, took up the story at a critical time, commissioning, supervising, and defending my one-hour prime-time *Dispatches* film, "MMR— What They Didn't Tell You." There, Dorothy Byrne, head of news and current affairs, green-lighted the project, while her deputy, Kevin Sutcliffe, supervised it for much of the time on a daily basis. At the independent company Twenty Twenty Productions, the executive producer, Claudia Milne, set the tone and style with producer and director Tim Carter. Hugo Godwin, associate producer, contributed phenomenal research, while Peter Casely-Hayford kept an eye on the management side. A key segment, when I confronted Wakefield at the Indianapolis Convention Center, was filmed by Iki Ahmed, whose skill at keeping up with a moving target revealed to viewers the nature of the man we sought.

At *The BMJ*, formerly known as the *British Medical Journal*, the editor-in-chief, Dr. Fiona Godlee, was inspired to invite me to lay out my findings for a professional audience, generating what I believe to be the most-read report in her journal's history. She personally supervised the project, "Secrets of the MMR Scare," which took our journalism most vitally into the United States. She was supported by her deputy, Jane Smith, tasked with fact-checking key elements of the evidence, while editors Trevor Jackson, Tony Delamothe, Deborah Cohen, Rebecca Coombes, Jackie Annis, and Trish Groves all contributed to discussing, querying, checking, and getting the copy into the pages and online.

I'm naturally indebted to the supervising publisher of this book, Johns Hopkins University Press, Baltimore. At Aevitas Creative Management in New York City, my primary agent was Becky Sweren, supported especially by Esmond Harmsworth in Boston and Chelsey Heller, director of foreign rights.

On matters potentially impacting on public health and the safety of children, as well as the reputation of individuals, none of my journalism would have been possible without legal advice, checking, and support at every stage. At the *Sunday Times*, the editorial team and I were advised by solicitors Pat Burge and Alastair Brett as well as several ad hoc opinions from counsel.

At Channel 4, Prash Naik, then deputy head of legal and compliance, worked on the story alongside the production team, ensuring accuracy and fairness commensurate with the network's statutory duties. Jan Tomalin, head of legal and compliance, drove forward a "defend like a claimant" strategy, in which we obtained court orders against Wakefield to compel him to produce medical records. Wise people don't seek litigation, but we relished the possibility of seeing him at trial in London, but he threw in the towel, and paid our costs. At our solicitors, Wiggin LLP, we were advised and supported by Amali De Silva, Caroline Kean, Farida Mansoor, and Ross Sylvester. External counsel, retained from the London chambers of 5RB, were Adrienne Page QC, Matthew Nicklin (later Mr. Justice Nicklin QC), and Jacob Dean.

At *The BMJ*, Kim Lenart provided in-house legal support, and advice on copy came from Godwin Busuttil (5RB). From external solicitors Farrer & Co of London were Julian Pike and Harriet Brown. In the United States, our external advisers were Vinson & Elkins, where my point man was Marc A. Fuller (Dallas, Texas), with Thomas S. Leatherbury (Dallas), Sean W. Kelly (Dallas), Lisa Bowlin Hobbs (Austin, Texas), and David P. Blanke (Austin).

Peer review was contributed at numerous points along the way, including two rounds to meet the requirements of Johns Hopkins

University Press. Additionally, I'm grateful especially to Dr. Harvey Marcovitch (pediatrics) and Professor Karel Geboes (gastrointestinal pathology) for providing that function for the *BMJ* series. Reading a late version of this book's full manuscript, Professor Ingvar Bjarnasson (gastroenterology) picked me up on some important points of detail that a qualified reader might have spotted.

I benefited, too, from a personal seminar by consultant histopathologist Dr. Salvador Diaz-Cano at the Department of Pathology, King's College Hospital, London, and from endoscopies performed on me, for purely clinical reasons of course, by Miss Lindsay Barker (lower) and Dr. Jeremy Nayagam (upper). Professor Ian Bruce (molecular biology) read my chapters featuring the polymerase chain reaction.

Many others lent kind support, advice, documents, and help. Most critically were the many parents of children with developmental and other issues who were involved with Wakefield, or various vaccine campaigners, and approached me with information. To protect them from abuse, I don't name them here. And along with everyone who reads this book (and a good many who don't), I gained immensely from the contribution of my special source inside Wakefield's circle, who, turning double agent, supplied me with evidence, documents, and briefings over the better part of a decade. There is so much more that I could say about that, and I probably will elsewhere.

I'm deeply grateful to Sir Harold Evans, one of the most respected newspapermen of modern times, who not only recommended me to an agent, but whose seminal series of books on newspaper editing and design made it possible for me in the 1980s to bluff my way through my first months at the *Sunday Times*. On that theme, I owe the break of my life to Tony Bambridge (1937–1997) when, as editor of the *Sunday Times Business News*, he gave me a chance and, as a result, put up with more aggravation than he ever deserved. So, too, with Tony Rennell, whose advice to me as a young headline writer has remained with me as a beacon: "No, try again." Such wisdom.

For practical help, I thank so many people, including Paulo Henrique Nico Monteiro and Vivian Lederman, São Paulo, Brazil; Gabriel León, Andrés Bello National University, Santiago, Chile; the staff of the British Library, science section; the Imperial War Museum, London; and Ronald J. O'Brien, at Thermo Fisher Scientific, Waltham, Massachusetts, for arranging a briefing on the ABI Prism 7700 PCR machine.

My friends Nick Downing and Ryan G. Wilson contributed vital advice and support, as well as the forbearance of listening to me going on about all this for years at a stretch. When writing, I was supported by the hour by Rádio NovaBrasil FM 89.7 São Paulo, with Hunny, the Clockwork Dog, mostly a chow chow, sleeping beside my chair. During her periods on duty, I can reveal I was never attacked from behind.

The investigation that became *The Doctor Who Fooled the World* was funded entirely by the *Sunday Times*, London; the Channel 4 TV network; *The BMJ*; publishers' advances for this book; and a check from Wakefield's lawyers, on his behalf, to cover legal expenses for my website.

INDEX

- - - - - - - - - - - - - - - - - - - -

ABI Prism 310 capillary sequencer, 152, 209. *See also* sequencing (DNA)

ABI Prism 7700 RT-PCR machine, 151–55, 171, 173, 183, 203–7, 209, 249–50, 385

Advocates for Children's Health Affected by Mercury Poisoning, 224

Ahmed, Marian, 309

AidsVax, 121, 193, 320

Akita University (Japan), 107, 155

Allergy-Induced Autism, 39, 43, 138

American Academy of Pediatrics, 139, 375

American Journal of Gastroenterology, 160, 308

American Journal of Surgical Pathology, 266

Anthony, Andrew, 264

Anti-Vaccination League of America, 169, 347

Appelman, Henry, 261

Asperger's syndrome/disorder, 168, 276, 351; diagnosis distinct from autism, 148–49, 238–40; not regressive, 240, 272

Association of the British Pharmaceutical Industry, 300

Association of University Teachers, 157

autism, 6–7, 23, 38, 54, 60, 72, 105, 119, 138–39, 230, 239, 252, 276, 309–10, 329, 351–52, 358; claimed link with measles virus, 111, 114, 139, 149, 151–52, 180–84, 210, 246, 248–50, 253; regressive, 4, 33–34, 38, 52–54, 129, 148, 172, 234, 240–41, 264, 270, 277, 322, 329

autism and vaccines, 6, 8, 55, 67–71, 100, 119, 139, 152, 168, 180, 230–31, 247–48, 295–96, 302, 306, 344–45, 375

Autism Media Channel, 310, 317

Autism Research Institute, 229–30

Autism Research Review International, 231, 246

Autism Society of America, 232

Autism Unlocked, 169

autistic enterocolitis, 135, 141, 148, 180, 204, 247, 285, 297; claimed measles virus link, 146, 151, 155, 158; not established to exist, 308; Wakefield asked to prove existence of, 144. *See also* enterocolitis

Aventis Pasteur. *See* Pasteur-Merieux

Bactrim, 192

Ball family, 227; Charlie, 228; Colton, 228; Marshall, 228; Troylyn, 227–28

Barclay, Sarah, 171

Barr, Richard, 54, 58, 61, 89–90, 108, 130, 137–38, 140–41, 149, 153, 158, 163, 168, 174, 177–81, 183–85, 187, 197, 246, 253, 256, 263, 270–71, 281, 288–89, 294, 323, 355–56, 358; Coombe Women's Hospital and, 201–2, 206–10, 375; fact sheets and newsletters, 95, 132, 136–38, 168, 178, 187, 231, 341, 368–69; first MMR client, 90–92; as Society of Homeopaths board member, 187; Wakefield deal and, 94–103, 114, 118, 122, 128, 132, 134–36, 167, 175, 214, 218–19, 221, 223, 231, 244, 309, 373

Barts Hospital, 40, 42–43, 45, 59, 130, 160, 183, 313, 367

Berelowitz, Mark, 47, 68, 240, 264

Best, Margaret, 78–81

Betteridge's law of headlines, 31
Bignall, John, 63
Bigtree, Del, 332–34, 336–38, 345, 354, 364; claims to be Emmy winner, 332
Birt, Elizabeth, 224–25, 227, 229
Bjarnasson, Ingvar, 384
Blatch, Bryan, 115–16, 162
Blaxill, Mark, 342, 345
BMJ (British Medical Journal), 261, 297–99, 301, 306, 334, 376, 379, 382, 384–85
Bocelli, Andrea, 51
Booth, Ian, 258, 263
Bradstreet, James Jeffrey, 225–27, 229, 232
Brant, Sarah, 157, 160–62, 165
Brett, Alastair, 234, 383
British Medical Journal. See *BMJ*
Brittain, Amy, 334
Bustin, Stephen, 202, 206, 208, 250–51, 254

Calman, Kenneth, 65, 87–88
Canadian Journalism Foundation, 301
Candy, David, 63
Carmel Healthcare, 140–44, 204; and John O'Leary, 153–54
Casson, David, 46
"CDC whistleblower." *See* Thompson, William
Cedillo, Michelle, 245–46, 248–49, 251–53, 359
Cedillo, Theresa, 245–49, 251, 253, 278
Cedillo v. Secretary of Health and Human Services, 245–54
Centers for Disease Control and Prevention (CDC), 71, 316–17, 319–22, 324, 326, 331, 333, 344, 346, 364, 376; AidsVax, 121, 193, 320; congressional committee, 154; MRC meeting, 123
Centro de Vigilância Epidemiológica (São Paulo), 343
Chadwick, Nick, 48–49, 99, 109–12, 117, 135, 149–51, 154–55, 158, 185, 226, 232, 250, 365
Chan, Margaret, 340
Channel 4 Television, 232, 234–36, 239, 243, 276, 300, 382–83, 385
Chester Beatty Laboratories, 104, 112

Clifford, Max, 291–92
CNN, 299–301, 376
Coates, Adele, 98
Cohen, Zane, 19
Coleman, Mary, 119
colitis, nonspecific, 59–60, 66–67, 69, 135, 158, 188, 225, 257–61, 272, 350. *See also* enterocolitis
colon, 46–49, 67, 258–59, 266, 271
colonoscopy (*including* ileocolonoscopy, scoping), 40, 45–46, 50–52, 57–59, 61, 65, 94, 99, 105, 116, 128, 130, 134–35, 158, 177, 212, 225, 231, 249, 253, 255, 270, 279, 311–12, 350, 356, 376; as performed by Simon Murch, 56, 47–49, 161; as performed by Mike Thompson, 216; research procedure, 45, 99
Committee on Publication Ethics, 214
constipation, 45–46, 225, 230, 253, 262–63, 286, 350
Coombe Women's Hospital (Dublin), 150, 154, 174, 178, 184, 201–11, 248–50
Coonan, Kieran, 306
Cooper, Anderson, 299–301, 376
Cotter, Finbarr, 184
Cowie, Joanne, 100–101
Crohn, Burrill B., 20, 114
Crohn's disease, 19–20, 50, 71; Wakefield and, 23–26, 28–31, 35, 38, 40–41, 43–44, 50, 95, 99, 107–10, 114, 116, 124–26, 155, 345, 373
"Cry Shame" (public campaign), 289–90
Cure Autism Now, 224

Dada, Gillian Aderonke, 202, 204, 207–9, 211
Dahl-Regis, Merceline, 339–40
Daily Mail, 62, 91, 163, 220–21, 315
Davies, Susan, 66, 257–60, 265–67
Deakin University (Australia), 192
Dean, Sylvia, 265
Defeat Autism Now!, 230, 247
De Niro, Robert, 334–35, 344–45, 376
deoxyribonucleic acid. *See* DNA
De Silva, Amali, 236, 243–44, 383
DeStefano, Frank, 71, 326, 331
Dhillon, Amar, 260–61, 264, 266
disintegrative disorder, 67, 238–39, 277

DNA, 149, 158, 203-4, 209, 250, 357

Domizio, Paola, 260

DTP (diphtheria, tetanus, pertussis) vaccine, 78, 80, 83-85, 91, 93, 98-100, 169, 180, 193-95, 202, 224, 240, 242-43, 246-48, 278, 315, 326

Eady, Mr. Justice (Sir David Eady), 235, 243, 300

Edwards, Heather, 287, 292

Edwards, Josh, 287, 292

Eight, Child, 271

Eleven, Child, 105, 108-11, 279. See also Eleven, Mr.

Eleven, Mr., 104, 105-6, 108-9, 111-12, 119, 255, 279-80, 298. See also Eleven, Child

Else, Martin, 102

Endogen Research, 115

enteritis, 258

enterocolitis, 62, 129, 151, 171, 180, 260, 264, 277, 285; defined, 258. See also autistic enterocolitis

Evans, Harold, 193, 385

Families for Early Autism Treatment (FEAT), 169-70

Ferguson, Anne, 123, 125, 127-30, 132-33, 213, 263

Fisher, Barbara, 224

Five, Child, 58, 131

Fletcher, Jackie, 36-38, 43, 49, 52, 54, 58, 61, 72, 87, 94, 100, 126-30, 197, 218, 237, 275, 358-59, 373-74. See also JABS

Fombonne, Eric, 240, 246, 252

Four, Child, 52-59, 67, 105, 129, 237, 259, 271, 277, 281. See also Four, Ms.

Four, Ms., 52-58, 60, 67, 89, 186, 255, 274, 281-82, 288, 323. See also Four, Child

Fraser, Lorraine, 49, 61, 147, 152, 161, 163, 166, 225

Freemedic, 115, 117-18, 143-44

Fudenberg, Hugh, 106, 108, 118-21, 226, 231-32

Geboes, Karel, 260, 384

Geist, Willie, 334

General Medical Council (GMC), 165, 198, 281; findings on Wakefield, 293-94, 297, 376; public hearing, 34, 217, 225-67, 283-84, 286, 356, 367; reinvestigation of Deer's evidence, 217, 235, 255; Walker-Smith appeal, 312-13

Generation Rescue, 322

Gershon, Michael, 172-74

GlaxoSmithKline (GSK). See Smith-Kline Beecham

GMC. See General Medical Council

Godlee, Fiona, 298, 301, 382

Goldblatt, David, 125

Golding, Alan, 286-87

Golding, Wendy, 265

Great Ormond Street. See Hospital for Sick Children

Griffin, Diane, 249

Griffith, Arlwyn, 85

Grillo, Beppe, 343, 346

The Guardian, 35, 66, 70, 85, 275, 296, 308

guilt, 3-4, 61, 132, 169, 174, 181, 228, 254, 294, 305, 345, 367-69, 371, 379

Guiver, Malcolm, 202, 204, 208

Hadden, Abel, 199, 214, 217

Haemophilus influenzae type b vaccine, 87, 247

Haga, Yoichi, 108

Hall, Celia, 91-92

Hamilton, Justice Liam, 80

Harris, Evan, 212, 220

Hastings, George L., Jr., 248, 251, 253-54

Hazlehurst, William, 254

Heinonen, Olli, 353-54

Helicobacter pylori (H. pylori), 23, 62, 364

hepatitis B vaccine, 4, 84, 247-48, 336

Hickey, Henry, 80

Hightower, Grace, 334

Hinchliffe's rule, 31

Hirosaki University, 108, 155

Histogene, 115

histopathology, 49, 58, 129, 146, 162, 237, 259, 265, 384

Hodgson, Humphrey, 217, 219

Hooker, Brian, 317–18, 320–26, 332–33, 376

Horton, Richard, 44, 63, 211–13, 216–18, 219–20, 308, 367

Hospital for Sick Children, Great Ormond Street, 81–82, 86, 125, 195, 201, 224

human papillomavirus (HPV) vaccine, 4

Hutchinson, Philippa, 64, 69

Iizuka, Masahiro, 107

ileal-lymphoid-nodular hyperplasia (*including* ileal lymphoid hyperplasia, lymphoid hyperplasia), 57–58, 66–67, 109, 135, 158, 160, 258–59, 286

ileocolonoscopy. *See* colonoscopy

ileoscopy. *See* colonoscopy

ileum, 26, 40, 44, 48–49, 57, 109, 160, 171, 249, 258–59, 261–62

Immravax, 88

immunohistochemistry, 28, 62, 107, 124

Immunospecifics Biotechnologies, 117, 120–22, 140, 153, 158

Inceltec, 115

indeterminate colitis, 59

inflammatory bowel disease. *See* Crohn's disease; indeterminate colitis; ulcerative colitis

in situ hybridization, 28, 108

Institute of Medicine, 320

International Child Development Resource Center, 225–27

JABS (Justice, Awareness, and Basic Support), 36–39, 43, 49, 52, 54, 58, 72, 127–30, 197, 237, 275, 358. *See also* Fletcher, Jackie

Johnson, Jane, 229–31

Journal of Medical Virology (*J Med Virol*), 28, 39, 64, 88–89, 93, 107–9, 125, 215, 366

Journal of Virological Methods, 110

Kawashima, Hisashi, 117, 158–59, 171, 185

Kennedy, Robert F., Jr., 8, 354

Kinnear, Johnnie, 83

Kinnear, Susan, 83

Kirby, David, 224–25, 227

Koplik spots, 26

Korda, Alex, 114, 117, 121–22, 140–41

Krigsman, Arthur, 253, 311

Kulenkampff, Marcia, 82

Kumar, Surendra, 265, 293–94

Lancaster, Angela, 90–92, 95

The Lancet, 15, 24–25, 30, 44, 51, 107, 109, 152, 155, 159, 353; response to Deer's early findings, 211–14, 216–20. *See also* Wakefield, Andrew, *Lancet* paper 1989, 1995, *and* 1998

large bowel/large intestine. *See* colon

Lauer, Matt, 97, 293–96, 298

Laurance, Jeremy, 10, 20, 25–26

Legal Aid Board (Legal Services Commission), 91, 92, 109, 110–11, 114, 128, 132, 139, 149, 218; ends money for lawsuit, 181, 185–86; funds Wakefield MMR research, 92, 99–103, 134–35, 150, 186–87, 212, 215, 255, 294, 296, 305, 373–74; funds Wakefield personally, 97, 187, 219; planned customer for Wakefield's company, 141

Limb, Kirsten, 95–96, 130, 136–38, 168, 178–79, 183, 202, 231, 253, 368; brain-injured daughter of, 96; as homeopathic practitioner, 187. *See also* Barr, Richard

Linderman, Curt, 335

Liu, Ying, 107

Livingstone, Ken, 181

Llewellyn Smith, Chris, 144, 157, 160, 161

Loveday, Susan. See *Loveday v. Renton*

Loveday v. Renton, 84–85, 98, 242

MacDonald, Tom, 160

Macpherson, Elle, 361–64

March, John, 179–80, 182–83

Marques, Cristiano Corrêa de A., 343

Marshall, Barry, 23–24, 62, 114, 364

Maskrey, Simeon, 181

Matanoski, Vincent, 250

Matthews, Bridget d'Estouteville (Mrs. Wakefield), 14–17, 370

Matthews, Edward, 16–17, 370
McCarthy, Jenny, 8, 270, 299, 322, 358
measles outbreaks, 8, 29, 31, 36, 69,
    113, 137, 193, 270, 315, 339–41;
    Albania, 342; Brazil, 343–44;
    Britain, 342, 367; California, 327;
    Europe, 342; France, 342; Georgia,
    342; Greece, 342; India, 342,
    343; Italy, 342; Kazakhstan, 342;
    Minnesota, 310, 341–42; Myanmar,
    342; New York, 346–47; Philippines,
    342; Poland, 342–43, 346; Romania,
    253, 342; Serbia, 342; Thailand, 342;
    Ukraine, 342, 346; United States,
    346; Venezuela, 343; Vietnam, 342
measles vaccines, 29–31, 38, 45, 52, 55,
    65, 89, 93–95, 114, 116–18, 126–28,
    135, 140–41, 164, 172–73, 175, 242,
    363–64
measles virus, 26, 28, 29, 31, 35, 38–39,
    41, 43, 87–88, 93, 106, 109, 114, 121,
    125, 131, 133, 139, 149, 158, 170, 173,
    181–82, 188, 206, 209, 246, 248, 273,
    360, 364–65; tests for, 48, 52, 89,
    99, 107–8, 110–12, 116–18, 134–35,
    140–41, 143, 150–52, 155, 158, 171–73,
    178, 180–85, 203, 206, 208, 227,
    248–49, 250, 268, 355, 366
Medical Interventions for Autism, 225
Medical Research Council, 28, 180;
    meeting to discuss Wakefield's
    claims, 123; Wakefield's withdrawal
    from event, 175
Merck Inc., 30, 88, 174, 179, 202, 215, 235
mesalazine prescribing, 59–60
Micropathology, 178
Miller, Clifford, 199–200, 290–92
Minor, Philip, 27
Mirchandani, Vinod, 205–6
Mitting, Mr. Justice (Sir John
    Mitting), 313
M-M-R II, 88
Moms on a Mission for Autism, 51
Montgomery, Scott, 30, 125–26, 132,
    159, 163–65, 175
Moodley, Parimala, 265
mumps, 88, 89–90, 111, 137, 208, 242,
    373
Murch, Simon, 56, 68, 161–62, 177,
    215–19, 221, 255, 257, 262, 264, 293,
    355; performance of colonoscopy,
    48–49; recollection of doubt over
    pathology, 265–67; research on
    autistic children, 45

National Autism Association, 224
National Childhood Encephalopathy
    Study, 84
National Institute of Biological
    Standards and Control, 27
National Vaccine Information Center,
    224
NBC, 97, 224, 246, 293, 334, 344, 376
Neuroimmuno Therapeutics
    Research Foundation, 118. See also
    Fudenberg, Hugh
New Autism Initiative, 289–90
New Indian Express, 4, 348
Newsnight, 35–37, 54, 61, 126–28, 157,
    237, 350
New York Times, 2, 7, 169, 301, 316, 319
Nine, Child, 256, 277
nonspecific colitis. *See* colitis
nucleotides, 124, 135, 149, 152, 158–59,
    183, 203, 209
Nuki, Paul, 191–95, 199, 214–17,
    220, 381

O'Donovan, Carmel Philomena, 19,
    23, 29, 52, 143, 237, 281
Office of Special Masters of the US
    Court of Federal Claims. *See*
    "vaccine court"
Oldstone, Michael, 173–74
O'Leary, John, 146–48, 150–55, 215,
    355, 375; Barr deal, 153; Carmel
    Healthcare, 153–54; in *Cedillo v.
    Secretary of Health and Human
    Services*, 248–52; at Coombe
    Women's Hospital, 201–10;
    criticism of, during congressional
    hearing, 173–74; Immunospecifics,
    153; *Molecular Pathology* paper, 171;
    Unigenetics, 153, 248
olsalazine prescribing, 59–60
One, Child, 46, 48, 274
opioid excess hypothesis, 39, 68,
    138–39, 148, 173, 178, 180, 182–83,
    253
opioid suppression hypothesis, 183

Pan American Health Organization (PAHO), 339-41, 343-44
Panksepp, Jaak, 138
Pasteur-Merieux (Aventis Pasteur/Sanofi Pasteur), 88, 179, 202
Pattison, John, 125, 133
Paxman, Jeremy, 36
PCR. *See* polymerase chain reaction
Pegg, Michael, 101-2
Peltola, Heikki, 353-54
Pepys, Mark, 142-45, 153, 156-57, 165, 172-73
Peyer's patches, 261
Plusarix, 88
polymerase chain reaction (PCR), 107-9, 112, 115, 150, 154, 155, 183, 185, 149-50, 310, 384-85; at Coombe Women's Hospital, 202, 206-9
Pounder, Roy, 30, 62-63, 65, 68-70, 110, 115, 121-22, 140-41, 144, 265-66, 366
proteins, 28, 107, 124-25, 135, 150, 155

"refrigerator" mother, 230, 369
regressive autism, 4, 62, 114, 117, 129, 148, 172, 180-81, 234, 240-41, 264, 270-73, 277, 285
Reibel, Ken, 358
Research Assessment Exercise, 25, 65, 115, 266
Revolta Contra Vacina (Rio de Janeiro), 347
ribonucleic acid. *See* RNA
Ricciardella, Lynn, 247, 251
Rima, Bertus, 205-6, 208-9, 249
Rimland, Bernard, 229-32, 246-47
rinderpest, 26, 180, 340
RNA, 26, 28, 110, 149, 152, 158, 173, 184, 203, 204, 208, 249-50, 340, 365
Rouse, Andrew, 132
Royal College of Pathologists, 308
Royal College of Surgeons, 124, 159, 162, 213, 263, 308
Royal Free Hospital, 22-23, 35, 43, 45-47, 49, 56, 61, 63-66, 97, 101-2, 104, 110, 225
Royal Free Medical School, 22-23; press conference for Wakefield's question-marked measles vaccine-Crohn's paper, 35; press conference for Wakefield's MMR-autism paper, 61-71
rubella, 88, 111, 137, 242, 273, 339, 352, 359-60; congenital rubella syndrome, 87
Rutter, Michael, 289

SafeMinds, 224
Salisbury, David, 86-89, 92-93, 124, 156, 168, 242, 306
Sato, Helena, 343
Schafer, Lenny, 169-73, 176, 188, 202, 209, 224, 234, 284, 291, 310
Schwartzman, José Salomão, 82-83, 240, 344
Science Museum, London, 182
Scripps Research Institute (La Jolla), 173-74
secretin, 226, 229, 311, 357
Selz, Bernard and Lisa, 334-35, 345
Septra, 192
Septrin, 192
sequencing (DNA), 99, 134, 143, 149, 152, 158-59, 171-72, 174, 185, 209-10, 249; in outbreak, 310
Seven, Child, 256
Simmonds, Peter, 205, 208
Six, Child, 237-38, 240-43, 272. *See also* Six, Ms.
Six, Ms., 241-43, 275, 281, 285, 287, 289, 290, 291, 355-56. *See also* Seven, Child; Six, Child
60 Minutes (CBS), 161, 202, 332, 375
Skidmore, Thomas, 348
Sleat, Robert, 114, 117, 121-22, 140-41, 150
Smith, Sally, 259, 264, 297
SmithKline Beecham (GlaxoSmithKline/GSK), 30, 88, 179, 202, 208, 284, 355
Snyder, Colten, 254
Somali Parents Autism Network, 309
Spourdalakis, Alex: death of, 311, 376-77
SSPE, 87, 93, 195
stoned rodent model of autism, 139-40, 178, 230, 253, 262
Stott, Carol, 288-91
Stuart-Smith, Jeremy, 180-81

Stuart-Smith, Lord Justice (Sir Murray Stuart-Smith), 76, 80, 83-85, 224, 256; vaccine damage checklist, 98, 100, 135, 138, 181, 251, 277

Stutt, Colin, 187

subacute sclerosing panencephalitis (SSPE), 87, 93, 195

sulphasalazine (sulfasalazine) prescribing, 59-60

Sun, Lena, 334

Sunday Times, 3, 61-62, 75-78, 85, 94-95, 117, 129, 132, 191-95, 197, 199, 220-21, 234, 243, 269, 290, 294, 306-7, 358, 375-76, 379, 381, 383, 385

Swaminathan, Soumya, 342

TaqMan. *See* ABI Prism 7700 RT-PCR machine; polymerase chain reaction

Tarhan, Cengiz, 114-18, 121, 123, 144

Taylor, Brent, 152-54

Tebb, William, 169, 347

Ten, Child, 256

terminal ileum, 44, 160, 259, 261-62

thalidomide, 193, 196-97

thimerosal, 139-40, 233, 248, 285, 322, 325, 336, 375

This Week, 81-82

Thompson, Mike, 216-17

Thompson, William, 317-26, 331, 333, 376

Thorsen, Poul, 320

Thoughtful House Center for Children, 227-31, 234, 238-39, 247, 253, 276, 289, 308, 311

Three, Child, 275, 349-53, 359. *See also* Three, Ms.

Three, Ms., 275, 349-51, 354, 357, 359-60. *See also* Three, Child

Thrower, David, 284-85, 289

Tommey, Polly, 310-11, 318, 333-34, 336-37, 345, 354, 357-58, 368

Toronto Star, 19

transfer factor, 118, 120-21, 231

Trump, Donald, 1-3, 5-8, 321, 337, 342, 363

Twelve, Child, 58. *See also* Twelve, Ms.

Twelve, Ms., 129, 305. *See also* Twelve, Child

Two, Child, 32-33, 37, 40-41, 46-50, 52-53, 56, 58-59, 61, 105, 116, 130, 148, 158, 182, 184, 195, 206, 210, 237, 257, 275, 359. *See also* Two, Ms.

Two, Ms., 32-33, 36-40, 43, 46-50, 67-68, 86-88, 107, 114, 126, 130, 138, 139-41, 147, 175, 180, 186, 194-200, 202, 209, 218, 222, 226, 237-38, 247, 262, 275-76, 277, 281, 287, 290-91, 313, 329, 354-56, 358. *See also* Two, Child

Tyer, Brad, 228

Tyrer, Robert, 214-17, 220, 381

ulcerative colitis, 19, 59, 116

Ullstein, Augustus, 96-100, 137, 180

Uniform Requirements for Manuscripts Submitted to Biomedical Journals, 127, 213, 215, 219, 264

Unigenetics, 153, 248

University College London, 25, 34, 140, 143, 156-57, 175

Urabe AM9 mumps strain, 88-89, 91-92

Vaccine Adverse Event Reporting System (VAERS), 358

"vaccine court," 245-54, 296, 310, 322, 338

Vaccine Roulette, 224, 246, 332

Vaccine Safety Council of Minnesota, 341

variolation, 82

VaxGen. *See* AidsVax

Vaxxed, 322-38, 344-45, 357, 364, 368, 376

Vioxx, 235-36

Visceral, 163, 171, 177, 289

Wakefield, Andrew, 13-23, 29, 52, 63; accuses scientists of conflicts, 174-75; appearance on *60 Minutes*, 161, 202, 375; claims of CDC "whistleblower," 316-26; claims to be winning vaccine "war," 342; denial of wrongdoing, 7, 215, 223, 294-95, 305-7, 341, 363; flees viva exam, 366; legal contract and, 97-103, 154, 214-16, 219-20, 272-73; libel actions and, 233-36, 244;

Wakefield, Andrew (*cont.*)
  minor falsified papers of, 157–60, 163–65; pharma funding of, 29–30, 143; praise for, 7, 44, 176, 216, 224, 227, 345, 356, 360, 361–62, 364, 369; purchase of blood from children, 295; refuge in anecdotes, 328–30; refusal to replicate MMR research, 143–45, 157, 160–61, 166; research ethically unauthorized, 44–52, 55, 99–103, 213, 219, 255; smears Deer, 288–89, 291, 299–300, 306, 312; withholding of William Thompson's statement, 321. *See also* Crohn's disease; *Vaxxed*
Wakefield, Andrew, business schemes, 113–18, 120–22. *See also* Carmel Healthcare; Immunospecifics Biotechnologies; Unigenetics
Wakefield, Andrew, findings of fraud and dishonesty against: by *BMJ*, 298–99, by General Medical Council, 293–94; by *Lancet*, 308; by parents of research children, 279–82
Wakefield, Andrew, medical opinions: on aluminum, 336; anti-vaccine, 341; on government intention to damage brains of millions, 336; on hepatitis B vaccine, 336; on importance of listening to patient, 330; on measles as benign, 364; on MMR as cause of autism, 168, 184, 296, 345; on MMR suspension, 65, 69; on mother's instinct, 329–30; on thimerosal, 336; on vaccines dumbing down boys, 336
Wakefield, Andrew, *Lancet* paper, 1989 (Crohn's and blood vessels), 24–25
Wakefield, Andrew, *Lancet* paper, 1995 (question-marked, measles vaccine, and Crohn's), 30–31, 34–36, 126
Wakefield, Andrew, *Lancet* paper, 1998 (twelve child, MMR, and autism), 4–5, 61–63, 65–72, 112–13, 115, 224, 237–38, 242, 256–59, 262–63, 266–67, 270–74, 276–82, 296–97, 344, 365, 374; changes to claimed temporal link, 277–78; clinicians'

diagnoses altered, 276–77; GI pathology misreported, 258–67; misreporting, overview, 269–72; normal blood tests reported abnormal, 306; parental claims misreported, 273–76; patient selection concealed, 69, 127–33, 135, 213, 218, 296–97; retraction of interpretation section, 221; retraction of paper, 5, 308; sponsorship by Legal Aid Board, 102, 255
Wakefield, Andrew, patents, 232, 266, 277, 294; September 13, 1994, nucleotide primers, 115; December 1, 1994, "Wakefield's box," 115; March 28, 1995, Medicament for inflammatory bowel disease, and "measles vaccine," 116; June 6, 1997, "combined vaccine/therapeutic agent," 117, 121–22, 374; and Royal Free medical school, 140, 144, 165, 168
Wakefield, Graham, 15–16, 68, 82
Walker-Smith, John, 40–43, 59–61, 63, 67, 117, 198, 216–19, 239, 255–57, 262–66, 274–75, 287, 367; appeal, 312–13; GMC verdict, 293; opinion of Wakefield, 44, 215, 264, 313–14; research on autistic children, 44–48, 50, 58–59, 99, 128–29, 131; retraction of *Lancet* "Interpretation," 221; views on Australian independence, 43
Warren, Robin, 23–24, 27, 62, 364
Washington Post, 195, 220, 334
Watts, Susan, 36
Webster, Stephen, 265
Wellcome Trust, 29, 192
Wiggin LLP, 236, 240, 243–44, 383. *See also* De Silva, Amali
Wilson, John, 81–83, 85–87, 93, 169, 195, 224, 240, 242, 246, 278, 315, 364
Witherow, John, 199, 290, 381
Wiznitzer, Max, 252
World Health Organization (WHO), 64, 148, 239, 340–42, 346, 377

Zuckerman, Arie, 25, 28, 34, 64, 66, 68–69, 101–2, 217, 366–67